NON-INVASIVE
CARDIAC DIAGNOSIS

NON-INVASIVE CARDIAC DIAGNOSIS

EDWARD K. CHUNG, M.D., F.A.C.P., F.A.C.C.

Professor of Medicine
Jefferson Medical College of
Thomas Jefferson University
and
Director of the Heart Station
Thomas Jefferson University Hospital
Philadelphia, Pa.

LEA & FEBIGER   *Philadelphia • 1976*

Library of Congress Cataloging in Publication Data

Main entry under title:

Non-invasive cardiac diagnosis.

   Includes index.
   1. Heart—Diseases—Diagnosis. I. Chung, Edward K.
[DNLM: 1. Heart diseases—Diagnosis. WG141 N811]
RC683.N65   1976   616.1′2′075   75-38915
ISBN 0-8121-0541-9

Published in Great Britain by Henry Kimpton Publishers, London

PRINTED IN THE UNITED STATES OF AMERICA

To My Wife, Lisa
and
To Linda and Christopher

Preface

The majority of cardiac problems can be diagnosed with relative certainty by non-invasive means if the physician has sufficient and appropriate knowledge. The clinical diagnosis entertained by non-invasive means can be confirmed later by invasive diagnostic methods, if necessary, as for the preoperative evaluation of various heart diseases. Therefore, the non-invasive diagnostic approach is extremely important in evaluating various cardiac problems, particularly when the invasive diagnostic facilities are not available—the usual situation for many practicing physicians.

The purpose of this book is *not* to discuss in depth various subjects in medicine or to describe in detail all possible problems in the field of Non-Invasive Cardiac Diagnosis. The primary intention is to describe common non-invasive cardiac diagnostic problems that are frequently encountered in our daily practice.

This book presents 16 chapters, including Examination of the Cardiovascular Systems, Carotid Sinus Stimulation, Electrocardiography, Electrocardiographic Stress Testing, Holter Monitor Electrocardiography, Computer Electrocardiography, Vectorcardiography, Echocardiography, Phonocardiography, Pulse Tracings

and Apexcardiography, Systolic Time Intervals, Ballistocardiography, Non-Invasive Roentgenographic Studies in Cardiovascular Diseases, Serum Digitalis Level Determination, Interpretation of Antiarrhythmic Drug Levels and Laboratory Studies in Cardiovascular Diseases.

The contents are intended to be clinical, concise and practical so that all physicians will be provided with up-to-date materials that will assist them directly in the daily care of their patients with common cardiac problems.

The book will be extremely valuable to all practicing physicians, particularly internists, cardiologists, family physicians and emergency room physicians along with house staff and cardiology fellows. In addition, medical students and coronary care unit nurses will also greatly benefit by reading this book and learning a general approach to various cardiac problems.

I am sincerely grateful to all the authors for their valuable contributions to this book, Non-Invasive Cardiac Diagnosis. I also wish to thank my personal secretary, Miss Theresa McAnally for her devoted and cheerful secretarial assistance. She has been most valuable in handling correspondence to all contributors, in addition to typing several chapters of mine for this book. It has been my pleasure to work with the staff of Lea & Febiger. In particular, I would like to express my sincere thanks to Mr. R. Kenneth Bussy, Executive Editor, for his cooperation and invaluable assistance.

Philadelphia   EDWARD K. CHUNG, M.D.

Contributors

J. Thomas Bigger, Jr., M.D., F.A.C.P.,
  F.A.C.C.
Professor of Medicine and Pharmacology
Columbia University College of Physicians
  & Surgeons
Attending Physician
Presbyterian Hospital
New York, New York

Cesar Augusto Caceres, M.D., F.A.C.C.
Professor, Department of Electrical
  Engineering
University of Maryland
School of Engineering
College Park, Maryland

Edward K. Chung, M.D., F.A.C.P.,
  F.A.C.C.
Professor of Medicine
Jefferson Medical College of
Thomas Jefferson University
and
Director of the Heart Station
Thomas Jefferson University Hospital
Philadelphia, Pennsylvania

Lisa S. Chung, M.D.
Chief Medical Officer and Medical
  Director
U.S. Public Health Service
Philadelphia, Pennsylvania

William Dock, M.D., F.A.C.P., M.A.C.P.,
  F.A.C.C.
Professor of Medicine, Emeritus
State University of New York
Chief, Cardiac Laboratory
Lutheran Medical Center
Brooklyn, New York

Gordon A. Ewy, M.D., F.A.C.C.
Professor of Medicine
University of Arizona
College of Medicine
Director of Diagnostic Cardiology
Arizona Medical Center
Tucson, Arizona

Elsa-Grace V. Giardina, M.D., F.A.C.P.
Assistant Professor of Medicine
Columbia University College of Physicians
  & Surgeons
New York, New York

Marun S. Haddad, M. D.
Fellow in Cardiology
Thomas Jefferson University
Philadelphia, Pennsylvania

Claude R. Joyner, M.D., F.A.C.P.,
F.A.C.C.
Clinical Professor of Medicine
University of Pittsburgh
School of Medicine
Director, Department of Medicine
Allegheny General Hospital
Pittsburgh, Pennsylvania

Eugene C. Klatte, M.D.
Professor and Chairman
Department of Radiology
Indiana University
School of Medicine
Medical Staff
Indiana University Hospital
Indianapolis, Indiana

William Likoff, M.D., F.A.C.P., F.A.C.C.
Professor of Medicine
Director of the Cardiovascular Institute
Hahnemann Medical College and Hospital
Philadelphia, Pennsylvania

Frank I. Marcus, M.D.
Professor of Medicine
Director, Division of Cardiology
University of Arizona
College of Medicine
Tucson, Arizona

Ernesto E. Salcedo, M.D.
Clinical Associate
Department of Clinical Cardiology
Cleveland Clinic Foundation
Cleveland, Ohio

L. Thomas Sheffield, Jr., M.D., F.A.C.C.
Professor of Medicine
Director of University Hospital
Electrocardiographic Laboratory and
Allison Laboratory of Exercise
Electrophysiology
The University of Alabama in Birmingham
School of Medicine
Birmingham, Alabama

Wayne Siegel, M.D., F.A.C.P., F.A.C.C.
Head, Cardiac Function Laboratory
Department of Clinical Cardiology
Cleveland Clinic Foundation
Cleveland, Ohio

Morton E. Tavel, M.D., F.A.C.P.,
F.A.C.C.
Associate Professor of Medicine
Indiana University School of Medicine
Associate Director of Heart Station
Methodist Hospital
Indianapolis, Indiana

Calvin L. Weisberger, M.D.
Cardiologist
Kaiser Foundation Hospital
West Los Angeles, California

Heun Y. Yune, M.D.
Professor of Radiology
Indiana University
School of Medicine
Medical Staff
Indiana University Hospital
Indianapolis, Indiana

Contents

Chapter 1

Examination of the Cardiovascular Systems

WILLIAM LIKOFF

A complete cardiac diagnosis should include the anatomic or structural abnormality, its cause, the resulting functional impairment, the natural history of the ailment and its prognosis under the most effective treatment. To reach these conclusions, the physician depends upon information obtained from the medical history, physical examination and special investigative studies, which, depending upon the presenting problem, may include x-ray examination, electrocardiography, echocardiography, phonocardiography, catheterization and angiography. In the vast majority of patients a correct, complete diagnosis cannot be reached without utilizing all parameters of inquiry.

Symptoms are subjective manifestations of abnormal physiology. Their type, severity, onset and the manner in which they evolve comprise the essential elements of a medical history. The extraction of this information from an individual beset with the uncertainties of ill health is a distinct art, the mastery of which depends upon the examiner's training, knowledge, experience, discipline, compassion, sensitivity and tact. There is no greater obligation in the practice of medicine than to develop and exploit the art of history taking to its fullest account.

Physical abnormalities are the objective signs of disease. Their form and severity are documented by means of the physical examination, which may confirm what the medical history already implies or may be the only means of establishing a diagnosis. Skill in performing the examination is as pertinent to a correct, complete cardiac diagnosis as the art of history taking.

The search for physical abnormalities should take place according to an established routine that directs attention to all parts of the body. The particular format followed is relatively immaterial as long as the examiner remains consistent in his approach. Obviously it is most convenient to examine the patient from head to feet, and from front to back, in that order, delaying more intimate inquiries such as the rectal examination until everything else has been accomplished. Unless a systematic approach is followed, the risk of errors of omission increases materially even in the most experienced hands.

The discovery of physical abnormalities resides in large measure with the technical skill of the examiner. If the physician fails

1

to place the patient in the appropriate position an abnormal jugular venous pulse cannot be recognized. Renal artery stenosis may not be suspected if the examiner does not listen for the auscultatory hallmark. However, it also holds that skill alone does not determine the productivity of the examination. Other factors include knowledge of all the pertinent findings apt to result from any specific disorder and the dedication to seek them out. The most rewarding examination results from uncovering predictable physical signs rather than from the discovery of unsuspected abnormalities.

The detection of abnormal physical findings is a clear implication that an organ or system is deranged in structure or function. In many instances the exact nature of the derangement and its severity can be determined from the objective signs. When the second heart sound is greatly attenuated in patients with aortic stenosis the valve leaflets are believed to be relatively immobile, and the lesion is considered hemodynamically significant. Further confirmation may be obtained from a painfully slow rising carotid pulse that is also distinguished by a marked dicrotic notch. Similarly a wide peripheral pulse pressure and distinctly palpable left ventricle mark aortic insufficiency as being quantitatively significant. Regrettably, simple, effective correlations such as these are not made as frequently as they should be at the bedside. This default of our times has developed with the introduction of instruments and laboratory procedures capable of providing a precise analysis of anatomic distortion and functional impairment. Without unrealistically bemoaning the availability of these instruments and procedures, it holds that our reliance upon them can be reduced materially if the pathogenesis of physical signs is understood and properly applied by the physician at the time the examination is being conducted.

Although dependence upon instruments and complex procedures for diagnosis is to be discouraged, if for no other than economic reasons, the continued use of outmoded unreliable methods of examination is to be condemned with equal vigor. Most notorious among these techniques is percussion of the chest to outline cardiac size. The disparity between the results of percussion and actual size is so great as to render the procedure worthless.

The fundamental objective of the physical examination is to collect data. However, the examiner must have the capability to select, discard and correlate the information obtained. It is the latter function, in particular, that identifies extraordinary competence.

Examination of the cardiovascular systems includes peripheral circulation, venous and arterial pulses and the heart itself. The patient should be adequately exposed in the supine position. The physician should be comfortably stationed and should proceed from general inspection to palpation and auscultation in practiced, disciplined steps.

PERIPHERAL CIRCULATION

The color of skin, lips, ears, nose and extremities should be judged in natural daylight. By simply passing the dorsal surface of the hand lightly across the body and extremities, skin temperature can be estimated at the same time. In order to obtain as much information as possible from this initial phase of examination, identical portions of upper and lower extremities should be compared.

Vasoconstriction. Generalized coldness and pallor of the skin signify vasoconstriction, which, unless a physiologic response to environmental conditions or stress, occurs when cardiac output is depressed. A number of primary disorders of the heart may be responsible, including ischemic heart disease, rheumatic valvular disease and cardiomyopathy.

Localized coldness and pallor point to

vascular obstruction. This may be transient, as is witnessed in arteriolar spasm or Raynaud's phenomenon, or a constant finding when caused by obliterative arterial disease.[1,2]

Severe, prolonged vasoconstriction results in increased peripheral oxygen extraction and a distinct bluish discoloration of the lower extremities in particular. This kind of cyanosis differs from the central type caused by right-to-left intracardiac shunts in that it appears in exposed areas of the body, is associated with coldness and disappears when the part is warmed.[3] Occasionally vasoconstriction may be severe enough to interfere with nutrition of the skin and bring about indolent, trophic lesions.

Vasodilatation. Unusually warm skin suggests peripheral vasodilatation. When not a normal reaction to heat, it implies increased cardiac output. The usual causes include pregnancy, arteriovenous fistulas, thyrotoxicosis and anemia. In each instance cutaneous vasodilatation is a physiologic accommodation for increased peripheral blood flow.

When vasodilatation is generalized the skin of the entire body is warm and flushed, except in the presence of severe anemia when it is warm and pale.[4] Capillary pulsations are commonly observed with generalized vasodilatation. They can be demonstrated by pressing upon the edge of a fingernail or toenail until a small segment of the subungual area blanches. The area is then observed to decrease and increase in size during systole and diastole respectively. A similar phenomenon can be observed when the tip of the finger is transilluminated with a small light, each capillary pulsation causing the fingertip to darken with systole. If a glass slide is placed against the forehead with just enough pressure to obliterate superficial vessels, normal skin color will return with each systole when capillary pulsations are present.

Localized vasodilatation may result from uneven application of heat, infection, occlusive disease of deep veins or arteriovenous communication. The demarcation between areas of normal and abnormal blood flow usually is not difficult to recognize.

General Cyanosis. Cyanosis of both skin and mucous membranes without appropriate skin temperature changes is central in type and implies a serious cardiorespiratory disorder such as right-to-left intracardiac shunt, reversed flow in an arteriovenous communication, pulmonary hypoventilation and oxygen diffusion block due to advanced, diffuse pulmonary intestinal fibrosis. It usually appears when oxygen saturation falls below 75%, and approximately 4 to 5 gm. of reduced hemoglobin per 100 ml. of blood is being circulated. However, the percentage of oxygen desaturation may be much greater in individuals with severe anemia and considerably less in those with polycythemia. Central cyanosis is never confined to exposed areas, is not associated with abnormal skin temperature, does not disappear when the part is warmed and is always accompanied by subnormal arterial oxygen saturation.

Digital Clubbing. Diagnosis is based upon the contour and color of fingers and toes. Early, the skin is glossy at the nail root, the normal angle between skin fold and nail is obliterated, and the longitudinal convexity of the nail itself is exaggerated. When clubbing is fully developed the digits are expanded, thickened and spatulate.

Although clubbing does occur as a familial abnormality in otherwise normal subjects, it is encountered most commonly when a significant cardiorespiratory disorder and central cyanosis coexist.[5] It also has been observed in patients with cirrhosis of the liver, ulcerative colitis and regional enteritis. If clubbing and cyanosis are limited to the toes the finding is diagnostic of patent ductus arteriosus with reversed flow from pulmonary artery to aorta.

Peripheral Pulsations. Abnormal vascular pulsations may be seen anywhere on the body or extremities and may arise from a superficial or deep vessel. Failure to obliterate the pulsation with gentle pressure implies the latter is at fault.

An arterial pulsation along the margins of the lower ribs suggests the presence of coarctation of the aorta. It is seen and felt particularly on the posterior surface of the chest and originates in dilated intercostal vessels.

Diffuse, circuitous, collateral venous channels are commonly seen on the lower extremities when they compensate for varicosities of superficial veins. They are much more prominent when congestive heart failure coexists. Collateral vessels are also observed on the surface of the chest when the superior vena cava is obstructed.

VENOUS AND ARTERIAL PULSES

No portion of the physical examination is more informative than the analysis of the venous and arterial pulses. It should take place after evaluation of the peripheral circulation and prior to examination of the precordium or auscultatation of the heart.

Jugular Venous Pulse. To study the jugular venous pulse the physician should inspect both sides of the neck just above the middle third of the clavicle, the suprasternal notch and the supraclavicular fossa, while the patient sits at a 45-degree angle.

When there are prominent pulsations in the neck the jugular venous pulse can be distinguished from the carotid arterial pulsations by its quality and wave form as well as the effect of position, respirations and abdominal pressure.

The venous pulse can be seen but not felt. It is a soft, undulating, diffuse movement in contrast to the sharp, forceful arterial wave—a distinction that is quite apparent when the carotid pulse is examined simultaneously by placing the thumb under the angle of the jaw on the same or opposite side. Furthermore, it consists of three distinct waves, instead of the single carotid pulse, and can be obliterated easily by applying light pressure against the root of the vein above the medial end of the clavicle.

In patients changing from the recumbent to sitting position the pulsation and distention of veins, rather than arteries, tend to diminish, except in patients with extremely high venous pressure and engorged jugular veins in whom distinct pulsations may not be visible even when they are lying quite flat.

In contrast to its effect on the arterial pulse, respiration alters venous pulsation. Inspiration decreases intrathoracic pressure, increases venous return to the heart and hence lowers distention and the level of venous pulsations. The opposite occurs during expiration. Patients with severe heart failure and elevated venous pressure or with constrictive pericarditis may respond by increasing venous distention with deep inspiration. The Valsalva maneuver increases venous pressure and distention by increasing intrathoracic pressure and impeding the return of blood to the heart.

When moderately firm pressure is applied with the palm of the hand over the site of the liver for a brief interval, both arterial and normal jugular venous pulsations are not significantly altered. However, in the presence of right heart failure, jugular venous distention and pulsations may increase markedly, probably because the heart is unable to accommodate the additional volume load.

Wave Forms. Normally, there are three positive waves in the jugular venous pulse tracing, which are designated a, c and v, and two negative troughs, x and y (Fig. 1-1). These pulsations essentially are related to pressure and volume changes in the right atrium that are transmitted to the jugular vein.

The a wave is produced by right atrial contraction. It begins before the first heart sound and about 0.05 to 0.08 second after the peak of the P wave.

The x descent follows the a wave and develops as a result of atrial relaxation and traction on the atrioventricular septum by the contracting ventricle. The trough persists throughout most of systole, reflecting the aspirating effect on the blood in the veins when blood is being expelled from the thoracic cavity.

The second positive wave, or c wave, interrupts the x descent and is a slight peak synchronous with the closure of the tricuspid valve at the outset of ventricular systole and with the rise of the carotid pulse.[7] The beginning of the upstroke of the c wave falls approximately 0.14 second later than the onset of the QRS complex. Although regularly recorded the c wave cannot be seen in the neck.

The third positive wave, or v wave, is caused by the rise in volume and pressure in the right atrium as the chamber fills during late systole and early diastole, just prior to the opening of the tricuspid valve and after the first heart sound. In normal subjects it is slightly less prominent than the a wave.[8]

The y descent, which succeeds the v wave, represents the fall in pressure as blood flows from right atrium into right ventricle. The slope of this trough reflects the rate of filling of the right ventricle.

Components of the venous pulse wave usually can be recognized without difficulty in adults when the pulse rate is normal. They are less easily defined when the heart rate is rapid and in infants and children.

Abnormalities of a Wave. Amplitude of the a wave is increased by any condition in which there is increased resistance or an obstruction to right ventricular filling (Fig. 1-2). Tricuspid stenosis, severe pulmonary stenosis and pulmonary hypertension are among the more common causes. A large a wave does not develop when pulmonary hypertension accompanies an atrial septal defect because the energy generated by

right atrial contraction is dissipated through the defect.

Whenever the right atrium contracts against a closed tricuspid valve the a wave becomes greatly exaggerated and is designated a cannon wave. It is presystolic, abrupt and collapsing in quality and is frequently accompanied by a loud presystolic sound heard over the jugular vein and increasing in intensity with inspiration. Abdominal compression increases its amplitude. Irregularly occurring cannon waves, the most common type, are produced by premature contractions arising in the atria, the atrioventricular node or the ventricles. They are also observed in subjects with normal sinus rhythm and complete heart block and in individuals with ventricular tachycardia.

Regularly occurring cannon waves are recorded in nodal rhythm, nodal tachycardia and first- or second-degree atrioventricular block when the P-R interval is exceptionally long.

The amplitude of the a wave may be diminished in sinus tachycardia because it

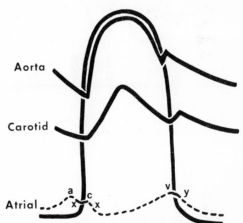

Figure 1-1. Jugular venous pulse and right atrial, carotid and aortic pulses. The a wave caused by atrial contraction precedes the first heart sound. It is followed by x descent that occurs with atrial relaxation. The c wave is too small to be seen. The v wave occurs after the first heart sound and develops with filling of the right atrium. The y descent represents the fall in pressure as the right atrium emptied into the right ventricle.

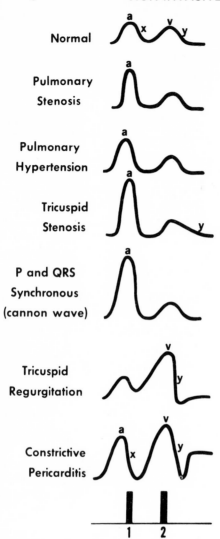

Normal

Pulmonary Stenosis

Pulmonary Hypertension

Tricuspid Stenosis

P and QRS Synchronous (cannon wave)

Tricuspid Regurgitation

Constrictive Pericarditis

Figure 1-2. a Wave patterns in clinical conditions marked by increased resistance to right ventricular filling. In tricuspid regurgitation and constrictive pericarditis the v wave also is dominant.

simulates the ventricular tracing as if a common chamber exists.

Atrial fibrillation itself lessens the negative x wave only to a minor degree. A broad, positive systolic wave is not inscribed unless considerable tricuspid regurgitation coexists.

The amplitude of the negative x wave may be increased in subjects with constrictive pericarditis alone or associated with acute pericarditis.

Abnormalities of the v Wave. An exaggerated v wave is observed in tricuspid regurgitation because the incompetent valve allows reflux of blood into the right atrium and great veins during ventricular systole.[9] It can be distinguished from the presystolic a wave of tricuspid stenosis by timing it against the carotid pulse. The v wave follows the initial rise of the carotid pulse and the first heart sound and is well transmitted to the liver and to the femoral venous pulse.

Abnormalities of the y Descent. A sharp y descent indicates rapid filling of the right ventricle. It is encountered in patients with chronic constrictive pericarditis and in subjects with severe heart failure in whom venous pressure is quite high. Filling stops abruptly in constrictive pericarditis because dilatation of the ventricle is arrested by the rigid pericardium. As a result, pressure rises and remains high through the end of diastole. Graphically, the pulse wave is distinguished by an initial sharp y trough, followed by a sustained plateau (Fig. 1-2). A similar venous pulse wave develops in patients with severe congestive failure and subendocardial fibroelastosis owing to restriction of right ventricular filling.[10]

Venous Pressure. Estimation of venous pressure can be accomplished by examining arm and hand veins or the external and internal jugular veins.

When the veins on the dorsum of the hand are utilized the patient should be sitting or lying at a 30-degree elevation with

may be fused with the preceding v wave or lost in the y descent. No a wave is found in atrial fibrillation or flutter since the atria are not contracting.

Abnormalities of the x Wave. The x descent is materially influenced by the presence of tricuspid regurgitation, the trough becoming less significant as the valve dysfunction increases. In advanced lesions the contour of the right atrial pulse

the hand held below the level of the heart until the veins overfill. The physician then raises the subject's arm slowly, observing the point at which the veins collapse. If this should take place at a point higher than the angle of Louis, venous pressure may be considered to be elevated. A number of conditions other than heart failure may be responsible for a positive response, including local or thoracic inlet venous obstruction and subcutaneous edema.

The technique utilizing the external jugular vein requires the trunk of the body to be elevated 30 to 60 degrees, with the head rotated away from the vessel being examined. After the forefinger is placed just above and parallel to the clavicle, gentle pressure is exerted so as to occlude the vein for 15 to 45 seconds, after which the vessel is allowed to fill, and the apparent height of the fluid column within the vein is observed. Normally the level does not rise beyond a few millimeters above the superior border of the clavicle. If venous pressure is increased above normal the level of venous filling is correspondingly elevated.

As an alternative method of examination the jugular venous pulse may be observed, and the highest point to which it rises may be recorded. The latter marks the level of venous filling and, consequently, measures venous pressure.

The most common cause of elevated venous pressure is right heart failure. Other causes include cardiac tamponade, tricuspid stenosis, right atrial myxoma and superior vena cava obstruction. Since the jugular venous pressure also usually rises with increased intra-abdominal pressure (ascites), increased intrathoracic pressure (cough), a slow heart rate, hyperkinetic states and increased blood volume, all of these possibilities must be eliminated before it is concluded that cardiac decompensation is present.

Arterial Pulse. The purpose of examining the arterial pulse is to determine rate, rhythm, quality and wave form. The examination should be performed with the patient reclining and the trunk elevated 15 to 30 degrees. The carotid artery usually is evaluated first. To facilitate the procedure the head of the patient is turned to the ipsilateral side as the physician places the pulp of the forefinger lightly over the artery. When the examination is extended to the peripheral pulses, it is important to palpate the radial and femoral arteries simultaneously for a brief interval to determine the relative time of onset of the pulse at the two locations.

The normal carotid arterial pulse wave consists of an ascending limb, peak and descending limb (Fig. 1-3). The upstroke or ascending limb begins about 80 msec. after

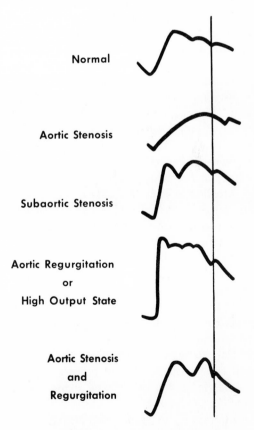

Normal

Aortic Stenosis

Subaortic Stenosis

Aortic Regurgitation
or
High Output State

Aortic Stenosis
and
Regurgitation

Figure 1-3. Normal carotid pulse compared with altered patterns in left ventricular outflow tract obstruction, and aortic regurgitation alone and in combination with aortic stenosis.

the initial component of the first heart sound and represents isovolumetric contraction and the interval required for transmission of the pulse wave to the carotid artery. It arises rapidly and terminates in a smooth, rounded peak. The descending limb is not as abrupt and is marred by an incisura, caused by closure of the aortic valve, that is palpated, if at all, as a change in direction of down slope. The pulse wave arrives later in peripheral vessels where it is characterized by a steeper initial ascending limb and a higher peak.

Rate. Even in health there is considerable variation in pulse rate. Exercise, emotional stress, febrile states, hypertension, hyperkinetic disease, paroxysmal ectopic rhythms, constrictive pericarditis and congestive heart failure are some of the conditions under which unusually rapid pulse rates are encountered. Abnormally slow rates may result from vagotonia, increased intracranial pressure, myxedema and various forms of heart block.

Rhythm. Normally the pulse is quite regular. Ectopic contractions, atrial flutter, with varying degrees of atrioventricular block, and atrial fibrillation, with changing atrioventricular conduction, are common causes of irregularity.

Amplitude. The amplitude or volume of the pulse is determined by left ventricular stroke output, rate of ejection, distensibility of arterial bed, peripheral vascular resistance, difference between systolic and diastolic pressures and distance between the vessel being palpated and the heart.

The pulse is small when stroke output is diminished, pulse pressure is narrow, and peripheral vascular resistance is increased. Mitral stenosis, constrictive pericarditis and left ventricular failure following myocardial infarction are classic causes of a small or weak pulse.

Conversely, the pulse becomes full and bounding when stroke volume is increased, pulse pressure is wide and peripheral resistance is decreased. This combination is encountered in stress, exercise, pregnancy, hyperkinetic conditions, febrile states, aortic regurgitation and arteriovenous shunts. A full pulse implies that the stroke volume is adequate.

Other Characteristics. When left ventricular ejection is delayed by an obstruction such as aortic stenosis, the upstroke of the pulse wave, frequently the site of vibrations, rises slowly to a sustained peak. Because the notch on the upstroke cannot be palpated, this pulse wave has been designated as anacrotic.

A sharp upsurge of the pulse wave followed by an abrupt collapse is observed in all conditions in which there is excessive diastolic filling of the left ventricle. Aortic and mitral regurgitation, ventricular septal defect and patent ductus arteriosus are prime causes for such a wave, which is commonly designated a *water-hammer pulse.* Other causes include exercise, pregnancy, alcoholism, hyperkinetic states and cor pulmonale.

When a double impulse during systole replaces the normal single upstroke, the finding is called *pulsus bisferiens* and most commonly is encountered in combined aortic stenosis and regurgitation.[14]

Pulsus paradoxus refers to a marked decrease in amplitude during inspiration. Normally the fall in intrathoracic pressure during inspiration brings sufficient blood into the right heart to compensate for the expanded pulmonary vascular capacity, thereby preventing a fall in cardiac output and in the amplitude of the pulse. Inability of the right ventricle to receive an augmented load, as in pericardial effusion, constrictive pericarditis or congestive failure, defeats the compensatory mechanism so that the pulse diminishes during inspiration.

Pulsus alternans is the term applied to regularly spaced upstrokes of alternately smaller and larger volume. The mechanism responsible for this phenomenon is obscure. However, pulsus alternans is observed in cardiac decompensation and in patients with aortic stenosis who do not have significant elevation of end-diastolic pressure in the left ventricle. The presence of pulsus alternans may be confirmed by observing the difference in the systolic pressure between the alternate beats while recording the blood pressure.

EXAMINATION OF THE PRECORDIUM

Examination of the precordium should precede auscultation of the heart. Inspection and palpation are much more meaningful than percussion. Included among pertinent observations are chest deformities that could lead to erroneous conclusions regarding heart size, forward bulging of the anterior chest wall indicating the possibility of a congenital cardiac defect and right ventricular hypertrophy and a rocking motion of the precordium suggesting enlargement of either ventricle.

Normally, and particularly in children as well as lean adults, the apex beat is seen at the fifth left interspace in the midclavicular line. When the left ventricle is enlarged, the apex beat is more pronounced and is displaced downward and to the left. Right ventricular hypertrophy results in a visible precordial lift at the third, fourth or fifth interspace to the left of the sternum.

Palpation of the precordium is carried out to determine the nature of the apical pulsation and its location and size, as well as the presence of impulses and vibrations at the base of the heart, the lower parasternal area, the midprecordium and the epigastric region. Palpation is first performed with the palm of the hand placed over the area under inquiry. The finger may be used to define subtle details of the abnormal finding that is discovered.

The apex beat is felt at the fifth left intercostal space in the midclavicular line; the right ventricle, over the third and fourth intercostal spaces at the left parasternal area; the aorta, in the right parasternal area over the second and third interspaces; and the pulmonary artery, at the same level but at the left parasternal area.

The impulse felt at the apex usually is that of the left ventricle. The movement is a brief, outward, well-localized thrust that is felt in all but very obese subjects.[15]

Left ventricular hypertrophy produces a more forceful, longer and somewhat more diffuse movement that lifts the palpating fingers of the examining hand with each systole.

Left ventricular dilatation causes the apical thrust to be displaced laterally and to a lower intercostal space where the point of maximum intensity becomes difficult to localize. In instances of extreme dilatation the pulsation may be felt in the midaxillary line and in the sixth and seventh left interspaces. Among the most common causes of marked left ventricular dilatation are aortic and mitral regurgitation, ventricular septal defect, ventricular aneurysm and patent ductus arteriosus.

Normally, pulsation of the right ventricle cannot be felt. However, when the chamber is hypertrophied or in pulmonary stenosis, a localized, forceful thrust is palpable immediately to the left of the sternum at the fifth intercostal space. The movement of a dilated right ventricle is distributed widely over the precordium to the left of the sternum.

Under normal conditions, vascular pulsations cannot be felt at the precordial area. When pulmonary artery pressures are elevated the systolic pulsation of the vessel may be palpated in the third interspace just to the left of the sternum.

Palpation may be helpful in defining abnormal heart sounds and murmurs. The short, high-pitched first heart sound of mitral stenosis may be palpable at the apex as a sharp, highly localized tap that is easily differentiated from the sustained thrust of left ventricular hypertrophy or the diffuse lift of left ventricular dilatation.

Pulmonary valve closure may be detected in the third interspace to the left of the sternum when pulmonary hypertension is present and the valve leaflets are pliable.

The presence of a loud, prolonged pathologic murmur is suggested when a thrill is felt at the apex or base of the heart. The murmurs that are usually responsible for thrills are those of mitral regurgitation, aortic senosis, ventricular septal defect, pulmonary stenosis and mitral stenosis.

The thrill of mitral regurgitation is systolic and is felt at the apex. The thrill of aortic stenosis also is systolic but is palpated in the second right interspace and is transmitted in the direction of the neck vessels. A ventricular septal defect thrill is felt in the fourth and fifth left interspaces

and radiates transversely. The systolic thrill of pulmonic stenosis is palpated at the second left interspace and radiates to the infraclavicular area. Mitral stenosis frequently produces an apical diastolic thrill.

AUSCULTATION OF THE HEART

Auscultation is an art that, except for those with defective hearing, matures with training and experience. To develop it fully the physician must be familiar with current concepts regarding the genesis of heart sounds and murmurs and the manner in which they relate to structure and function, must master the routine mechanics of performing a proper auscultatory examination and, above all, must be willing to attain

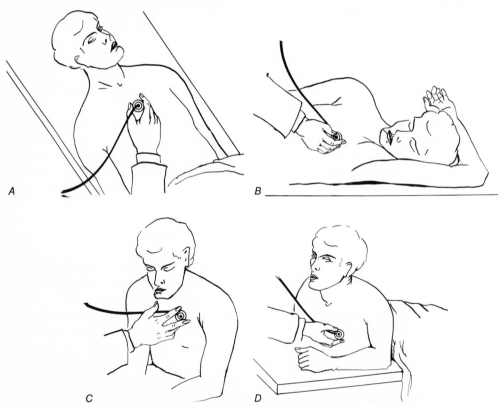

Figure 1-4A. Initial position for auscultation of the heart. Patient should be in the semirecumbent position, 45 degrees to the horizontal. *B.* The left lateral position is preferred for palpation of the left ventricle and hearing the diastolic rumble of mitral stenosis. *C.* The sitting position accentuates the high-frequency murmur of aortic regurgitation. Splitting of the second sound also is heard better in this position. *D.* The knee-chest position may increase the intensity of distant heart sounds and the murmur of aortic insufficiency.

competence through repeated, meaningful clinical experiences. There is no substitute for listening to sounds and murmurs over and over again.

Technique. Auscultation requires a quiet environment. An ideal examining room is isolated from all ordinary sources of noise, including the telephone, typewriter, air-conditioner and conversation.

The patient may be asked to assume different positions and, therefore, should be free of all encumbrances (Fig. 1-4A–D). Sitting in the semirecumbent position, 45 degrees to the horizontal, resting supine, lying on the left side and bending forward are the classic positions used. Each, except the supine position, increases the contact of the apex with the chest wall and is helpful in bringing out left ventricular sounds and mitral valve murmurs. The left lateral position accentuates the diastolic murmur of mitral stenosis. The supine position is best for pulmonic and tricuspid murmurs, while bending forward improves the audibility of aortic diastolic murmurs. Regardless of the position the patient assumes, the precordium should be completely exposed, and the physician should stand to the right of the patient since, in this position, the stethoscope lies in the most direct line from the examiner's ears to the subject's chest wall.

Auscultation should begin at the apex with the patient in the semirecumbent position. Each auscultatory area is then studied by advancing the stethoscope slowly across the precordium (Fig. 1-5).

The apical area is the best location to hear mitral valve murmurs, atrial and left ventricular gallop sounds and the aortic component of the second sound. Not uncommonly the murmurs of aortic stenosis and aortic insufficiency also are heard quite distinctly in this area and are confused with mitral valve murmurs.

At the fourth and fifth interspaces, 2 to 4 cm. to the left and 2 cm. to the right of the sternum, is the area where the mur-

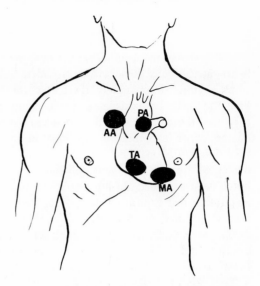

Figure 1-5. Auscultatory areas. The aortic area is at the second right interspace, pulmonic area at the second left interspace, tricuspid area at the lower left parasternal border and mitral area at the apex.

murs of tricuspid stenosis and tricuspid insufficiency, ventricular septal defect and pulmonary insufficiency, as well as atrial and right ventricular gallop sounds, are heard best.

The aortic area includes the second right and the third left interspaces. Here the murmurs of aortic stenosis and aortic insufficiency, dilatation of the aorta and carotid artery stenosis, as well as the aortic ejection click and the aortic component of the second heart sound, are heard clearly.

The pulmonary area is formed by the second and third interspaces just to the left of the sternum and the adjacent infraclavicular region. This is the location where the murmurs of pulmonary stenosis and insufficiency, pulmonary artery dilatation, the pulmonary component of the second sound and the pulmonary ejection click are heard most distinctly.

Only one auscultatory event is listened to at a time. To attempt to do otherwise simply overwhelms perceptive and interpretive senses. Accomplished examiners proceed from one observation to another in a disciplined routine, blocking out all but the event to which they are listening.

The first step in auscultation is to record heart rate and any departures from normal sinus rhythm. Immediately thereafter the first and second sounds at each auscultatory area must be identified. The accuracy of the entire examination depends upon this differentiation. The sounds are then evaluated for intensity and splitting. The latter is best judged during partial to full inspiration and expiration. Once identified, the systolic and diastolic periods are first examined for abnormal sounds, such as ejection and gallop sounds, and then for the presence of murmurs.

The use of a disciplined auscultatory routine not only conserves time and energy, but provides the physician with the best opportunity to observe, analyze, correlate and interpret meaningful findings.

Heart Sounds. There are five types of heart sounds: (1) valve closure sounds, (2) valve opening sounds, (3) ventricular filling sounds, (4) ejection sounds and (5) extracardiac sounds.

The first and second heart sounds are valve closure sounds. The first heart sound is produced by closure of the mitral and tricuspid valves.[21] It is lower in pitch and longer in duration than the second sound. The interval between it and the second sound is shorter than the interval between the second sound and the next succeeding first sound.

The best area for hearing the first sound is the apex and midprecordium. The intensity is increased in mitral stenosis, systemic hypertension and in hyperkinetic states. It is decreased in myocardial infarction, mitral insufficiency, aortic insufficiency, hypothyroidism and myocarditis (Fig. 1-6).

Splitting of the first sound is relatively common in normal adolescents. However, in adults, splitting often is confused with an atrial gallop sound (S_4), which is never heard in normal hearts.

The second sound is produced by closure of the aortic and pulmonic valves. The components of the sound are heard best at the second and third interspaces to the right and left of the sternum.

Loudness of the aortic component is increased in systemic hypertension, coarctation of the aorta and aortitis. It is diminished in aortic stenosis when flexibility of the leaflets is seriously impaired.

The intensity of the pulmonic component is increased in pulmonary hypertension, regardless of cause. There is decreased intensity loudness in pulmonary stenosis.

Splitting of the second sound is encountered frequently during inspiration in normal children and adolescents. Abnormal splitting occurs when right bundle branch or right ventricular volume overload delays pulmonary valve closure. Left bundle branch block is responsible for a delay in aortic valve closure and paradoxical splitting (Fig. 1-7).

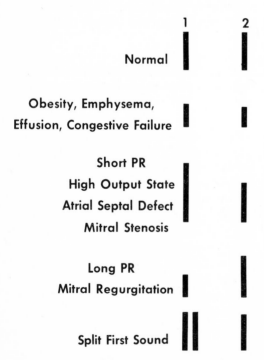

Figure 1-6. Variations in intensity and splitting of the first heart sound (S_1).

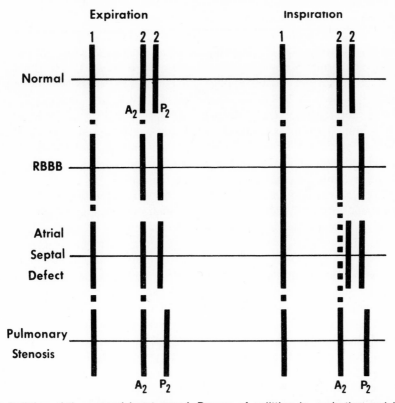

Figure 1-7. Splitting of the second heart sound. Degree of splitting in expiration and inspiration under normal conditions compared with right bundle branch block, atrial septal defect and pulmonary stenosis.

Normally, valve opening sounds are inaudible, but under pathologic conditions such as mitral or tricuspid stenosis, they become accentuated. In mitral stenosis the opening sound (opening snap) is heard best at the fourth left interspace just to the left of the sternum. It appears as a short, high-pitched sound. The total auscultatory effect is that of a widely split second sound. Occasionally the mitral valve opening snap can be heard in left ventricular diastolic overload as in mitral insufficiency and patent ductus.

The opening snap of tricuspid stenosis is audible at the fourth and fifth interspaces to the left and right of the sternum. It can be heard in some instances when there is right ventricular diastolic overload as in tricuspid insufficiency, atrial septal defect and ventricular septal defect.

Ventricular filling sounds (S_3 and S_4) arise when impaired distensibility produces abnormal vibrations of the wall or the chordae. They are low in frequency and intensity and are heard in diastole.

The third sound (S_3) is heard best at the fourth and fifth interspaces to the right and left of the sternum and at the apex. It occurs approximately 0.12 to 0.16 second after the second heart sound. It may be heard in normal children and young adults. However, it usually is a hallmark of heart failure.

The fourth heart sound (S_4) occurs prior to the first sound and is heard most commonly at the apex. It, too, may be audible at the fourth and fifth interspaces to the right and left of the sternum. Myocarditis, atrial flutter, various degrees of atrioventricular block, systemic hypertension and aortic stenosis are among its more common causes. Pulmonary stenosis or pulmonary hypertension may be responsible for a right ventricular S_4 sound.

The term gallop rhythm often is applied indiscriminately when an S_3 or S_4 sound is heard. It is more appropriate to restrict the term to a lilting rhythm, occasioned by the appearance of a loud S_3 or S_4 sound, usually associated with a rapid ventricular rate. Gallop rhythms generally occur in patients with myocardial failure.

Ejection sounds are attributed to sudden distention of a dilated aorta or pulmonary artery or forceful opening of the aorta or pulmonic cusps in the presence of aortic or pulmonary stenosis. They have a sharp, clicking quality and occur early in systole.

The pulmonic ejection sound is best heard at the second and third interspaces to the left of the sternum. In addition to mild valvular pulmonary stenosis, it is encountered in idiopathic dilatation of the pulmonary artery and pulmonary hypertension accompanied by a dilated pulmonary artery.

The aortic ejection sound is best heard over the apical area. It may be heard whenever the aorta is dilated, regardless of cause.

Systolic clicks and ejection sounds are often confused. The former occur later in systole, moving with inspiration closer to the first sound. They have no known clinical significance. In most instances they are believed to arise from extracardiac structures.

Pleural and pericardial friction rubs, as well as pericardial knocks, are among the most common extracardiac sounds that may be mistaken for abnormal cardiac auscultatory findings. In contrast to the pleural friction rub, which usually is heard in both upright and supine positions, the pericardial rub must be searched for with the breath expelled and the patient sitting upright, leaning forward, lying down and even turned to either side.

Heart Murmurs. Heart murmurs are noises that are produced as a result of turbulent blood flow, eddy formation and possibly cavitation.[22,23] The most important features of murmurs, and the basis for their classification, are timing and duration in relation to the cardiac cycle, and intensity. Other characteristics such as pitch, quality, area of maximum intensity and transmission are helpful, but not essential, in defining their cause.

Murmurs are either systolic or diastolic in time or they may be heard during both intervals.

Systolic murmurs are classified as: (1) ejection murmurs, which occur after the first sound, predominantly in midsystole; (2) pansystolic murmurs, which occur with the first sound and extend throughout systole; (3) early systolic murmurs, which are limited to the first part of systole, and (4) late systolic murmurs, which are restricted to the last part of systole[18] (Fig. 1-8).

An ejection systolic murmur is commonly encountered in most infants, many children and even some adults who do not have heart disease. This physiologic or benign murmur probably is caused by turbulent blood flow in the right ventricular outflow tract and main pulmonary artery.

Important structural abnormalities producing an ejection systolic murmur include narrowing of either the left or right ventricular outflow tract by valvular stenosis or constriction above or below the valve, dilatation of the aorta or pulmonary artery and increased blood flow through either vessel. In atrial septal defect with left-to-right shunting the increased flow through the pulmonary artery commonly produces an ejection systolic murmur.

Pansystolic murmurs are produced by the passage of blood from a high to a low pressure chamber throughout systole. This occurs in mitral regurgitation, tricuspid regurgitation and ventricular septal defects. Pansystolic murmurs never occur in normal hearts.

Early systolic murmurs are not heard commonly. They are caused by ventricular septal defects, limited to the muscular septum, that close in midsystole as a result of contraction of the septum.

Late systolic murmurs almost invariably are caused by mild mitral regurgitation, which in turn may result from structural abnormalities of any portion of the mitral valve complex, including posterior left atrial wall, mitral annulus, leaflets, chordae tendineae, papillary muscles and left ventricular wall.

The numbers I to VI are usually used in grading the intensity of systolic murmurs, grade I being just audible and grade VI being loud enough to be heard with the stethoscope barely lifted from the chest wall.

Diastolic murmurs almost always indicate heart disease. They occur early, mid-late or late in diastole.

Early diastolic murmurs are caused by aortic or pulmonary regurgitation. They are produced immediately or very soon after valve closure. The aortic murmur may be very soft in intensity. It is typically decrescendo. The pulmonic murmur, whether secondary to pulmonary hypertension or an actual structural deformity of the valve, is also high pitched and decrescendo, but usually more intense.

Mid-late diastolic murmurs are due to turbulent flow of blood across the mitral or tricuspid valves, usually when their orifices are actually stenosed. They are also heard in rheumatic carditis and in mitral regurgitation. In the latter instance there is increased flow of blood across the valve due to the regurgitation that occurred during the previous systole. Mid-late diastolic mitral murmurs due to increased flow of blood are also heard in ventricular septal defect and patent ductus arteriosus, with left-to-right shunts. Finally, a mid-late mitral diastolic murmur is frequently present in moderate or severe aortic regurgitation. The mechanism of this murmur, de-

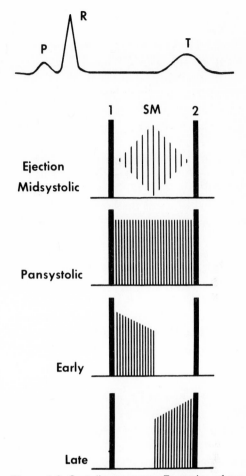

Figure 1-8. Systolic murmurs. Examples of systolic cycle and their relation to S_1 and S_2.

scribed by Austin Flint, is probably that the aortic regurgitant jet presses the anterior leaflet of the mitral valve backward so that it impedes the flow of blood from left atrium to ventricle.

Late diastolic or presystolic murmurs are caused by the turbulent flow of blood across a narrowed mitral or tricuspid valve. It is high pitched and has a crescendo character leading to the first sound. Similar to the mid-late diastolic murmur, it may be heard particularly at the tricuspid area, when there is increased flow through a normal valve as in left-to-right shunts at the atrial level.

Continuous murmurs are present in both

systole and diastole. They usually have a crescendo pattern in systole and are decrescendo in diastole, followed by a short, silent period. Patent ductus arteriosus is the most common pathologic cause. Other structural causes are arteriovenous communications in the lungs and coronary and systemic circulations. Venous hum is the most frequent explanation for a continuous murmur in the neck of normal children.

LUNGS

Examination of the lungs is an essential detail in the evaluation of the circulatory system since pulmonary congestion, pulmonary consolidation and pleural effusion may be direct expressions of cardiovascular disease. The traditional methods of examination, inspection, palpation, percussion and auscultation should be utilized in the appraisal even though chest x-ray examination is contemplated for definitive conclusions.

ABDOMEN

The abdominal examination is conducted to detect the presence of organ enlargement, particularly the liver, spleen and kidneys, to ascertain whether there is an unusual configuration of the aorta, to eliminate the possibility of fluid accumulation and to inquire about abnormal pulsations.

Hepatic enlargement is frequently present in right heart failure, regardless of cause. Gross splenomegaly is rare except if subacute bacterial endocarditis is associated with the failure. While the liver edge is easily detected during deep inspiration with the patient lying flat, the spleen is difficult to palpate below the left costal margin. Indeed, it has to enlarge to approximately twice its normal size before it can be felt. An enlarged spleen is often best felt with the patient lying comfortably on the right side; during deep inspiration the exploring hand of the examiner is placed under the left costal cage.

Renal enlargement must be excluded during the cardiac examination, since polycystic kidneys or bilateral hydronephrosis can lead to hypertension. Because renal artery stenosis is another cause of hypertension, auscultation should be carried out in the midline just above the umbilicus and then more laterally on both sides over the flanks.

Careful palpation of the abdomen should determine whether aneurysmal dilatation of the aorta is present and whether there are unusual vascular pulsations.

Distention of the abdomen may be due to ascites, which in turn may be the result of heart failure. Under such circumstances, liver enlargement is almost invariably present.

PERIPHERAL EDEMA

Peripheral edema may indicate severe right heart failure. In its initial stage it appears just below the ankles and over the lower tibia where small indentations may be made with the examining fingers. Later the swelling may extend throughout the legs and appear over the sacrum, the scrotum and the lower abdominal wall. Disproportionate accumulations to one side or the other are usually positional in origin.

GENERAL EXAMINATION

The examination of heart and blood vessels is not complete without a thorough general examination of the patient. The information obtained in most instances, together with a competent history, usually is sufficient to reach a reasonable diagnostic conclusion before additional information is obtained from objective methods of study such as electrocardiography and chest x-ray examination.

SUMMARY

In the total appraisal of patients suspected of having heart disease it is generally agreed that the physical examination is second in importance only to the medical history. This holds, despite the numerous

history. This holds, despite the numerous diagnostic advances that have taken place, including the development of echocardiography, cardiac catheterization and angiography. However, one should not attempt to evaluate the cardiac status of any patient without using every type of examination that may be considered necessary or helpful.

Subjective manifestations usually appear in conjunction with objective signs of cardiovascular disease. The most notorious exception is coronary heart disease, which may present with crippling angina and absolutely no indication of structural abnormality. It is under such circumstances that specialized techniques of examination such as exercise electrocardiography and coronary arteriography are most likely to be used.

A remarkably accurate perspective of a diagnostic problem can be developed if coexisting symptoms and signs are analyzed in terms of their pathogenesis. Examples are legion: (1) What is the comparative importance of peripheral edema in mitral and aortic stenosis? In mitral stenosis, right ventricular failure alone accounts for the edema, while in aortic stenosis biventricular failure must be suspected. (2) Does the disappearance of recurrent hemoptysis in mitral stenosis represent improvement? It does not. Increased pulmonary vascular resistance is responsible for the lessening of hemoptysis, but it causes further and continued hemodynamic embarrassment to the right ventricle.

The bedside techniques by which the cardiovascular systems are appraised are invaluable in reaching a complete cardiac diagnosis. Particular note is made of the usefulness of auscultation in clinical medicine. The diagnosis of most forms of congenital heart disease and rheumatic valvular afflictions can be accomplished with ease and considerable accuracy by means of the stethoscope. In addition, the finding of a diastolic gallop rhythm may precede the discovery of any subjective expression of cardiac decompensation. Endless other examples of the importance of auscultation in diagnosis may be cited, including the recognition of dysrhythmias.

The basic technique for the examination of the cardiovascular systems requires attention to what appear to be pedestrian details, such as the comfort of the examiner, the position and exposure of the patient and the physical qualities of the examining room. Yet by honoring these requirements, the physician is likely to garner the fullest rewards.

REFERENCES

1. Allen, E., Barker, N., and Hines, E.: Peripheral Vascular Diseases. Philadelphia. W. B. Saunders Co., 1962.
2. Winsor, T.: Peripheral Vascular Diseases. Springfield, Ill., Charles C Thomas, 1959.
3. Wood, P.: Diseases of the Heart and Circulation, ed. 2. Philadelphia, J. B. Lippincott Co., 1956.
4. Beck, L., and Brody, M. J.: Physiology of vasodilatation. Angiology 12:202, 1961.
5. Fisher, D. S., Singer, D. H., and Feldman, S.: Clubbing: A review with emphasis on hereditary acropachy. Medicine 43:459, 1964.
6. Cossio, P., and Buzzi, D.: Clinical value of venous pulse. Am. Heart J. 54:127, 1957.
7. Mackay, I. F. S.: An experimental analysis of the jugular pulse in man. J. Physiol. 106:113, 1947.
8. Groedel, F. M.: The Venous Pulse and Its Graphic Recording. New York, Brooklyn Medical Press, 1946.
9. Lottenbach, C., and Shellingford, J.: Functional tricuspid incompetence in relation to the venous pressure. Br. Heart J. 19:395, 1957.
10. Korner, P., and Shellingford, J.: The right atrial pulse in congestive heart failure. Br. Heart J. 16:447, 1954.
11. Robinson, B.: The carotid pulse. Relation of external recordings to carotid, aortic and brachial pulses. Br. Heart J. 25:61, 1963.
12. Robinson, B.: The carotid pulse, Diagnosis of aortic stenosis by external recordings. Br. Heart J. 25:51, 1963.
13. Benchimal, A., Dimond, E. G., and Shen, Y.: Ejection time in aortic stenosis and mitral stenosis, Am. J. Cardiol. 5:728, 1960.
14. Segal, B. L., and McGarvy, T. F.: The venous and arterial pulse. J.A.M.A. 187:323, 1963.
15. Eddleman, E. E., Jr., Hiefner, L., Reeves, T. J., and Harrison, T. R.: Movements and forces of the human heart. Arch. Int. Med. 99:401, 1957.
16. Levine, S. A., and Harvey, W. P.: Clinical

Auscultation of the Heart. Philadelphia, W. B. Saunders Co., 1959.

17. Segal, B. L., Likoff, W., and Moyer, J. J.: The Theory and Practice of Auscultation. Philadelphia, F. A. Davis Co., 1964.

18. Leatham, A.: Auscultation of the heart. Lancet 2:703, 1958.

19. Segal, B. L., and Likoff, W.: Phonocardiography: A valuable aid to clinical diagnosis. Dis. Chest 43:256, 1963.

20. Segal, B. L., Likoff, W., and Mason, D.: Cardiac auscultation in health and disease. Pa. Med. J. 65:1237, 1962.

21. Leatham, A.: Splitting of the first and second heart sounds. Lancet 2:607, 1954.

22. Symposium on Cardiovascular Sound. Circulation 16:270, 1957.

23. Meisner, J. E., and Reishmer, R. F.: Eddy formation and turbulence in flowing liquids. Circ. Res. 12:455, 1963.

Chapter 2

Carotid Sinus Stimulation

EDWARD K. CHUNG AND LISA S. CHUNG

It has been known for many years that carotid sinus stimulation is very useful in distinguishing various tachyarrhythmias because the response to this procedure differs according to the origin and the nature of the arrhythmia. This is particularly true when one is dealing with regular and ectopic tachycardia and wide QRS complex in which the differential diagnosis is often urgently needed. In addition, carotid sinus stimulation is extremely valuable in terminating supraventricular (atrial or A-V junctional) tachycardia. Therefore, there are two major indications for carotid sinus stimulation—therapeutic and diagnostic (Table 2-1). On the other hand, the dan-

ger of applying carotid sinus stimulation to patients with suspected digitalis intoxication is well known: Ventricular fibrillation may be induced during or after carotid sinus stimulation in this circumstance.[1-5]

The purpose of this chapter is to review the literature concerning carotid sinus stimulation, with particular emphasis on its clinical usefulness as well as untoward response to the procedure. Various responses to carotid sinus stimulation are summarized in Table 2-2.

VARIOUS CLINICAL CIRCUMSTANCES

Sinus Tachycardia. In general, it is not necessary to apply carotid sinus stimulation for sinus tachycardia either diagnostically or therapeutically. However, the procedure is occasionally useful when the sinus rate is very rapid (around 150 to 160 beats per minute), and differentiation from atrial tachycardia is needed. Sinus tachycardia is only transiently slowed by carotid sinus stimulation, and the original sinus rate returns soon after the procedure is completed (Fig. 2-1). At times, prolongation of the P-R interval or slowing of the ventricular rate as a result of higher degree A-V block

TABLE 2-1

Indications for Carotid Sinus Stimulation

Indication	Arrhythmia
Therapeutic	Supraventricular (paroxysmal atrial or A-V junctional) tachycardia Unknown regular and rapid rate (150 to 250 beats per minute) whether QRS complex is normal or bizarre
Diagnostic	Unknown tachyarrhythmias whether QRS complex is normal or bizarre

19

TABLE 2-2

Various Responses to Carotid Sinus Stimulation

Arrhythmias	Responses
Sinus tachycardia	Transient slowing of sinus (atrial) rate
	Varying degree A-V block (less common)
Atrial tachycardia	Termination
	No response
	Slowing of ventricular rate due to increased A-V block (less common)
	Increased atrial rate (less common)
Atrial fibrillation or flutter	Slowing of ventricular rate due to increased A-V block
A-V junctional tachycardia Paroxysmal	Termination
	No response
Nonparoxysmal	No response
Ventricular tachyarrhythmias	No response (rare exceptions, see text)
W-P-W syndrome	Vary (see text)
Parasystole	Vary (see text)
Digitalis intoxication	Not recommended (see text)
Hypersensitive individuals	Not recommended (see text)

may be produced by carotid sinus stimulation.

Atrial Tachyarrhythmias. Carotid sinus stimulation is extremely valuable in terminating paroxysmal atrial tachycardia. When carotid sinus stimulation is applied for atrial tachycardia, there may be three different responses; namely, there may be no response at all; sinus rhythm may be restored (Fig. 2-2); or there may be slowing of the ventricular rate resulting from increased A-V block (Fig. 2-3), especially when the underlying cause is digitalis intoxication.[1, 6-9]

When carotid sinus pressure is applied in atrial fibrillation or flutter, a slowing of the ventricular rate is invariably produced because of the increased A-V block (Figs. 2-4 and 2-5). Not uncommonly, an extremely slow ventricular rate or even a long ventricular standstill may result when carotid sinus pressure is applied to elderly patients with atrial tachyarrhythmias (Figs. 2-3 and 2-4). Acceleration of the atrial rate from carotid sinus stimulation may be observed in atrial flutter or tachycardia, but the response is not so pronounced in most cases.[6-9]

A-V Junctional Tachycardia. It is often difficult or at times impossible to distinguish between paroxysmal atrial and A-V junctional tachycardias when only a conventional electrocardiogram is available. This is because the P wave may be superimposed on the S-T segment, T wave or QRS complex of the preceding or following beat in atrial and A-V junctional tachycardias. Therefore, the term supraventricular tachycardia is frequently used in this circumstance. Nevertheless, it is believed that the response of paroxysmal A-V junctional

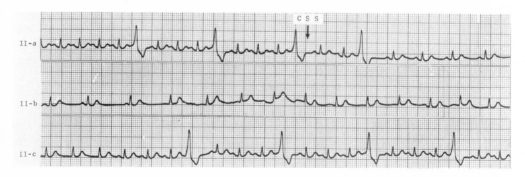

Figure 2-1. Leads II-a, b and c are continuous. Note transient slowing of sinus rate from carotid sinus stimulation (*arrow*) in sinus tachycardia. There are frequent ventricular premature contractions.

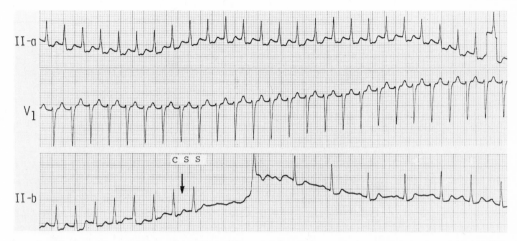

Figure 2-2. Leads II-a and b are not continuous. Supraventricular, most likely atrial, tachycardia (rate 187 beats per minute) is terminated by carotid sinus stimulation (*arrow*). Note occasional atrial premature contractions following restoration of sinus rhythm.

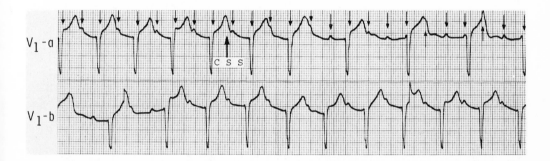

Figure 2-3. Leads V₁-a and b are continuous. Arrows indicate ectopic P waves. Slowing of the ventricular rate is produced by carotid sinus stimulation (*CSS*) because of increased A-V block in atrial tachycardia (atrial rate 168 beats per minute). The arrhythmia is considered to be digitalis induced.

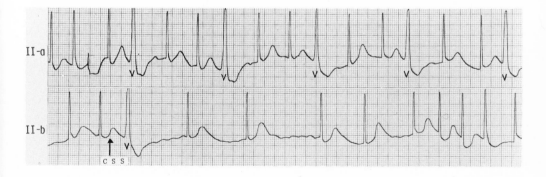

Figure 2-4. Leads II-a and b are continuous. Note marked slowing of ventricular rate from carotid sinus stimulation (*arrow*) in atrial fibrillation. There are frequent ventricular premature contractions (*V*).

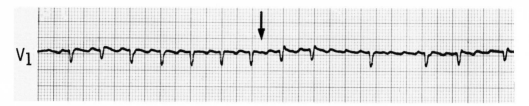

Figure 2-5. Slowing of the ventricular rate from carotid sinus stimulation (*arrow*) is observed in atrial flutter because of increased A-V block.

tachycardia to carotid sinus stimulation is similar to that of atrial tachycardia, that is, paroxysmal A-V junctional tachycardia may convert to sinus rhythm (Fig. 2-6), or it may not be influenced by the procedure. Nonparoxysmal A-V junctional tachycardia, however, is usually refractory to carotid sinus stimulation. (Paroxysmal A-V junctional tachycardia is defined as A-V junctional tachycardia with abrupt onset and termination, and this tachycardia always has a rapid rate [180 to 250 per minute]. On the other hand, nonparoxysmal A-V junctional tachycardia is defined as chronic A-V junctional tachycardia with a slower rate [70 to 150 per minute].[1,7,8]) Furthermore, the procedure may induce ventricular fibrillation when A-V junctional tachycardia is due to digitalis toxicity.[1-5] Thus, carotid sinus stimulation is not recommended for nonparoxysmal A-V junctional tachycardia, which is a common manifestation of digitalis toxicity.[1,9]

Ventricular Tachyarrhythmias. As a rule, ventricular tachyarrhythmias must be treated more actively when the diagnosis is made. However, carotid sinus stimulation is not uncommonly applied in order to differentiate ventricular tachycardia from supraventricular tachycardia, especially when the clinical situation is not urgent and the QRS complex is wide and bizarre. In contrast to supraventricular tachyarrhythmias, ordinary paroxysmal ventricular tachycardia does not respond to carotid sinus stimulation. Thus, absence of response to the procedure does not favor or exclude the diagnosis of supraventricular or ventricular tachycardia, but ventricular tachycardia is excluded if there is any response to carotid sinus stimulation. However, it should be noted that in ventricular tachycardia due to a parasystolic mechanism or in the nonparoxysmal form, carotid sinus stimulation may slow or even terminate or at times provoke recurrence of the

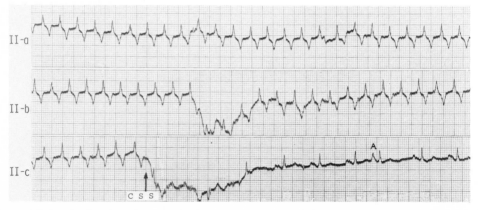

Figure 2-6. Leads II-a, b and c are continuous. Paroxysmal A-V junctional tachycardia is terminated by carotid sinus stimulation (*arrow*). Note an atrial premature contraction (*A*) following restoration of sinus rhythm.

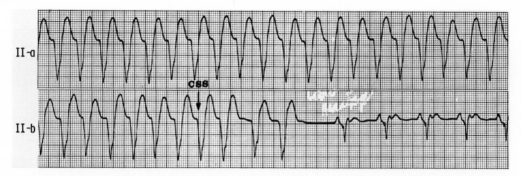

Figure 2-7. These rhythm strips were obtained from a patient with acute diaphragmatic myocardial infarction. Leads II-a and b are continuous. Nonparoxysmal ventricular tachycardia (rate 140 beats per minute) is terminated by carotid sinus stimulation (*arrow*).

arrhythmias[10] (Fig. 2-7). (Parasystole is defined as simultaneous activity of two [rarely more] independent impulse-forming centers, one of which is "protected" from the other, each competing to activate the atria or ventricles or both. Diagnostic criteria of parasystole include (1) varying coupling intervals, (2) constant shortest interectopic intervals and (3) frequent appearance of fusion beats.[7,8,10]

Nonparoxysmal ventricular tachycardia is defined as slow ventricular tachycardia [rate 70 to 150 beats per minute], which is common during 24 to 72 hours of acute myocardial infarction. Nonparoxysmal ventricular tachycardia is analogous to nonparoxysmal A-V junctional tachycardia[8]).

Wolff-Parkinson-White Syndrome. Carotid sinus pressure can abolish ventricular pre-excitation or, in occasional instances, may cause it to appear.[12-14] When carotid sinus pressure is applied in the presence of Wolff-Parkinson-White syndrome it can produce an A-V junctional rhythm with a normal QRS complex[15] since the vagal stimulation tends to prolong A-V conduction time or temporarily block the normal pathway and displace the pacemaker from the S-A node to the A-V junction.[16] Pick and Katz observed that, in one patient with paroxysmal atrial tachycardia with 1:1 conduction associated with the Wolff-Parkinson-White syndrome, carotid sinus pressure induced paroxysmal atrial

tachycardia with varying A-V block, which subsequently changed to atrial flutter and finally to atrial fibrillation.[17] Carotid sinus pressure is often effective in terminating atrial tachycardia associated with Wolff-Parkinson-White syndrome[7,8,18] (Fig. 2-8).

Parasystole. It is interesting to note that the atrial or A-V junctional parasystolic rate may be decreased by the application of carotid sinus stimulation.[19,20] This phenomenon never occurs in other forms of atrial or A-V junctional arrhythmias if the parasystolic mechanism is not present. Another interesting occurrence is the effect of carotid sinus stimulation on ventricular parasystole. It is generally known that carotid sinus stimulation has no or very little influence on the human ventricles in regard to contraction or impulse formation. However, in ventricular parasystole, carotid sinus stimulation may slow, terminate or even provoke recurrence of the arrhythmia.[21-24] The disappearance of ventricular parasystole, due either to the appearance of exit block or the disappearance of the protection block, due to the same mechanism, has been reported.[25] The disappearance of atrial parasystole as a result of carotid sinus stimulation has also been reported.[26] On the other hand, in certain cases, carotid sinus stimulation may not influence the arrhythmia.[10,23,27] This phenomenon was first described by Vedoya in a patient with A-V nodal rhythm.[28,29]

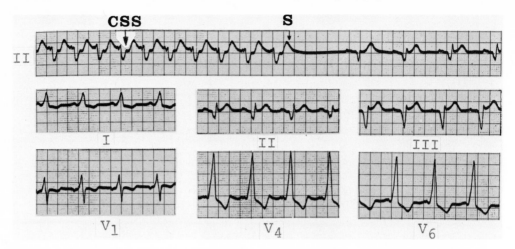

Figure 2-8. The first portion of the upper strip of lead II shows paroxysmal atrial tachycardia with a rate of 140 beats per minute, and then the rhythm is converted by carotid sinus stimulation (*CSS*) to sinus rhythm (*S*) with anomalous A-V conduction. Wolff-Parkinson-White syndrome type A is diagnosed during sinus rhythm because of a short P-R interval and wide QRS complex due to delta wave (initial slurring of upstroke of the QRS complex).

Digitalis Intoxication. Some investigators observed that carotid sinus stimulation frequently halts paroxysmal atrial tachycardia with A-V block not due to digitalis toxicity and is ineffective when digitalis is the etiologic factor.[30] On the other hand, slowing of the ventricular rate may result from increased A-V block from the procedure when the underlying cause is digitalis toxicity[1,6-9] (Fig. 2-3). However, we would like to emphasize the danger of applying carotid sinus stimulation to patients with suspected digitalis intoxication. Four deaths have been reported from ventricular fibrillation during or after carotid sinus stimulation.[2-5] All of the patients had been critically ill and had received cardiac glycosides. Based on these observations, ca-

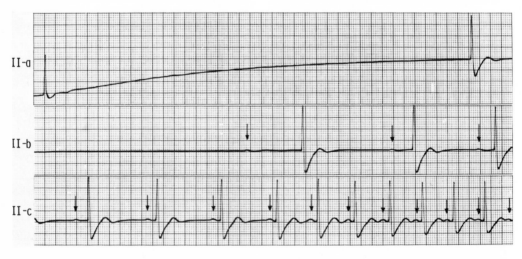

Figure 2-9. Leads II-a, b and c are continuous. Arrows indicate P waves. Marked slowing of atrial and ventricular rates with a long period of ventricular standstill is observed in a patient with a hypersensitive reaction to carotid sinus stimulation.

rotid sinus stimulation should be avoided as much as possible in patients who are taking even small amounts of digitalis.

Hypersensitive Reaction to Carotid Sinus Stimulation. On rare occasions certain individuals may show an extremely sensitive reaction to carotid sinus stimulation. Thus, minimum stimulation to the neck as from a tight shirt collar or shaving may cause dizziness or even a fainting episode as a result of extreme slowing of the heart rate[6,7] (Fig. 2-9). The extremely slow ventricular rate may be due to various mechanisms, including marked sinus bradycardia, sinus arrest, high degree A-V block and ventricular standstill (Fig. 2-9). Needless to say, carotid sinus stimulation of any degree should be avoided in individuals with a hypersensitive reaction to the procedure.

SUMMARY

Various responses to carotid sinus stimulation for diagnosis and treatment of various tachyarrhythmias have been described in detail. The response to carotid sinus stimulation differs according to the nature and origin of the various tachyarrhythmias. Carotid sinus stimulation is most effective in terminating paroxysmal atrial or A-V junctional tachycardia. The procedure is usually ineffective for ordinary paroxysmal ventricular tachycardia, but it may slow the ventricular rate if a parasystolic mechanism is involved. Nonparoxysmal A-V junctional tachycardia is usually refractory to carotid sinus stimulation. The danger of applying carotid sinus stimulation to patients with suspected digitalis intoxication has been emphasized. Similarly, carotid sinus stimulation should be applied with extreme caution to elderly individuals with atrial tachyarrhythmias because a long ventricular standstill may result. A hypersensitive reaction to carotid sinus stimulation in certain individuals is also stressed.

REFERENCES

1. Chung, E. K.: Digitalis Intoxication. Amsterdam, Excerpta Medica, 1969.
2. Alexander, S., and Ping, W. C.: Fatal ventricular fibrillation during carotid sinus stimulation. Am. J. Cardiol. 18:289, 1966.
3. Greenwood, R. J., and Dupler, D. A.: Death following carotid sinus pressure. J.A.M.A. 181:605, 1962.
4. Hilal, H., and Massumi, R.: Fatal ventricular fibrillation after carotid sinus stimulation. N. Engl. J. Med. 275:157, 1966.
5. Porus, R. L., and Marcus, F. I.: Ventricular fibrillation during carotid sinus stimulation. N. Engl. J. Med. 268:1338, 1963.
6. Friedberg, C. K.: Diseases of the Heart. Ed. 3. Philadelphia, W. B. Saunders Co., 1966.
7. Chung, E. K.: Principles of Cardiac Arrhythmias. Baltimore, Williams & Wilkins, 1971.
8. Chung, E. K.: Electrocardiography: Practical Applications with Vectorial Principles. Hagerstown, Md., Harper & Row, 1974.
9. Chung, E. K.: Cardiac Arrhythmias: Management (Tape Series). Baltimore, Williams & Wilkins, 1973.
10. Chung, E. K.: Parasystole. Prog. Cardiovasc. Dis. 11:64, 1968.
11. Wolff, L., and White, P. D.: Syndrome of short P-R interval with abnormal QRS complexes and paroxysmal tachycardia. Arch. Intern. Med. 28:446, 1948.
12. Wolff, L.: Electrocardiography; Fundamentals and Clinical Application, Philadelphia, W. B. Saunders Co., 1956.
13. Wolff, L., Parkinson, J., and White, P. D.: Bundle branch block with short P-R interval in healthy young people prone to paroxysmal tachycardia. Am. Heart J. 5:685, 1930.
14. Hecht, H. H., et al.: Anomalous atrioventricular excitation. Panel discussion. Ann. N. Y. Acad. Sc. 65:826, 1956.
15. Hejtmancik, M. T., and Herrmann, G. R.: The electrocardiographic syndrome of short P-R interval and broad QRS complexes: A clinical study of 80 cases. Am. Heart J. 54:708, 1957.
16. Wolff, L.: Anomalous atrioventricular excitation (Wolff-Parkinson-White syndrome). Circulation 19:14, 1959.
17. Pick, A., and Katz, L. N.: Disturbances of impulse formation and conduction in the pre-excitation (Wolff-Parkinson-White) syndrome—Their bearing on its mechanism. Am. J. Med. 19:759, 1955.
18. Chung, E. K., Walsh, T. J., and Massie, E.: Wolff-Parkinson-White syndrome. Am. Heart J. 69:116, 1965.
19. Scherf, D., Yildiz, M., and De Armas, D.: Atrial parasystole. Am. Heart J. 57:507, 1959.
20. Scherf, D., Bornemann, C., and Yildiz, M.: A-V nodal parasystole. Am. Heart J. 60:179, 1960.

21. Scherf, D., and Bornemann, C.: Parasystole with a rapid ventricular center. Am. Heart J. 62:320, 1961.

22. Golbey, M., Ladopoulos, C. P., Roth, F. H., and Scherf. D.: Changes of ventricular impulse formation during carotid pressure in man. Circulation 10:735, 1954.

23. Chung, E. K., Walsh, T. J., and Massie, E.: Ventricular parasystolic tachycardia. Br. Heart J. 27:392, 1965.

24. Muller, P., and Baron, B.: Clinical studies on parasystole. Am. Heart J. 45:441, 1953.

25. Scherf, D., and Boyd, L. J.: Three unusual cases of parasystole. Am. Heart J. 39:650, 1950.

26. Eliakim, M.: Atrial parasystole. Effect of carotid sinus stimulation, Valsalva maneuver and exercise. Am. J. Cardiol. 16:457, 1965.

27. Scherf, D., Choi, K. H., Bahadori, A., and Orphanos, R. P.: Parasystole. Am. J. Cardiol. 12:527, 1963.

28. Vedoya, R.: Parasistolia. Buenos Aires, A. Lopez, 1944.

29. Vedoya, R., Dumas, J. J., and Uradapilleta, V.: Comentarios sobre dos casos de parasystolia. Rev. Argent. Cardiol. 15:364, 1948.

30. Irons, G. V., Jr., and Orgain, E. S.: Digitalis-induced arrhythmias and their management. Prog. Cardiovasc. Dis. 8:539, 1966.

Chapter 3

Electrocardiography

EDWARD K. CHUNG

Obviously it is impossible to include all aspects of electrocardiography in this chapter. Therefore, the chapter contains some introductory remarks concerning the definition and value of the electrocardiogram, principles and order of electrocardiographic analysis, and historical considerations, and discussions of the normal electrocardiogram versus various common electrocardiographic abnormalities that are frequently misinterpreted in daily practice and the fundamental approach to cardiac arrhythmias.

Definition of Electrocardiogram.[1,2] An electrocardiogram is defined as a graphic

recording of electrical activity generated by the heart. The string galvanometer was initially introduced by Willem Einthoven in 1901. In 1933 unipolar electrocardiography was added by Frank N. Wilson and his associates. At present a routine electrocardiogram includes 12 leads.

Value of the Electrocardiogram. An electrocardiogram is the most important laboratory test in the diagnosis of various heart diseases, particularly myocardial infarction[2-5] (Fig. 3-1). In addition, the electrocardiogram is extremely helpful in diagnosing various noncardiac disorders such as thyroid, renal and pulmonary dis-

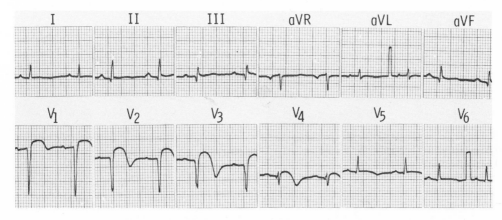

Figure 3-1. Acute anteroseptal myocardial infarction.

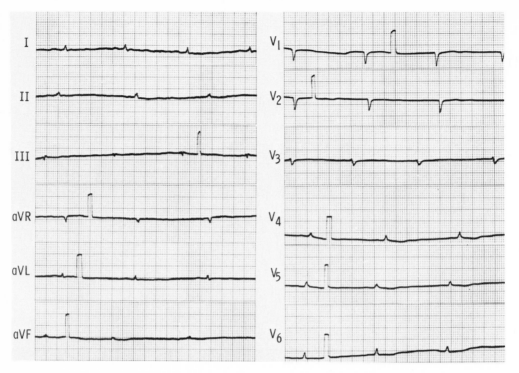

Figure 3-2. This ECG tracing was obtained from myxedema heart disease. Note the marked low voltage throughout. Sinus arrhythmia and bradycardia with a rate of 43 to 55 beats per minute. A pseudo anteroseptal myocardial infarction pattern is produced, but this patient did not suffer from myocardial infarction.

eases (Figs. 3-2 to 3-4) and various electrolyte imbalances, especially hypokalemia, hyperkalemia, hypocalcemia and hypercalcemia (Figs. 3-5 to 3-9). Furthermore, various abnormalities produced by cardiac as well as noncardiac drugs can be detected by the electrocardiogram (Figs. 3-10 and 3-11). One of the essential roles of the electrocardiogram is to recognize all types of cardiac arrhythmias (Figs. 3-12 and 3-13). It is obvious that function or malfunction of artificial pacemakers will be

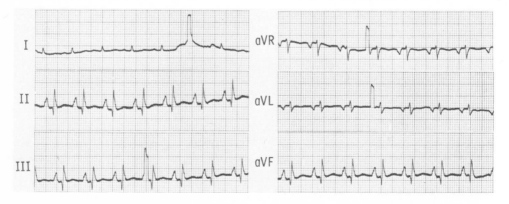

Figure 3-3. This ECG tracing was obtained from a patient with severe obstructive lung disease. The rhythm is sinus tachycardia with a rate of 110 beats per minute. Note peaked P wave indicative of P pulmonale.

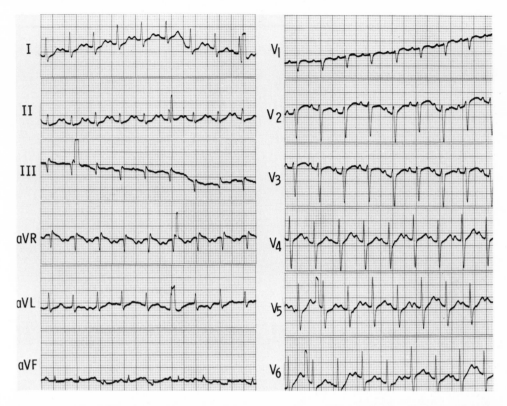

Figure 3-4. This ECG tracing was obtained from a patient with pulmonary embolism. Abnormal ECG findings include an S_1, Q_3 pattern and a pseudo diaphragmatic myocardial infarction pattern with posterior axis deviation compatible with pulmonary embolism. Marked sinus tachycardia with a rate of 148 beats per minute.

extremely difficult to assess without electrocardiographic analysis (Figs. 3-14 to 3-16).

Principles of Electrocardiographic Analysis. Electrocardiographic analysis should be as precise as possible. The electrocardiogram should be interpreted according to all available clinical information, including the patient's age, sex and body build, the clinical diagnosis and information on various drugs.[2-5] For example, the electrical axis varies according to the patient's age. The QRS axis of +90 degrees may be normal for a 20-year-old girl, but the same QRS axis will be abnormal for a 70-year-old man. Another example is that a very similar, if not identical, electrocardiographic finding may be observed in various clinical circumstances; namely, inverted T waves in leads V_{1-3} may be a normal variant ("juvenile T wave pattern" [Fig. 3-17]), but this finding may be due to various conditions, including anteroseptal myocardial ischemia; pulmonary embolism, infarction or both; myocarditis, pericarditis or both; electrolyte imbalance, especially hypokalemia, and cerebrovascular accident (Fig. 3-18).

One should not over-read or depend too much on electrocardiographic findings. It should be noted that a normal electrocardiogram is not necessarily indicative of a normal heart or vice versa. In addition, an electrocardiogram should not be interpreted by a *pattern* method; that is, the fundamental mechanism responsible for the production of a given electrocardiographic abnormality should always be con-

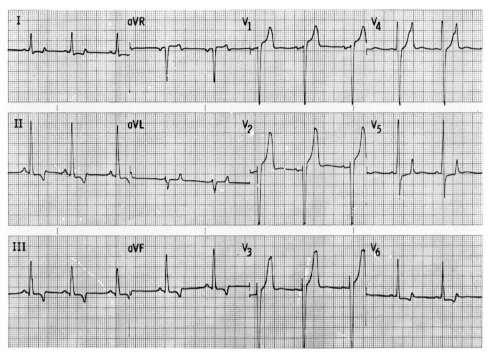

Figure 3-5. This tracing was obtained from a patient with uremia. The rhythm is sinus with a rate of 60 beats per minute. Note peaked and tent-shaped T waves compatible with hyperkalemia.

sidered. Therefore, a vectorial approach is essential to understand various electrocardiographic findings. Otherwise, an erroneous diagnosis can frequently be made. Furthermore, it is essential to compare the electrocardiogram with previous tracings if available. For instance, an old myocardial infarction pattern may disappear completely within a few months or years. This is especially true when one is dealing with diaphragmatic (inferior) or posterior myocardial infarction. Finally, one should ask

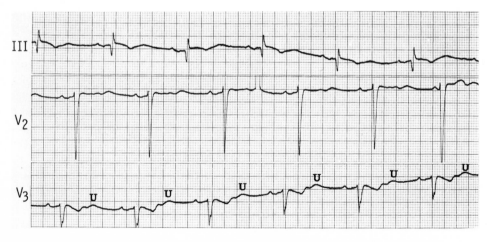

Figure 3-6. Sinus bradycardia with a rate of 48 beats per minute. Prominent U waves (*U*) indicate hypokalemia. In addition there is evidence of diaphragmatic myocardial infarction.

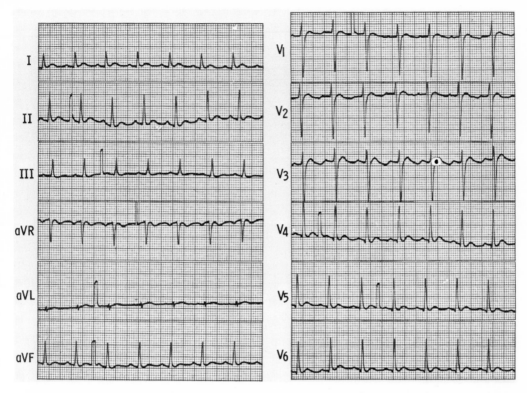

Figure 3-7. This tracing was obtained from a patient with metastatic carcinoma of the breast. Sinus tachycardia with a rate of 105 beats per minute. The short Q-T interval is due to absence of the S-T segment as a result of hypercalcemia.

oneself the following questions:

1. Is the electrocardiogram normal or abnormal?
2. If abnormal, what is the clinical significance?
3. Is treatment indicated?
4. What is the treatment of choice if treatment is indicated?

Order of Electrocardiographic Interpretation. The first and most important step in the analysis of any electrocardiographic tracing is determination of the mechanism(s) of the cardiac rhythm, that is, whether the basic rhythm is sinus or ectopic. It is not uncommon to observe two or more coexisting cardiac rhythms or beats. Following determination of the mechanism, the order of electrocardiographic interpretation should include determination of rates (P and QRS complexes), various intervals (P-R, QRS and Q-T [Fig. 3-19]) and axes of P, QRS and T complexes.[2-7]

The conclusion will be reached according to the description of each complex (P, P-R, QRS, Q-T, S-T segment and U wave) in addition to the above-mentioned items.

History of Electrocardiography.[2,5,8-15] The presence of an action current associated with the heart beat was demonstrated by Kolliker and Muller as early as 1856. By using a frog's nerve-muscle preparation that was connected to a beating heart, these investigators were able to demonstrate a twitching of a frog's muscle corresponding to each ventricular contraction. Later, in 1887, a measurable amount of current in the human body corresponding to the cardiac contraction was demonstrated by Waller and Ludwig by using the capillary electrometer. However, the current from the human heart beat was

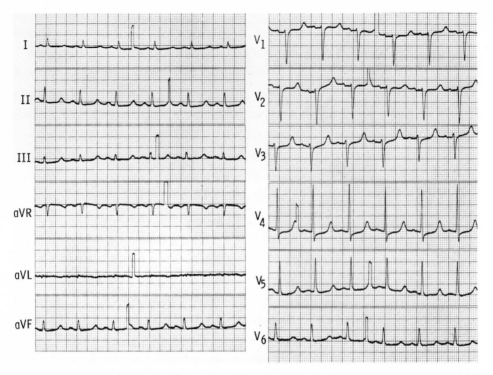

Figure 3-8. The rhythm is sinus with a rate of 92 beats per minute. The markedly prolonged Q-T interval is due to hypocalcemia.

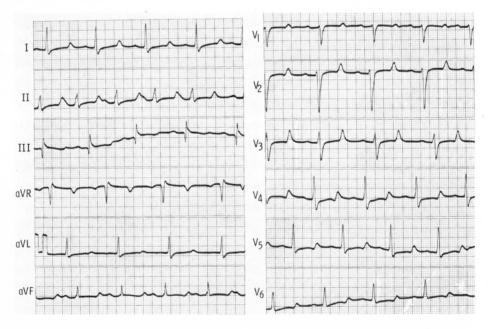

Figure 3-9. This ECG tracing was obtained from a patient with far-advanced uremia. Sinus arrhythmia and bradycardia (rate 52 to 70 beats per minute) with first-degree A-V block (P-R interval 0.24 second). ECG abnormalities produced by hyperkalemia include flat P waves, first-degree A-V block, peaked T waves and prolonged QRS intervals. In addition, the markedly prolonged Q-T interval is due to hypocalcemia.

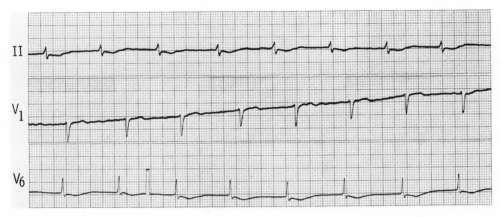

Figure 3-10. Atrial fibrillation with nonparoxysmal A-V junctional tachycardia induced by digitalis toxicity. Note prominent U waves compatible with hypokalemia.

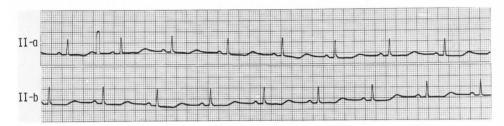

Figure 3-11. Sinus rhythm with a rate of 60 beats per minute. The markedly prolonged Q-T interval is effected by quinidine. Leads II-a and b are continuous.

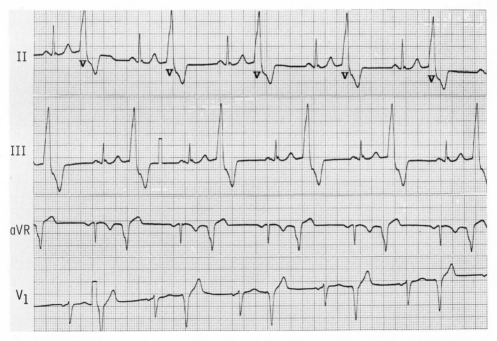

Figure 3-12. Sinus rhythm with frequent ventricular premature contractions (*V*) producing ventricular bigeminy.

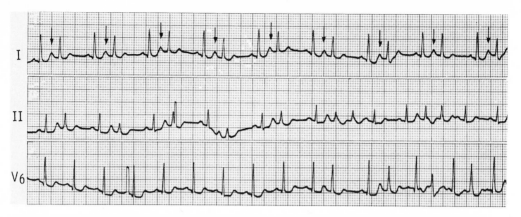

Figure 3-13. Sinus tachycardia (rate 115 beats per minute) with frequent atrial premature contractions (*arrows*) producing atrial bigeminy. Slightly bizarre QRS complexes of atrial premature beats are due to aberrant ventricular conduction.

registered in an accurate and quantitative manner for the first time in 1901 with introduction of the string galvanometer designed by Willem Einthoven.

The string galvanometer was initially used to record the heart beat in experimental studies, but later it was gradually utilized for routine clinical evaluation of human heart diseases. The principles of Einthoven's string galvanometer were based upon the fact that a magnet and a conductor of current will interact. This equipment consisted of a powerful electromagnet between whose poles was stretched a fine, metallic-covered quartz filament. By connecting the resting subject to the galvanometer string the electrical potentials generated by the heart were registered as a deflection of the quartz string. The string shadow was photographed on moving film by a system of lenses and a source of illumination. Other types of galvanometer

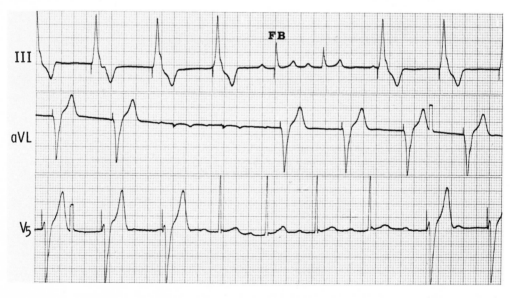

Figure 3-14. Sinus rhythm (rate 75 beats per minute) with first-degree A-V block and intermittent demand pacemaker–induced ventricular rhythm (rate 64 beats per minute) because of high degree A-V block. Note a ventricular fusion beat (*FB*).

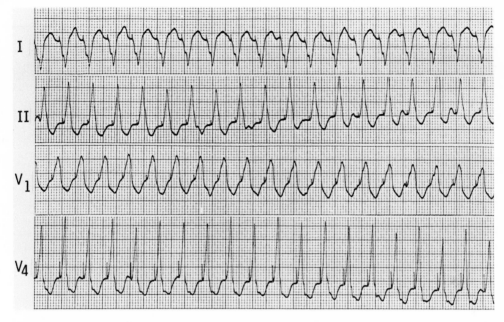

Figure 3-15. Runaway pacemaker as a manifestation of malfunction of artificial pacemaker. Pacemaker–induced ventricular tachycardia (rate 167 beats per minute) is termed runaway pacemaker. The preset pacing rate in this patient was 70 beats per minute.

equipment were devised, one of which was the oscillograph. This consisted of a small magnet to which a mirror was attached. The magnet was surrounded by coils of wire suspended by a fine thread. The electrical current moved through the coils of wire, and the magnet was deflected; a beam of light reflected by the mirror registered this movement.

Later, direct visualization of the electrical waves with a permanent record became possible by utilizing the cathode ray oscillograph. At present, immediate and direct recordings of the electrocardiogram are possible by using vacuum tube amplification equipment with a heated stylus that melts the wax on specially designed ECG paper. The ordinary paper speed for a rou-

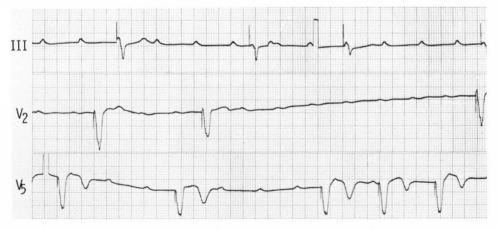

Figure 3-16. Malfunction of artificial pacemaker is manifested by extremely slow and irregular pacemaker rhythm with a long period of ventricular standstill.

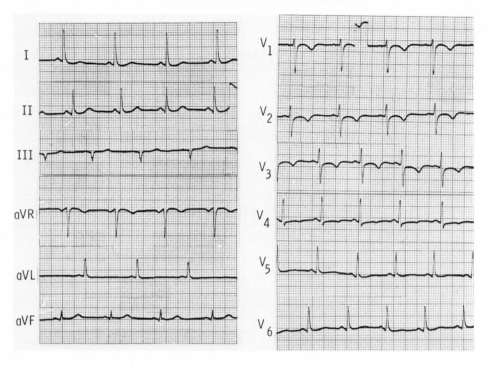

Figure 3-17. This ECG tracing was obtained from a youth without any demonstrable heart disease. Sinus arrhythmia. Inverted T waves in leads V_{1-4} are due to a juvenile T wave pattern, which is a normal variant in young individuals.

tine electrocardiogram is 25 mm. per second, but it is possible to record an electrocardiogram at much faster speeds (50, 75 or 100 mm. per second) for a special purpose.

During the first quarter of the 20th century, remarkable progress was made in the field of electrocardiography by Sir Thomas Lewis. The unipolar electrocardiogram was introduced by Frank N. Wilson in 1933. At present, the conventional electrocardiogram consists of twelve leads, including three bipolar limb leads, three unipolar limb leads and six unipolar precordial leads.

In the past decade, vectorcardiography has become an essential part of electrocardiography. Consequently the orthogonal-lead system (X, Y, and Z leads) is frequently utilized in addition to the conventional 12-lead systems. The X lead corresponds to lead I, whereas the Y lead corresponds to lead aVF of the conven-

tional electrocardiogram. The Z lead is a unique one that is almost like inverted conventional lead V_1 or V_2.

Deductive electrocardiography, advocated by Sodi-Pallares, is another approach to electrocardiographic interpretation. In this method the electrocardiogram can be analyzed by correlating the activation process in the heart with the morphology presented in all leads from a spatial view.

In addition to the conventional electrocardiogram the His bundle electrogram has been utilized recently in order to locate the precise site of an ectopic focus and the site of a block. In obtaining a His bundle electrogram an electrode catheter (bipolar, tripolar or multipolar) is introduced into a femoral vein and advanced under fluoroscopy into the right ventricular cavity via the tricuspid valve. The electrode catheter is then slowly withdrawn across the tricuspid valve until a sharp biphasic spike is recorded between the atrial and ventricular

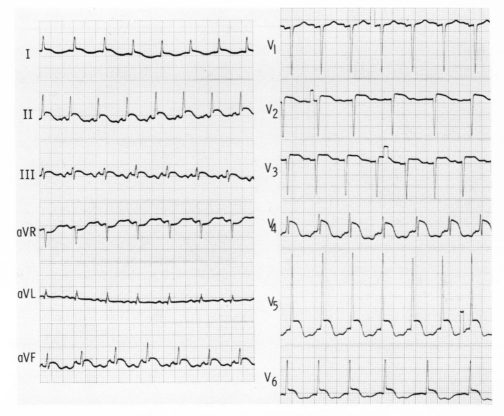

Figure 3-18. This ECG tracing was obtained from a patient suffering from subarachnoid hemorrhage. The marked S-T segment and T wave alterations are typical abnormalities observed in patients with subarachnoid hemorrhage. Anteroseptal myocardial infarction cannot be excluded in this ECG tracing.

deflections. The proximal terminals of the electrode catheter are led into the AC input of an ECG preamplifier to record bipolar electrograms.

In a His bundle electrogram, when the ventricular activity is preceded by a His bundle deflection the cardiac rhythm is supraventricular in origin. Conversely, in ventricular tachycardia or ventricular escape rhythm the ventricular deflection is not preceded by a His bundle deflection. The site of a block can thus be identified by the His bundle electrogram. For example, when the block occurs distal to the His bundle as in bilateral bundle branch block, the nonconducted P waves are followed by His deflections, and the QRS complexes are not preceded by His deflections. However, nonconducted P waves are not followed by His deflections when the block is in the A-V junction. In addition, the His bundle electrogram enables one to confirm the anomalous conduction pathway in Wolff-Parkinson-White syndrome. In this syndrome, His bundle deflection often occurs after the onset of the QRS complex. In addition to the intracardiac electrogram, the esophageal lead is often taken in order to clarify the atrial activity when one is dealing with complex arrhythmias.

Computerized electrocardiography has become popular in recent years at some medical institutions for routine electrocardiographic analysis. However, computerized electrocardiography has not been utilized universally.

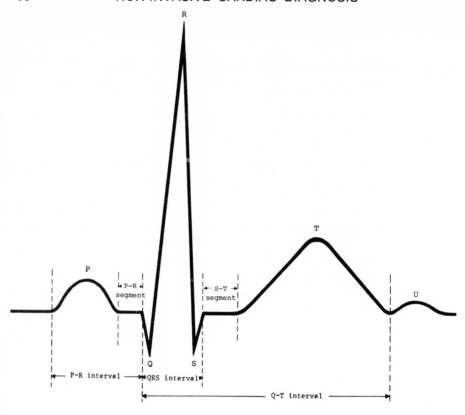

Figure 3-19. Diagram (lead II) showing various intervals.

NORMAL ELECTROCARDIOGRAM[2,5,10,11]

In the normal heart the impulse originating from the primary pacemaker (sinus node) passes the sinoatrial junction and spreads throughout the atria radially as if it were a wave formed on a pond after a stone was thrown into it. During atrial activation (at a rate of 800 to 1000 mm. per second) the P wave is inscribed on the electrocardiogram. The average time required for atrial depolarization in the normal heart varies between 0.08 and 0.10 second. The activation process spreads through the atrial muscle, finally reaches the atrio-A-V nodal junction and passes down the A-V nodal tissue. In the short stretch of the A-V node, with its complex interlacing structure and its slow conductivity, a delay in the activation process permits the atria to complete their systole before transmission of the activation process to the ventricles. The time required for this process is approximately 0.05 second. As the activation process passes from the A-V node directly to the A-V bundle, the conductivity markedly increases. The speed of conduction increases to 20 times that of the A-V junction when the bundle branches are reached. This rapid conductivity is maintained throughout the entire Purkinje system. Approximately 0.16 second is normally required for the cardiac impulse to travel from the sinus node, via the atria, the A-V node, the common bundle and bundle branches, the terminal Purkinje network and the transitional muscle fibers, to the first part of the ventricular myocardium. The time from the beginning of atrial depolarization to the beginning of ventricular depolarization is represented by the P-R interval (Fig. 3-19) on the electrocardiogram (A-V conduction time), and its average value in a normal adult varies from 0.12 to 0.20 second.

Activation of the ventricles originates in the septum. The initial septal force (vector) comes from the middle third of the left septal mass. The septal activation vector is directed to the right anteriorly and either inferiorly or superiorly, depending upon the position of the heart. This initial septal vector is responsible for the small q wave in the left precordial leads (leads V_{4-6}) and the initial r wave in the right precordial leads (leads V_{1-2} [Fig. 3-20]). After the initial activation of the ventricular septum, the free left ventricular wall undergoes depolarization. This force is directed toward the left posteriorly and either superiorly or inferiorly, depending upon the position of the heart. The endocardial surface is activated shortly before the epicardium in each portion of the ventricles because of a certain arrangement of the terminal Purkinje fibers. The connections of the terminal Purkinje network are such that the papillary muscles are activated earlier than the lateral wall of the ventricles. The activation process in the right ventricle is usually negligible in magnitude as compared with the left ventricle, although its activation occurs at the same time. The activation of the left ventricular free wall is responsible for the R wave in the left precordial leads and the S wave in the right precordial leads (Fig. 3-20). Following activation of the free wall of the ventricles, the basal portion of the heart is activated. The basal portions include the superior and posterior portions of the free walls and that part of the ventricular septum that primarily belongs to the right septal mass, including the crista supraventricularis. The vector of this terminal ventricular activation process is directed toward the right, slightly posteriorly and

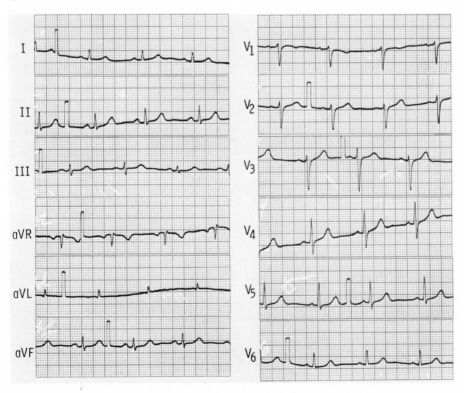

Figure 3-20. Typical normal electrocardiogram with normal sinus rhythm.

superiorly. This terminal vector is responsible for the terminal s wave in the left precordial leads and the terminal r or r' wave in the right precordial leads or lead aVR (Fig. 3-20). The interval required for ventricular activation (QRS interval) is usually between 0.06 and 0.10 second in normal hearts (intraventricular conduction time). The total duration of the activation process of the entire heart is approximately 0.25 second.

During ventricular depolarization in a normal heart the amplitude of the R waves in leads V_{1-3} progressively increases until the transitional zone is reached (Fig. 3-20). When the transitional zone is passed, small septal physiologic q waves begin to appear in leads V_{4-6} with the development of S waves in these leads (Fig. 3-20). This ventricular depolarization process is easily understandable from a vectorial approach. The vectorcardiogram uses es-

sentially the same principle in registering cardiac electrophysiologic events, but it is recorded from three dimensions—the horizontal (transverse), frontal and sagittal planes. The horizontal and frontal planes correspond respectively to the precordial and limb leads of the electrocardiogram. Since a vectorcardiogram records one more plane (sagittal) than the conventional electrocardiogram, the former is often able to show abnormalities that may not be detected by the latter. Vectorcardiography is discussed in detail in Chapter 7.

Depending upon the configuration of the QRS complexes, various terms have been used to describe such findings (Fig. 3-21). The term low voltage is used when the sum of the QRS complexes (both positive and negative components) in leads I, II and III is less than 15 mm. (Fig. 3-2). Low voltage may be due to various condi-

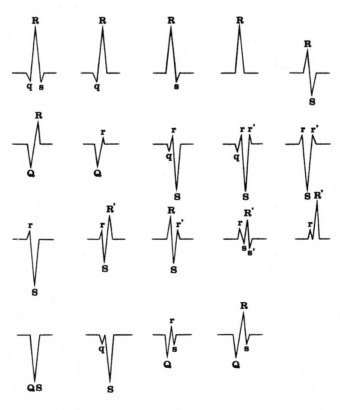

Figure 3-21. Diagram showing various QRS complexes.

tions, including obesity, emphysema, pericardial or pleural effusion, myxedema, marked congestive heart failure and acute myocardial infarction.

Following completion of ventricular depolarization, the ventricles undergo the repolarization process to produce T waves. As described previously, the direction of the repolarization process in a normal ventricle is from epicardium to endocardium, which is in reverse direction as compared to a muscle strip (Fig. 3-22). Therefore, a normal electrocardiogram usually shows upright T waves in leads V_{2-6} (Fig. 3-20). The configuration of T waves in the limb lead varies, depending upon the T axis. However, in general, the T wave is always inverted in lead aVR and upright in lead II (Fig. 3-20). The T wave in lead V_1 in a normal heart may be upright, inverted or biphasic.

Following the T wave there is another round upright wave of small amplitude that is called the U wave. Not uncommonly the U wave is superimposed on the last portion of the T wave. The exact mechanism for the production of the U wave is unknown, but it is thought to be produced by potentials elicited by the stretching of ventricular muscle during the period of rapid blood inflow. Alternatively the U wave is considered to be due to papillary muscle activation by some investigators. Clinically, recognition of prominent U waves (U wave $\geqq$ T wave) is extremely significant because they are almost always indicative of hypokalemia (Fig. 3-6). In addition, inverted U waves when occurring in leads I, II and V_{4-6} are usually due to myocardial ischemia. However, alteration of the U wave configuration is influenced by many other factors, including digitalis, quini-

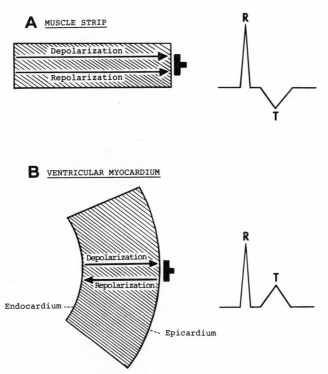

Figure 3-22. Depolarization and repolarization of a muscle strip (A) and ventricular myocardium (B). Note that the directions of depolarization and repolarization processes are the same in a muscle strip. In contrast to this, depolarization and repolarization processes are opposite in direction in ventricular myocardium. As a result the T wave is inverted in a muscle strip, whereas it is upright in the ventricular myocardium.

dine, epinephrine, hypercalcemia and thyrotoxicosis.

Normal Intervals.[2,5,10,11] Various intervals on the electrocardiogram are usually expressed in seconds, but the amplitude of the various complexes is expressed in millimeters (Fig. 3-19).

Various intervals in a normal electrocardiogram are relatively constant in a given individual unless the heart rate varies markedly from time to time. All intervals tend to be shorter in children than in adults. For example, the normal P-R interval is considered to be between 0.12 and 0.18 second in children and 0.12 and 0.20 second in adults. In all age groups the Q-T interval varies much more markedly in comparison with other intervals; it also varies according to the heart rate. Thus, the following formula for determination of the Q-T interval may be used to decide whether a given Q-T interval is normal or abnormal:

$$\text{Q-T calculation} = \frac{\text{Q-T (measured)}}{\sqrt{\text{R-R interval (second)}}}$$

For example, the Q-T calculation will be 0.44 second when the Q-T (measured) interval is 0.40 second and the R-R (measured) interval is 0.81 second.

$$\text{Q-T calculation} = \frac{0.40}{\sqrt{0.81}} = \frac{0.40}{0.9} = 0.44 \text{ second}$$

The Q-T interval is considered to be abnormal if the Q-T calculation is more than 0.42 second.

Determination of the Heart Rate. There are several ways to determine the heart rate.[2,3,5,6,11] When the atrial and the ventricular rates are different, as in second- or third-degree A-V block, both atrial and ventricular rates should be determined separately.

The easiest and the most practical method is to count the cardiac cycles between 6-second intervals and multiply by 10 since most electrocardiographic paper conveniently has vertical lines on the top of the paper at 3-second intervals. When such vertical markers are not available or the ECG tracing is cut short, other methods should be used. The ordinary ECG paper speed is 25 mm. per second or 1500 mm. (or 1500 small squares) per minute. Because the interval between two thin lines in the ECG paper is 1 mm., the R-R interval in a given tracing can be easily measured. The ventricular rate can be measured by dividing 1500 by the number of small squares. In the same manner, a rough estimation of the heart rate can be made by counting the number of large squares. Each large square (thick line) on the ECG paper consists of five small squares (thin lines). Thus, the ECG paper speed can be expressed as 300 large squares per minute (1500 ÷ 5 = 300). The heart rate is determined by dividing 300 by the number of large squares between R-R intervals. For example, when the R-R interval contains two large squares, the rate is 150 per minute; when the R-R interval contains three large squares, the rate is 100 per minute, and so on. When the heart rate varies markedly from time to time, as in atrial fibrillation or sinus arrhythmia, the two extreme values (slowest and fastest rates) should be determined.

Normal Sinus Rhythm. The first step in diagnosis of a normal electrocardiogram is confirmation of a normal sinus rhythm.[2–6,11]

The cardiac rhythm originating from the primary pacemaker (sinus node) is termed sinus rhythm. Most healthy individuals have sinus rhythm, but many patients with cardiac disease also have sinus rhythm. Therefore, the presence of sinus rhythm does not denote either a normal or diseased heart. The sinus rates in normal subjects differ among age groups. At birth, the rate is between 110 and 150 beats per minute; it gradually becomes slower, approaching the adult rate by 6 years. The sinus rate, at rest, in the majority of the adult population is usually between 65 and 85 beats per minute, but it varies from individual to individual; a rate between 60 and 100 beats per minute is arbitrarily considered to be the rate of a normal sinus rhythm. A sinus rate faster than 100 beats per minute is called sinus tachycardia, whereas a rate slower than 60 beats per minute is termed sinus bradycardia.

The rate of the sinus rhythm is influenced by various factors, including cardioinhibitory forces (vagal), cardio-acceleratory forces (sympathetic), chemical mediators, posture and position, exercise (either emotional or physical), various drugs, cardiac and noncardiac diseases, environmental and body temperature and the metabolic and nutritional state. Alteration of the sinus rate is often due to humoral or neurogenic effects rather than to actual anatomic alteration in the sinus node, even in diseased hearts.

When the basic rhythm is sinus, there may be occasional or frequent ectopic beats or even a bout of ectopic tachycardia. In these circumstances, the mechanism of the basic rhythm should always be mentioned as the dominant rhythm. Not uncommonly, sinus rhythm and ectopic rhythm may be present independently, as in A-V dissociation or parasystole. In these cases the atrial mechanism should be mentioned, and a sinus rhythm and an independent ectopic rhythm should be described accordingly.

Definition. Specifically, normal sinus rhythm is diagnosed only when the following criteria are present in the electrocardiogram (Fig. 3-20):

1. P wave of sinus origin (normal mean axis of P wave)
2. Constant and normal P-R interval (0.12 to 0.20 second)
3. Constant P wave configuration in each given lead
4. Rate between 60 and 100 beats per minute
5. Constant P-P (or R-R) cycle

Diagnostic Criteria for Normal Sinus Rhythm. P WAVE OF SINUS ORIGIN (NORMAL MEAN AXIS OF P WAVE). The first and most important step in the diagnosis of normal sinus rhythm is to prove that the mean axis of the P wave is within normal limits. This is because a normal mean P wave axis indicates that the P wave is of sinus origin. The mean axis of the P wave may be determined by utilizing Einthoven's triangle or the hexaxial reference frame.

The P, QRS and T complexes at birth show marked right and anterior axis deviation; they gradually move toward the left and posteriorly during aging. The mean axes of these complexes in most normal adults are between 0 and +90 degrees. Older individuals (over 60 years of age) may have mean axes between 0 and −30 degrees even without demonstrable heart disease. For this reason the mean axis of normal sinus rhythm must lie between 0 and +90 degrees in the adult population. The mean axis in young adults is usually between +60 and +90 degrees, while it is often between +30 and +60 degrees in older adults.

In order to satisfy the criteria for a normal P axis, the P wave must be upright in lead II and inverted in lead aVR. Other extremity leads (I, III, aVL and aVF) may show different configurations of the P wave, depending upon the direction of the P axis. For instance, if the P axis is +90 degrees the P wave will be isoelectric or biphasic in lead I, inverted in leads aVL and aVR and upright in leads II, III and aVF. Another extreme example is a P axis of 0 degree, which produces an isoelectric or biphasic P wave in lead aVF, inverted P wave in leads III and aVR and upright P wave in leads I, II and aVL. Thus, P waves are not necessarily upright in lead I or aVF in normal sinus rhythm although they are upright in most cases. For the same reason the P wave is frequently inverted in lead aVL in younger adults, whereas it is often inverted in lead III in older adults. These observations indicate that the most important leads to look for are lead II, which must show an upright P wave, and lead aVR, which must show an inverted P wave. To state that the P wave is upright in leads I, II, III and aVF and inverted in lead aVR in normal sinus rhythm is erroneous. In the precordial leads V_{1-2} the P wave of normal sinus rhythm is usually biphasic and sometimes is predominantly upright or inverted. The remaining precordial leads (V_{3-6}), in general, show an upright P wave in normal sinus rhythm, although this again varies, depending upon the mean axis of the P wave. The precordial leads are not usually recommended to determine normal sinus rhythm.

In addition, it should be noted that the P axis may be altered when there is atrial disease, as in mitral stenosis or cor pulmonale, just as the QRS axis changes according to alteration in ventricular depolarization due to left or right ventricular hypertrophy.

CONSTANT AND NORMAL P-R INTERVAL. When the mean axis of the P wave is within normal limits (0 to +90 degrees), each P wave should be followed by QRS and T complexes throughout the tracing (Fig. 3-20). In addition, the P-R interval, which is the A-V conduction time (the interval from the beginning of the P wave to the onset of the QRS complex), should be between 0.12 and 0.20 second in adults. In children the P-R interval tends to be shorter, primarily because of their faster heart rate. The P-R interval is measured in the extremity lead that shows the longest interval, because the P-R interval is falsely shorter in certain leads. This occurs when the mean axis of a portion of the P wave is perpendicular to that lead.

When the P-R interval is longer than 0.20 second, first-degree A-V block is present. Conversely, when the P-R interval is shorter than 0.12 second, it may be due

to Wolff-Parkinson-White syndrome, coronary nodal rhythm or Lown-Ganong-Levine syndrome. When long and short P-R intervals alternate, or occur intermittently, dual A-V conduction should be suspected. If the P-R intervals and P wave configuration vary considerably, but the P wave and QRS complex are still related, a wandering atrial pacemaker should be suspected. Needless to say, complete A-V dissociation is present when the P wave and QRS complex are independent. (In this case, the term P-R distance is substituted for P-R interval.)

CONSTANT P WAVE CONFIGURATION IN EACH GIVEN LEAD. The configuration of the P wave must be constant in each given lead in order to be diagnostic of normal sinus rhythm. However, it should be noted that the P wave configuration in some leads, particularly II, III and aVF, may change with respiration. The configuration of the QRS and T complexes also will be altered to a similar degree. This alteration of configuration due to respiration will be eliminated by momentary breath holding. When the configuration of the P wave changes from beat to beat or periodically, but a normal P axis with constant or slightly varying P-R interval (between 0.12 and 0.20 second) is present, a wandering pacemaker is said to be present in the sinus node. Even when the P wave is abnormal in contour, such as that seen in mitral stenosis (P mitrale) and in cor pulmonale (P pulmonale), normal sinus rhythm can be diagnosed as long as the above-mentioned criteria exist.

RATE BETWEEN 60 AND 100 BEATS PER MINUTE. As mentioned previously in this chapter, a sinus rate between 60 (P-P interval 1.00 second) and 100 (P-P interval 0.60 second) beats per minute is arbitrarily considered normal for healthy subjects. Thus the sinus rate must be from 60 to 100 beats per minute in normal sinus rhythm (Fig. 3-20).

CONSTANT P-P (OR R-R) CYCLE. Although it has been said that normal sinus rhythm should be regular the P-P (or R-R) cycle is not always precisely regular. In fact, by precise measurement, normal sinus rhythm in the cardiac cycle is often slightly irregular. Therefore, the P-P (or R-R) cycle is considered to be regular when the shortest and longest P-P (or R-R) intervals vary by less than 0.16 second. If the P-P cycle varies by more than 0.16 second, sinus arrhythmia is present. Sinus arrest (pause or standstill) and sinoatrial block produce marked irregularity and regular irregularity of the P-P cycle respectively.

COMMON ELECTROCARDIOGRAPHIC ABNORMALITIES

Nonconducted (Blocked) Atrial Premature Contractions. Atrial premature contractions (APCs) are one of the most common electrocardiographic findings. APCs may be blocked when the ectopic atrial impulses reach the A-V junction during an absolute refractory period. This is called a nonconducted or blocked APC[3,16] (Fig. 3-23). The occurrence of nonconducted APCs may be physiologic when the cou-

pling interval (the interval from the ectopic beat to the preceding beat of the basic rhythm) is very short. On the other hand, it is pathologic when the nonconducted APCs occur in the presence of a relatively long coupling interval. Nonconducted APCs obviously occur when there is a significant degree of A-V conduction disturbance even if the basic rhythm is a sinus mechanism with a normal P-R interval. Clinically, nonconducted APCs are not uncommon during mild digitalis intoxication. In addition, nonconducted APCs are fairly common in elderly individuals even without significant heart disease. Nonconducted APCs may be erroneously misinterpreted as other ECG abnormalities such as marked sinus arrhythmia, sinus bradycardia, sinus arrest or sinoatrial block, especially when the premature P waves are superimposed on the T waves of the preceding beats. Otherwise, nonconducted APCs may be misdiagnosed as 2:1 A-V block. Nonconducted atrial bigeminy closely simulates marked sinus bradycardia.

Wenckebach Sinoatrial Block. Sinoatrial (S-A) block occurs when the sinus impulses are unable to be conducted to the

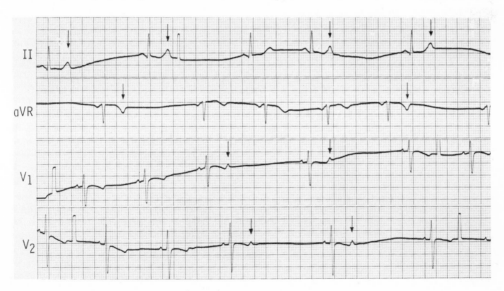

Figure 3-23. Arrows indicate ectopic P waves. Sinus bradycardia (rate 57 beats per minute) with frequent nonconducted atrial premature contractions.

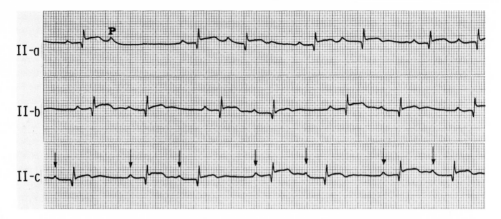

Figure 3-24. Arrows indicate sinus P waves. Sinus rhythm with 3:2 Wenckebach S-A block associated with 3:2 Wenckebach A-V block. Wenckebach A-V block is concealed because of coexisting Wenckebach S-A block except for the first portion of lead II-a (*P*). In addition, acute diaphragmatic myocardial infarction is present.

atria because of a block at the sinoatrial junction. S-A block is much less common than A-V block, and, at times, the former and the latter coexist on the same ECG tracing (Fig. 3-24). There are two types of S-A block. Mobitz type II S-A block is relatively easy to recognize because the long P-P interval due to S-A block is a multiple of the basic P-P cycle. Mobitz type I (Wenckebach) S-A block is one of the most difficult ECG findings to recognize even by experienced cardiologists. This is because the long P-P interval due to Wenckebach S-A block is *not* a multiple of the basic P-P cycle (Fig. 3-24).

The best approach to understanding Wenckebach S-A block is to study Wenckebach A-V block first (Fig. 3-25). As described in many excellent textbooks of electrocardiography, Wenckebach A-V block is characterized by progressive lengthening of the P-R intervals until a blocked P wave occurs.[3,5,6,16] During Wenckebach A-V block, the R-R intervals (ventricular cycle) become progressively shorter until a blocked P wave occurs because the degree of increment of the P-R interval prolongation becomes progressively less and less until a pause occurs (Fig. 3-25). Thus, Wenckebach A-V block

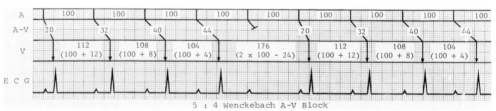

Figure 3-25. Mobitz type I (Wenckebach) A-V block. The numbers represent hundredths of a second. The numbers in the upper row represent the atrial cycle (P-P interval) with a rate of 60 beats per minute. The numbers within the oblique lines at the A-V level indicate the A-V conduction time (P-R interval). The progressive lengthening of the P-R intervals is apparent until a blocked atrial impulse (dropped P wave) occurs. Following this blocked atrial impulse the P-R interval shortens to its original value (0.20 second), and the sequence is repeated. The numbers in the lowest row represent the duration of successive ventricular cycles. The progressive shortening of the ventricular cycle length (R-R interval) is due to the progressive increment of A-V conduction before the blocked atrial impulse and the decrement immediately following the blocked P wave. The numbers in parentheses in the lowest row indicate the degree of increment or decrement in the ventricular cycle length.

characteristically shows progressive shortening of the R-R cycle.

When one applies the electrophysiologic phenomenon of the Wenckebach A-V block for interpretation of S-A block, it becomes obvious that Wenckebach S-A block produces progressive shortening of the P-P intervals (atrial cycle). When the Wenckebach S-A block shows 3:2 conduction, short and long P-P cycles alternate, but the long P-P interval is shorter than two short P-P intervals (Fig. 3-24). Wenckebach S-A block superficially resembles sinus arrhythmia, sinus bradycardia or atrial premature contractions. Clinically, S-A block is relatively common in digitalis toxicity and acute diaphragmatic myocardial infarction (Fig. 3-24). S-A block is also reported to be encountered frequently in patients with atrial myocardial infarction.

Differentiation of Supraventricular Tachyarrhythmias with Wide QRS Complexes and Ventricular Tachyarrhythmias. It is a well-known fact that ventricular tachyarrhythmias are closely simulated by supraventricular tachyarrhthmias associated with wide QRS complexes. In particular, one of the most difficult problems is differentiation between supraventricular tachyarrhythmias with aberrant ventricular conduction (Fig. 3-26) and ventricular tachyarrhythmias[3,6-8,17,18] (Fig. 3-27). Ventricular aberrancy occurs when supraventricular impulses (either sinus or ectopic) are conducted to the ventricles during a partial refractory period. Aberrant ventricular conduction tends to occur when the R-R interval preceding the coupling interval is long because the refractoriness of the heart beat is greatly influenced by the cardiac cycle of the preceding beats; namely, the longer the R-R interval of the preceding cycle, the greater is the ventricular aberrancy in the following beat. This finding is called Ashman's phenomenon; it can be observed in any basic supraventricular rhythm (Fig. 3-26). The evidence of aberrant ventricular conduction is supported by Ashman's phenomenon, a lack of post-tachycardiac pause, a right bundle branch block pattern and an identical initial vector between normal and abnormal beat. Ventricular premature beats or ventricular tachycardia shows a significant postectopic or post-tachycardiac pause, and no Ashman's phenomenon is observed (Fig. 3-27). In addition to the aberrant ventricular conduction, supraventricular tachyarrhyth-

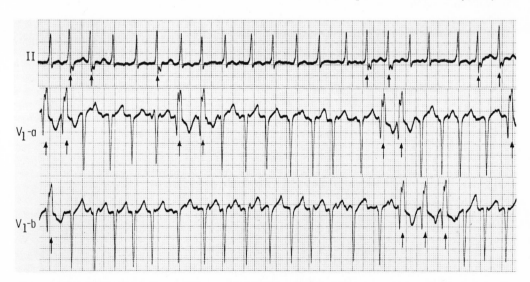

Figure 3-26. Leads V_1-a and b are not continuous. Atrial fibrillation with intermittent aberrant ventricular conduction (*arrows*) because of Ashman's phenomenon.

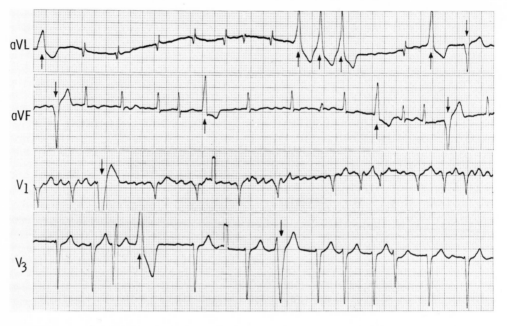

Figure 3-27. Atrial fibrillation with frequent multifocal ventricular premature contractions *(arrows)* with areas of ventricular group beats. Coarse atrial fibrillation indicative of left atrial hypertrophy.

mias may have wide QRS complexes when there is bundle branch block (Fig. 3-28) or intraventricular conduction delay due to hyperkalemia (Fig. 3-29). Supraventricular tachyarrhythmias associated with Wolff-Parkinson-White syndrome often exhibit wide and bizarre QRS complexes because of anomalous A-V conduction (Fig. 3-30).

Atrial Flutter with 2:1 A-V Response. Uncomplicated atrial flutter nearly always reveals 2:1 A-V conduction.[3,17] This is because the A-V junction is unable to conduct all of the rapid atrial impulses from a physiologically long refractory period. The term 2:1 A-V response is used rather than 2:1 A-V block since the 2:1 A-V ratio is merely a functional block rather than a true A-V block. Atrial flutter with 2:1 A-V response (Fig. 3-31) is often misinterpreted as A-V junctional tachycardia or even sinus tachycardia when other atrial

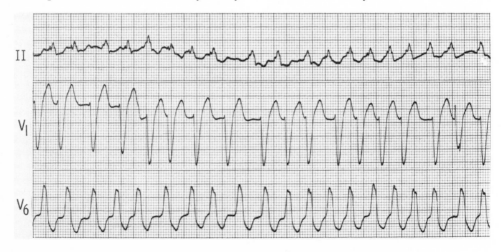

Figure 3-28. Atrial fibrillation with left bundle branch block.

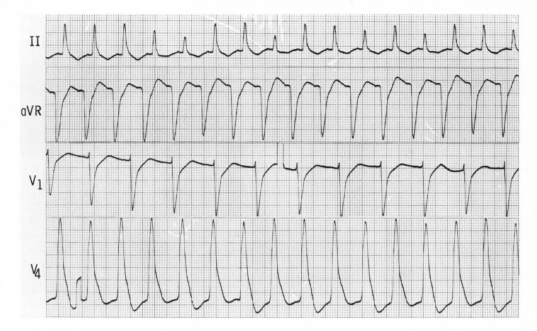

Figure 3-29. This tracing was obtained from a patient with terminal renal failure. Flat P waves with broad QRS complexes resemble ventricular tachycardia. The ECG abnormalities in this patient are produced by severe hyperkalemia. Sinus arrhythmia with areas of sinus tachycardia.

flutter waves are not recognized. In a practical sense, a ventricular rate around 150 beats per minute should always first suggest the possibility of atrial flutter with 2:1 A-V response. Carotid sinus stimulation is greatly helpful in diagnosis because the atrial flutter cycles will be clearly shown when the ventricular rate is slowed by the procedure (see Chapter 2).

Multifocal Atrial Tachycardia.[19] As can be expected, atrial tachycardia may be multifocal, although conventional atrial tachycardia is always unifocal. The diagnostic criteria and clinical significance differ greatly in multifocal atrial tachycardia and unifocal atrial tachycardia. The diagnostic criteria of multifocal atrial tachycardia (Fig. 3-32) include: (1) varying P wave configuration, (2) varying P-P cycles and (3) varying P-R intervals. In addition, the atrial rate is frequently slower (it may be as slow as 100 to 120 beats per minute) than that of unifocal atrial tachycardia, and varying degrees of A-V block often coexist. Multifocal atrial tachycardia is most commonly encountered

in chronic cor pulmonale and less commonly in pulmonary embolism, hypoxia due to various causes, pneumonia and coronary heart disease. Therapeutic approach to multifocal atrial tachycardia is a most difficult problem because none of the antiarrhythmic agents seems to be effective. Management of the underlying disease seems to be more beneficial than any particular antiarrhythmic agent. Multifocal atrial tachycardia is frequently misinterpreted as atrial fibrillation.

A-V Junctional Tachycardia in the Presence of Atrial Fibrillation. A-V junctional tachycardia or A-V junctional escape rhythm may occur as a pure form so that atrial as well as ventricular activation is controlled by the A-V junctional pacemaker.[3,17] However, more commonly, non-paroxysmal A-V junctional tachycardia or escape rhythm develops in the presence of pre-existing atrial fibrillation (Fig. 3-10) or flutter to produce A-V dissociation. This type of arrhythmia is almost always due to digitalis intoxication.[16] Nonparoxysmal A-V junctional tachycardia must be sus-

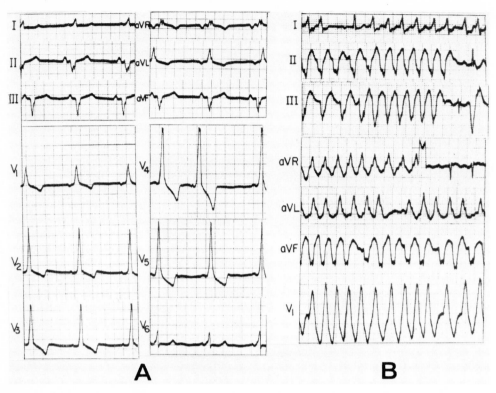

Figure 3-30. Tracings A and B were obtained from the same patient on different occasions. A, Wolff-Parkinson-White syndrome type A. B, atrial fibrillation with anomalous A-V conduction that closely simulates ventricular tachycardia.

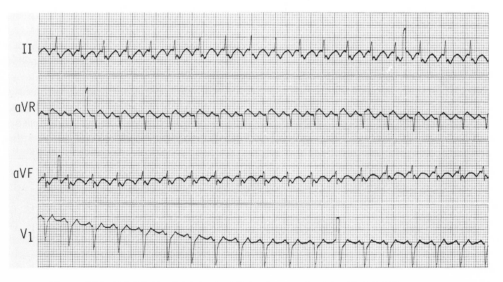

Figure 3-31. Atrial flutter (atrial rate 300 beats per minute) with 2:1 A-V response.

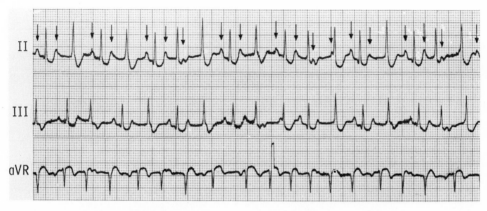

Figure 3-32. Arrows indicate P waves. Multifocal atrial tachycardia.

pected immediately when the R-R intervals become regular in the presence of atrial fibrillation. Under this circumstance the arrhythmia is often misdiagnosed as uncomplicated (pure) A-V junctional tachycardia or even sinus tachycardia. The usual rates of nonparoxysmal A-V junctional tachycardia range from 70 to 130 beats per minute.

Myocardial Infarction in the Presence of Bundle Branch Block. It is not uncommon for myocardial infarction to develop in the presence of bundle branch block or for bundle branch block to develop as a complication of myocardial infarction.[2,5,10,11] The diagnosis of myocardial infarction is relatively easy to make in the presence of right bundle branch block because the former involves the initial vector whereas the latter involves the terminal vector (Fig. 3-33). On the other hand, the diagnosis of myocardial infarction is often difficult and at times impossible when left bundle branch block (LBBB) is a preexisting abnormality. Nevertheless, acute myocardial infarction can be diagnosed in the presence of LBBB when unexpected S-T segment or T wave alterations or both occur. In other words, acute myocardial infarction is diagnosed when the S-T segment is elevated when it would be expected to be depressed or isoelectric. In addition, the primary T wave change usually replaces the secondary T wave change when acute myocardial

infarction develops in the presence of LBBB (Fig. 3-34). On rare occasions anteroseptal myocardial infarction can be diagnosed in the presence of LBBB on the basis of reappearance of small Q waves in the left precordial leads.

Ventricular Parasystole. Ventricular parasystole superficially mimics ventricular premature contractions although the basic mechanism involved and clinical significance are much different.[3,6,20] Ventricular parasystole is diagnosed when there are varying coupling intervals and constant shortest interectopic intervals. Because of the independence of the parasystolic rhythm, ventricular fusion beats are frequently observed (Fig. 3-35). Clinically, ventricular premature contractions are frequently digitalis-induced, whereas parasystole does not seem to be related to cardiac glycosides.

Pseudomyocardial Infarction in Wolff-Parkinson-White Syndrome. Wolff-Parkinson White (W-P-W) syndrome is characterized by a short P-R interval and a wide QRS complex due to a delta wave (initial slurring of the upstroke of the QRS complex).[1,8] A pseudomyocardial infarction pattern is commonly observed in W-P-W syndrome when the delta waves are directed superiorly (Fig. 3-36). In spite of the fact that W-P-W syndrome has been a well-recognized entity since 1931, the syndrome is frequently not recognized even

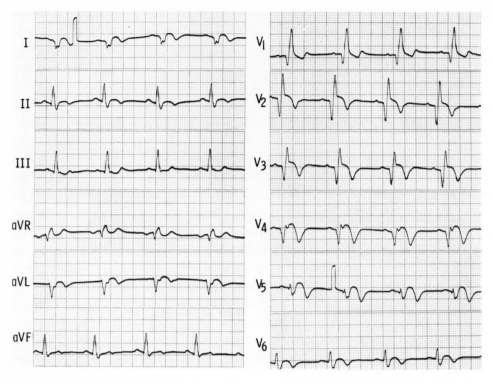

Figure 3-33. Recent extensive anterior myocardial infarction associated with right bundle branch block.

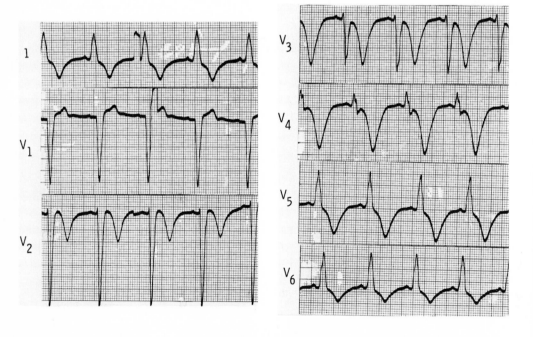

Figure 3-34. Acute anterior myocardial infarction associated with left bundle branch block. Note that the secondary T wave change is replaced by the primary T wave change.

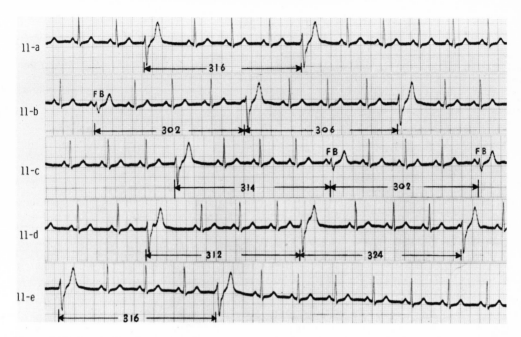

Figure 3-35. Leads II-a, b, c, d and e are not continuous. The rhythm is sinus with ventricular parasystole. Note varying coupling intervals with constant shortest interectopic intervals. There are frequent ventricular fusion beats (*FB*). (The numbers represent hundredths of a second.)

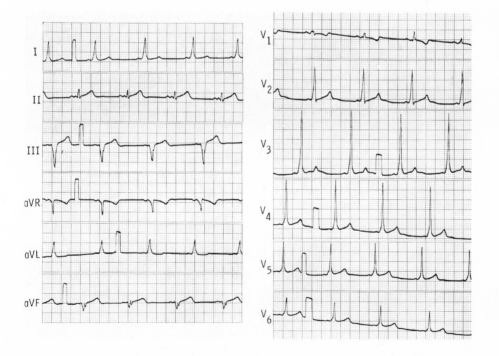

Figure 3-36. Wolff-Parkinson-White syndrome type A. A pseudo diaphragmatic myocardial infarction pattern is evident because of a delta wave that is directed superiorly.

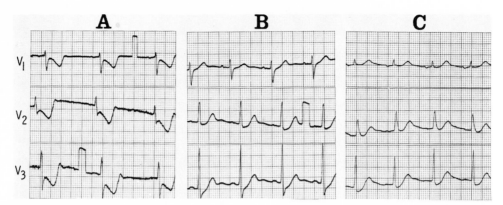

Figure 3-37. Tracings taken from the same patient at one-day intervals (*A, B, C*) show a typical finding of acute posterior myocardial infarction. Note progressive increment of R wave amplitude with loss of S wave in lead V₁.

by experienced physicians and often is misdiagnosed as myocardial infarction. Needless to say, it is extremely important not to overdiagnose or underdiagnose myocardial infarction. Furthermore, W-P-W syndrome should be diagnosed correctly. Otherwise, supraventricular tachyarrhythmias frequently associated with the syndrome (Fig. 3-30) may not be recognized and, accordingly, may not be properly treated.

Tall or Relatively Tall R Wave in Lead V_1. One of the most common problems in electrocardiographic interpretation is the occurrence of a tall or a relatively tall R wave (R : S ratio $\geqq 1$) in lead V_1.[2,10,11] The reason interpretation is a problem is that the tall R wave may have various causes, including posterior myocardial infarction (Fig. 3-37), right ventricular hypertrophy (Fig. 3-38), and septal hypertrophy as seen in idiopathic hypertrophic subaortic stenosis (Fig. 3-39), W-P-W syndrome type A, or it may be a normal variant. In young healthy individuals, the R wave in lead V_1 is frequently taller than usual, but the ECG is completely normal otherwise. Sinus arrhythmia is often present because of the youth of the group. A relatively tall R wave in lead V_1 due to posterior myocardial infarction is often associated with evidence of diaphragmatic myocardial infarction, lateral myocardial infarction or both. On the other hand, a relatively tall R wave in lead V_1 due to right ventricular hypertrophy is always associated with right axis deviation (Fig. 3-38). A vectorcardiogram will clarify the diagnosis when the R wave in lead V_1 is relatively tall (see Chapter 7).

THE FUNDAMENTAL APPROACH TO CARDIAC ARRHYTHMIAS[2,3,6,7,11,17]

For a precise diagnosis of a given cardiac arrhythmia, the following procedure should be followed:

1. Obtainment of all available clinical information
2. General inspection of the electrocardiogram
3. Determination of the dominant rhythm
4. Determination of the presence or absence of a P wave
5. Determination of the origin of the QRS complex when atrial and ventricular activities are independent
6. Determination of the nature and origin of beats occurring prematurely or later than usual
7. Final considerations

Obtainment of All Available Clinical Information. Available clinical information is of great help in the interpretation of car-

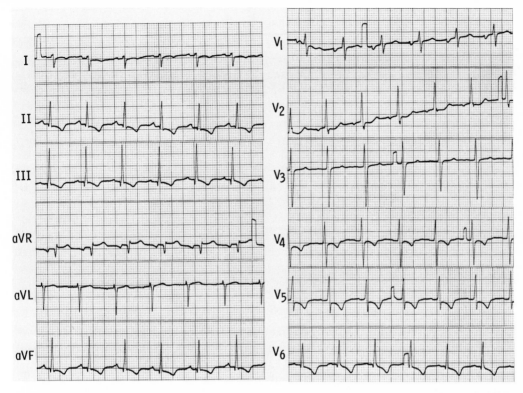

Figure 3-38. Right ventricular hypertrophy is diagnosed on the basis of right axis deviation with a relatively tall R wave in lead V_1. In addition, biventricular hypertrophy is suggested because of the markedly increased amplitude of the RS complex in leads V_3 and V_4 and the tall R wave in leads V_5 and V_6 with S-T, T wave change. (Leads V_{3-6} are half-standardized.)

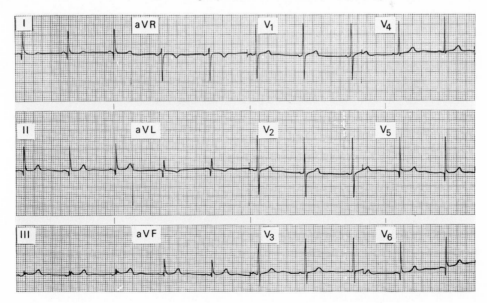

Figure 3-39. This tracing was obtained from a youth with idiopathic hypertrophic subaortic stenosis. Note the tall R wave in lead V_1 with somewhat deep and narrow Q waves in leads I, aVL and V_{5-6}.

diac arrhythmias. This information should include the patient's age; history of a previous similar arrhythmia, its onset and frequency; history of known heart disease; previous history of congestive heart failure and noncardiac diseases such as hyperthyroidism; and history of drug administration, particularly digitalis, and electrolyte imbalance. A detailed history of artificial pacemaker implantation, including the approximate date of implantation, type of pacemaker, etc., is important because malfunction of an artificial pacemaker may produce various serious arrhythmias (Figs. 3-15 and 3-16). In addition, one must review all available tracings in order to determine whether the patient in the past had any cardiac arrhythmia, left bundle branch block (Fig. 3-28), right bundle branch block (Figs. 3-40 and 3-41), bilateral bundle branch block, Wolff-Parkinson-White syndrome (Figs. 3-30 and 3-36), myocardial infarction (Figs. 3-1, 3-33 and 3-34), etc. This information is frequently invaluable in distinguishing between supraventricular and ventricular tachycardia and enhances the accuracy of the diagnosis.

General Inspection of the Electrocardiogram. By a general inspection of a given tracing it is possible to determine whether the basic rhythm is a normal sinus rhythm or a type of cardiac arrhythmia. If any arrhythmia is present one should determine whether it occurs occasionally, frequently, continuously, regularly or irregularly, repetitively or with various combinations. Various artifacts, which may simulate cardiac arrhythmias, must also be detected (Fig. 3-42). It is also possible to determine whether the arrhythmia is simple or complex, clinically benign or serious.

Determination of the Dominant Rhythm. After general inspection of a given electrocardiogram, determination of the dominant rhythm is the next step. The dominant rhythm may be sinus (Fig. 3-20), but it could be any type of ectopic rhythm. If an ectopic rhythm is dominant one should

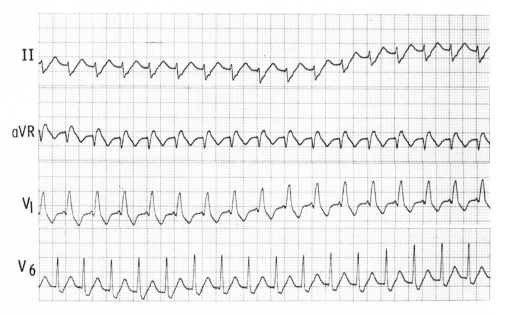

Figure 3-40. Figures 3-40 and 3-41 were obtained from the same patient on different occasions. Figure 3-40 shows regular tachycardia (rate 150 beats per minute) with a wide QRS complex that can be diagnosed as either ventricular tachycardia or supraventricular (probably A-V junctional) tachycardia with right bundle branch block. In this case the diagnosis of supraventricular tachycardia is confirmed because a pre-existing right bundle branch block is obvious in Figure 3-41.

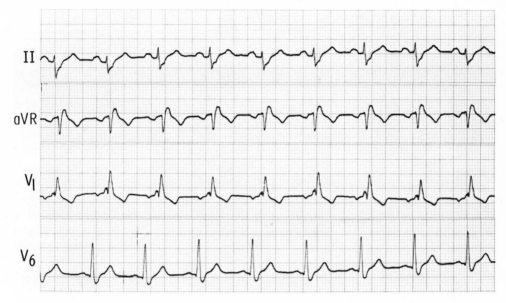

Figure 3-41. Sinus rhythm (rate 78 beats per minute) with right bundle branch block.

determine whether it is due to active or passive impulse formation. However, in most common and simple arrhythmias the dominant rhythm is of sinus origin. The second most common dominant rhythm is atrial fibrillation (Figs. 3-10, 3-26, 3-28, and 3-30); less common is atrial flutter (Fig. 3-31).

Occasionally the dominant rhythm may change from one mechanism to another

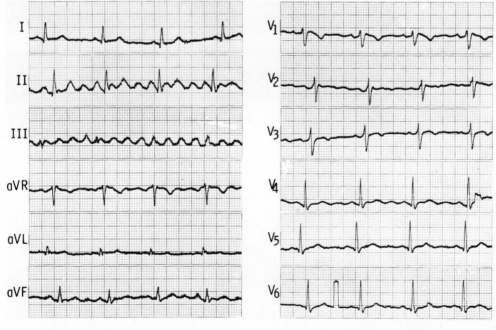

Figure 3-42. This ECG tracing was obtained from a patient with Parkinson's disease. Artifacts produced by muscle tremor closely simulate atrial flutter. The actual rhythm is sinus with a rate of 75 beats per minute.

(from sinus to ectopic or vice versa or even from ectopic to ectopic) on the same electrocardiogram. At times it is difficult to determine the dominant rhythm, particularly with complex arrhythmias. Even if the dominant rhythm is ectopic in origin, as a rule one begins with sinus beats, if present even occasionally. It is immensely helpful to determine whether sinus beats are present.

Determination of the Presence or Absence of a P Wave. By knowing whether a P wave is present or absent one can narrow the differential diagnosis significantly. When a P wave seems to be present, one should be certain that it is a true P wave and not one of various other waves as in atrial fibrillation or flutter; one should ascertain that it is not a T wave or U wave or even an artifact that looks like a P wave. If a true P wave is definitely present, one should determine whether the P wave and QRS complex are related or independent.

Presence of P Wave. When a P wave is present, one should determine whether the P wave is of sinus or ectopic origin. The following steps should be carried out:

1. Determination of origin of P wave (mean axis of P wave)
2. Inspection of P wave configuration
3. Inspection of regularity of P-P cycle
4. Measurement of P wave rate
5. Determination of the relationship between P wave and QRS complex

If the P wave is found to be of sinus origin, one can conclude whether normal sinus rhythm, sinus tachycardia, sinus bradycardia, etc., is present. If the P wave is not of sinus origin, it must be originating from an ectopic focus in the atria or A-V junction or, rarely, the ventricles. When the P wave originates in the atria, it may resemble or at times be almost identical to the sinus P wave, but the rate is usually faster when impulses originate in the atria. The P wave may be conducted in a retrograde fashion if it originates from either the A-V junction or ventricle. If this occurs the P wave will be inverted in lead II but upright in lead aVR and thus have a direction opposite to that of a sinus P wave. When the atria are activated in a retrograde fashion from the A-V junction (Fig. 3-43) the P wave may appear before or after the QRS complex, depending upon whether the atria or ventricles are activated first. If the atria and ventricles are activated simultaneously, the P wave will be superimposed on the QRS complex, leading to absence of the P wave. When the P wave configuration changes from beat to beat in the presence of a constant P-R interval, a wandering pacemaker is present in the sinus node (Fig. 3-44). The pacemaker may wander in the atria. This may be diagnosed when one observes a changing P-R interval with fluctuations in the P wave configuration; retrograde P waves are absent. A wandering pacemaker is present between the sinus node and A-V junction when the P wave configuration changes from upright to inverted in the same lead with or without a changing P-R interval. It should be noted that respiration may slightly change the P wave configuration in some leads, and this should be distinguished from a wandering atrial pacemaker; in addition to its influence on the P wave, respiration may also affect the QRS complex and T wave in a similar fashion. An electrocardiogram taken during sustained inspiration or expiration will eliminate this problem. On rare occasions the P wave configuration may change only after ectopic beats. This is due to aberrant atrial conduction (Chung's phenomenon, Fig. 3-45). A varying P wave configuration is also observed when atrial fusion beats of varying degree appear on the electrocardiogram.

An irregular P-P cycle is usually due to sinus arrhythmia but may also occur with intermittent sinoatrial block (Fig. 3-24), sinus arrest or even sinus premature beats. Ectopic atrial beats (Figs. 3-13 and 3-45)

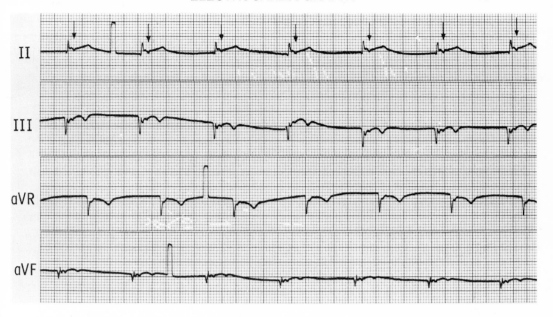

Figure 3-43. Arrows indicate retrograde P waves. A-V junctional escape rhythm with a rate of 57 beats per minute. This patient suffered from acute diaphragmatic myocardial infarction.

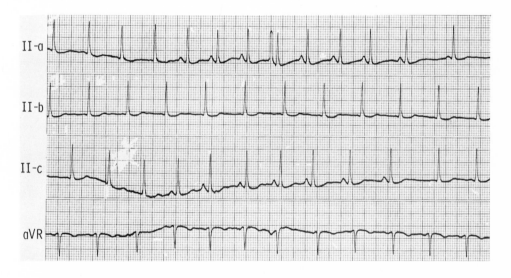

Figure 3-44. Sinus arrhythmia with wandering atrial pacemaker. Note varying configurations of P waves. Leads II-a, b and c are continuous.

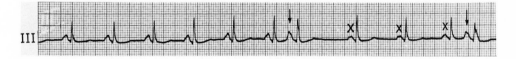

Figure 3-45. Sinus rhythm with two atrial premature contractions (*arrows*), followed by aberrant atrial conduction (Chung's phenomenon [*X*]). Note that atrial premature beats reveal slight aberrant ventricular conduction.

that appear during sinus rhythm also result in an irregular P-P cycle, but the configuration of the ectopic P wave is usually different from that of the sinus P wave. The rate of the P wave helps to determine the cardiac rhythm with relative accuracy. A P wave rate between 60 and 100 beats per minute with the P wave conducted in a forward direction is usually indicative of normal sinus rhythm (Fig. 3-20). Nonparoxysmal A-V junctional tachycardia often produces the same rate as normal sinus rhythm, but the P wave during the former is conducted in a retrograde fashion. In general, nonparoxysmal A-V junctional tachycardia produces retrograde P waves with a rate between 70 and 130 beats per minute. When the rate of the P wave is between 180 and 250 per minute, the ectopic rhythm present is usually either atrial tachycardia or paroxysmal A-V junctional tachycardia. The P wave is conducted in a forward fashion in the former but in a retrograde fashion in the latter. A-V junctional escape rhythm may produce retrograde P waves but at a much slower rate (40 to 60 per minute) than A-V junctional tachycardia. Rarely, idioventricular rhythm (ventricular escape rhythm) may show retrograde P waves. These P waves usually occur after the QRS complex. It is not uncommon to find a retrograde P wave following artificial pacemaker–induced ventricular rhythm. A retrograde P wave also

can be produced in reciprocal rhythm or reciprocating tachycardia.

The final step in the subgroup is to appreciate the relationship between atria and ventricles. If the P-R or R-P intervals are constant, all of the above-mentioned diagnostic possibilities (normal sinus rhythm, sinus bradycardia, sinus tachycardia, atrial tachycardia, A-V junctional tachycardia, A-V junctional escape rhythm and idioventricular rhythm) should be considered. This list should be narrowed after careful observation of the direction and rate of P waves. If the P-R interval varies one must be certain whether or not the atria and ventricles are related in the cardiac cycle. The degree of frequency of the above relationship must be determined. When no relationship exists between the atria and ventricles complete A-V dissociation is said to be present. The underlying disorders responsible for A-V dissociation may be (1) marked slowing of sinus impulse formation, (2) acceleration of ectopic impulse formation in the A-V junction or ventricles and (3) complete A-V block (Fig. 3-46).

Complete A-V dissociation need not always be present, for the atria and ventricles may at times become related (atrial or ventricular captured beats), and this rhythm is known as incomplete A-V dissociation (Fig. 3-47). Various complex mechanisms, including supernormal A-V conduction, concealed conduction and uni-

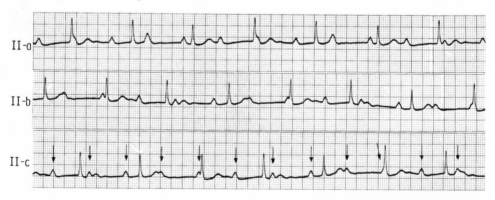

Figure 3-46. Leads II-a, b and c are continuous. Arrows indicate P waves. The rhythm is sinus with A-V junctional escape rhythm (rate 52 beats per minute) due to complete A-V block.

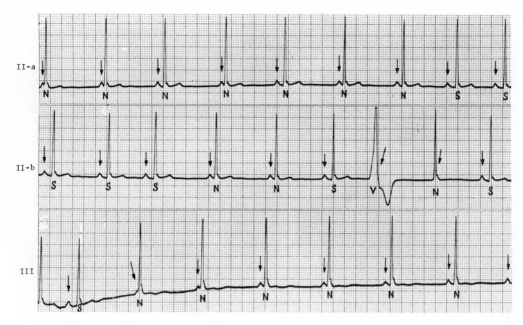

Figure 3-47. Leads II-a and b are not continuous. Arrows indicate sinus P waves. Sinus arrhythmia (S) with intermittent A-V junctional escape rhythm (N) producing incomplete A-V dissociation. Note a ventricular premature beat (V).

directional block, are often responsible for the production of captured beats, particularly when A-V block exists.

When the atrial rate is found to be a multiple of the ventricular rate, a second-degree or advanced (high-degree) A-V block, such as 2:1, 3:1, etc., is usually present (Fig. 3-48). Wenckebach A-V block (common type, Mobitz type I) is characterized by gradual lengthening of the P-R interval until a P wave is present with-

out a QRS complex after it. This pattern may then repeat itself. Thus the atrial/ventricular ratio becomes 3:2, 4:3, etc. (Fig. 3-49). A less common form of second-degree A-V block, namely, Mobitz type II (uncommon type), also produces a 3:2, 4:3, etc., A-V block, which may resemble the Wenckebach type, but the P-R intervals remain constant except when a blocked (nonconducted) P wave occurs.

First-degree A-V block has a constant

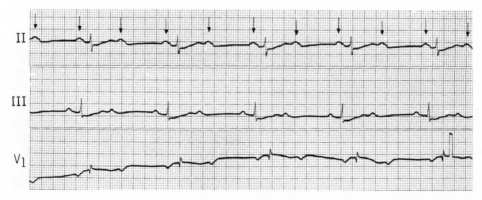

Figure 3-48. Arrows indicate sinus P waves. The rhythm is sinus with 2:1 A-V block induced by digitalis toxicity. In addition there is evidence of left atrial hypertrophy.

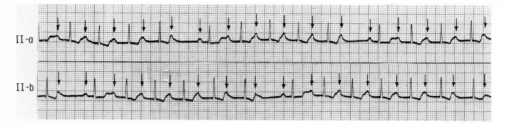

Figure 3-49. Leads II-a and b are continuous. Arrows indicate sinus P waves. The rhythm is sinus with varying degree Wenckebach (Mobitz type I) A-V block.

but prolonged (0.21 second or more) P-R interval. The relationship between atria and ventricles may occasionally be reversed; Wenckebach retrograde ventriculoatrial block may be the resulting abnormality.

Absence of P Wave. When the P wave is not discernible one should determine whether the P wave is truly absent or falsely absent.

It is not uncommon to observe a P wave superimposed on a portion of the QRS complex, S-T segment or T wave of the preceding or subsequent cycle. This occurs frequently during atrial tachycardia or A-V junctional tachycardia and may occasionally be observed during sinus tachycardia. Various maneuvers such as carotid sinus pressure, breath holding, etc., may enable one to delineate the P wave from other complexes by reducing the heart rate.

If after the above techniques the P wave is still not observed, the atrial mechanism must be determined. The most common cause of absence of a P wave is atrial fibrillation (Figs. 3-26 and 3-28); less common is atrial flutter (Fig. 3-31). In these cases an atrial fibrillation or flutter wave is present in place of the P wave. Untreated atrial fibrillation usually has a rapid ventricular rate (more than 120 to 160 per minute), unless a significant A-V conduction defect is present. In untreated atrial flutter the ventricular rate is usually one-half that of the atrial. This block is not anatomic in nature. Its presence is due to the fact that the A-V junction is unable to conduct the

very rapid atrial rate. Thus the ventricular rate is frequently around 150 to 180 per minute. In A-V junctional tachycardia or escape rhythm the P wave may be totally superimposed on the QRS complex, leading to absence of P waves. This occurs when atrial and ventricular depolarization occur simultaneously. In rare circumstances, notably in severely diseased hearts, atrial activity may be completely absent because of atrial standstill.

Determination of the Origin of the QRS Complex When Atrial and Ventricular Activities Are Independent. When the P wave and QRS complex are either temporarily or continuously independent, incomplete or complete A-V dissociation is said to exist (Figs. 3-46 and 3-47). When this occurs, either the atrial or ventricular mechanism may equally dominate. In other words, the atria may be controlled by the sinus node or any other atrial ectopic focus (atrial fibrillation, flutter or tachycardia), whereas the ventricles may be controlled by either the A-V junction or a ventricular ectopic focus (Figs. 3-10, 3-46 and 3-47).

When the QRS complex is unrelated to the P wave, the fundamental genesis of the impulse that activates the ventricles should be determined. It is essential to determine whether the QRS complex is produced by active or passive impulse formation. In addition, it should be determined whether the QRS complex originates from the A-V junction or the ventricle. If there is active impulse formation in the above examples, A-V junctional or ventricular tachycardia, respectively, will result. In contrast to this, passive impulse formation from the A-V junction or ventricle results in A-V junctional or ventricular escape rhythm respectively. The QRS complex that originates from the A-V junction is ordinarily of normal configuration (Figs. 3-46 and 3-47) although it may be slightly bizarre and wider than usual because of aberrant ventricular conduction. Aberrant ventricular conduction may occur when there is an extremely rapid rate or Ashman's phenomenon. The QRS complex that originates in the ventricle is usually wide and has a bizarre configuration (Fig. 3-50).

Determination of the Nature and Origin of Beats Occurring Prematurely or Later Than Usual. Various fundamental mechanisms may produce a P wave or QRS complex that occurs prematurely. The most common example of this is the ordinary premature beat (extrasystole), which may originate from the atria, A-V junction or ventricles (Figs. 3-12, 3-13 and 3-45) or rarely from the sinus node. When a premature beat is found, one should determine its origin. The origin of a premature P wave is determined by the electrical axis and configuration of the P wave and its relationship to the QRS complex. The configuration of the P wave of a sinus premature beat is identical to the P wave of the underlying sinus rhythm, whereas the P wave of an atrial premature beat is usually slightly different in configuration from the sinus P wave. An atrial premature beat is ordinarily followed by a normal QRS complex (Fig. 3-13). When a short coupling interval, Ashman's phenomenon or both are present the QRS complex following an atrial premature beat may appear bizarre because of aberrant ventricular conduction (Fig. 3-45). At times a premature P wave may not be followed by a QRS complex, and this is termed a nonconducted or blocked atrial premature contraction (Fig. 3-23). When the P wave is conducted in a retrograde fashion it should be deter-

mined whether the P wave is related to the preceding QRS complex or the one that followed or both. The P wave of an A-V junctional premature beat may be preceded or followed by the QRS complex, depending upon whether the atria or ventricles were activated first. When a retrograde P wave is related to both the preceding and the following QRS complex and becomes placed between them, a reciprocal beat is usually present.

The QRS complex of A-V junctional premature or reciprocal beats may show a bizarre form because of aberrant ventricular conduction. The QRS complex of a ventricular premature beat is usually wide and bizarre (Figs. 3-12 and 3-27). Rarely, as previously mentioned, a P wave may follow the QRS complex of a ventricular premature beat.

Recognition of an artifical pacemaker–induced ventricular rhythm is obvious because of the presence of the artificial electrical artifact preceding each QRS complex (Fig. 3-14).

Rare types of prematurely appearing P waves may be due to atrial or A-V junctional parasystole, atrial dissociation, A-V dissociation or cardiac transplantation.

Ventricular parasystole produces prematurely appearing QRS complexes with varying coupling intervals (Fig. 3-35).

In the presence of A-V dissociation, atrial or ventricular captured beats may produce prematurely appearing P waves or QRS complexes respectively. Fusion beats (summation beats), atrial or ventricular in origin, produce variations in the shape of the P waves and QRS complexes. Fusion beats are very common in parasystole. When a QRS complex appears later than usual in the basic rhythm it is usually either an A-V junctional or ventricular escape beat. The QRS complex of an A-V junctional escape beat ordinarily appears normal, but not uncommonly it may be wide and bizarre because of aberrant ventricular conduction. Ventricular escape (idioven-

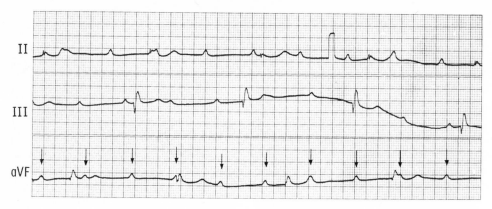

Figure 3-50. Arrows indicate sinus P waves. The rhythm is sinus with ventricular escape (idioventricular) rhythm (rate 32 beats per minute) due to complete A-V block.

tricular) beats are always wide and bizarre (Fig. 3-50). Escape beats, either A-V junctional or ventricular in origin, follow a long pause and are seen with various arrhythmias, including S-A block, sinus arrest, marked sinus bradycardia, sinus arrhythmia, second- or third-degree A-V block and premature beats (extrasystoles).

Final Considerations. After complete clinical and electrophysiologic impressions are obtained one should summarize all findings and ask oneself the following questions:

1. What is the origin of the dominant rhythm?
   a. Is it normal sinus rhythm?
   b. Is it an ectopic rhythm?
2. What is the fundamental genesis of the arrhythmia?
   a. Is it abnormal impulse formation?
      —(1) Is it active impulse formation? (2) Is it passive impulse formation? (3) Is it atrial, A-V junctional or ventricular in origin?
   b. Is it a conduction disturbance?
   c. Is it a combination of both?
3. Is the P wave present in the dominant rhythm?
   a. What is the origin of the P wave?
   b. What is the rate of the P wave?
   c. Is the P wave related to the QRS complex?

d. If related, what is the mode of relationship between the P wave and the QRS complex?
   e. If unrelated, what is the basic disorder producing A-V dissociation?
4. What is the atrial mechanism if the P wave is absent?
   a. Is it truly absent or superimposed on a portion of the QRS complex, S-T segment, T or U wave?
   b. Is it atrial fibrillation?
   c. Is it atrial flutter?
   d. Is it A-V junctional escape rhythm or tachycardia?
   e. Is it atrial standstill?
5. What are the origin and nature of the QRS complex if atrial and ventricular activities are independent?
   a. Is it active impulse formation in the A-V junction?
   b. Is it passive impulse formation in the A-V junction?
   c. Is it active impulse formation in the ventricles?
   d. Is it passive impulse formation in the ventricles?
   e. Is it artificial pacemaker–induced ventricular rhythm?
6. What are the nature and origin of the beats that occur prematurely?
   a. Is it atrial, A-V junctional, or ventricular, or perhaps sinus in origin?

b. Is it an ordinary premature beat (extrasystole)?

c. Is it sinus arrhythmia?

d. Is it parasystole?

e. Is it a reciprocal beat?

f. Is it a captured beat? (in the presence of A-V dissociation?)

g. Is the wide and bizarre QRS complex due to aberrant ventricular conduction of a supraventricular beat, or is the beat of ventricular origin?

7. Is this a simple or complex, common or uncommon cardiac arrhythmia?

a. Are there any complex mechanisms such as concealed conduction, unidirectional block, supernormal A-V conduction, etc., involved?

b. Is the interpretation of the arrhythmia entirely satisfactory?

c. Are there any alternative interpretations?

8. What is the clinical significance of the arrhythmia?

a. Is treatment indicated?

b. What is the treatment of choice if treatment is indicated?

REFERENCES

1. Wilson, F. N.: A case in which the vagus influenced the form of two ventricular complexes of the electrocardiogram. Arch. Intern. Med. 16:1008, 1915.

2. Chung, E. K.: Electrocardiography: Practical Applications with Vectorial Principles. Hagerstown, Md., Harper & Row, 1974.

3. Chung, E. K.: Principles of Cardiac Arrhythmias. Baltimore, Williams & Wilkins Co., 1971.

4. Chung, E. K., and Chung, D. K.: ECG Diagnosis: Self Assessment. Hagerstown, Md., Harper & Row, 1972.

5. Marriott, H. J. L.: Practical Electrocardiography, ed. 5. Baltimore, Williams & Wilkins Co., 1973.

6. Schamroth, L.: The Disorders of Cardiac Rhythm. Oxford, Blackwell Scientific Publications, 1971.

7. Pick, A.: Mechanisms of cardiac arrhythmias: From hypothesis to physiologic fact. Am. Heart J. 86:249, 1973.

8. Massumi, R. A., Vera, Z., and Mason, D. T.: The Wolff-Parkinson-White syndrome. A new look at an old problem. Mod. Concepts Cardiovasc. Dis. 42:41, 1973.

9. Lewis, T.: Mechanism and Graphic Registration of the Heart Beat, ed. 3. London, Shaw & Son, 1925.

10. Chung, E. K.: Vectorcardiography: Self Assessment. Hagerstown, Md., Harper & Row, 1974.

11. Massie, E., and Walsh, T. J.: Clinical Vectorcardiography and Electrocardiography. Chicago, Year Book Medical Publishers, 1960.

12. Sodi-Pollares, D., et al: Deductive and Polyparametric Electrocardiography. Mexico, Instituto Nacional de Cardiologia de Mexico, 1970.

13. Rosen, K. M., et al: Site of heart block as defined by His bundle recording. Pathologic correlations in three cases. Circulation 45:965, 1972.

14. DeJoseph, R. L., and Zipes, D. P.: His bundle electrocardiography—Its clinical value. In Controversy in Cardiology, edited by E. K. Chung. New York, Springer-Verlag, 1976.

15. Pordy, L.: Computerized electrocardiography. In Controversy in Cardiology, edited by E. K. Chung. New York, Springer-Verlag, 1976.

16. Chung, E. K.: Digitalis Intoxication. Amsterdam, Excerpta Medica, 1969.

17. Chung, E. K.: Clinical Electrocardiography, Cardiac Arrhythmias: Differential Diagnosis, New York, Medcom, 1974.

18. Ashman, R., and Hull, E.: Essentials of Electrocardiography, New York, The Macmillan Co., 1941.

19. Chung, E. K.: Appraisal of multifocal atrial tachycardia. Br. Heart J. 33:500, 1971.

20. Chung, E. K.: Reappraisal of parasystole. Heart and Lung 2:81, 1973.

Chapter 4

Electrocardiographic Stress Testing[*]

L. THOMAS SHEFFIELD, JR.

Exercise ECG testing is a highly valuable mode of clinical evaluation, aiding in the detection of coronary artery disease, cardiac arrhythmias of varied etiology and functional capacity evaluation. For arrhythmia detection the exercise test complements the long-term Holter monitor examination; however, once an arrhythmia is discovered, the prognostic import is usually uncertain except when the arrhythmia complicates coronary heart disease.[1] Exercise testing has proved useful for estimating functional capacity, thus helping the physician to determine whether a patient with valve disease should be referred for surgery or to evaluate the effects of medical or surgical therapy.[2] The main clinical value of the exercise ECG test, however, is in the diagnosis and evaluation of coronary artery disease. For this purpose the exercise ECG has no serious competitor among noninvasive procedures, although studies of the resting ECG,[3] systolic time intervals,[4] precordial vibrations[5] and echocardiographic recordings[6] have been carefully evaluated for possible diagnostic usefulness. Rapidly

* Supported in part by Cardiovascular Program Project Grant HE-11310 of the National Heart and Lung Institute and by Lipid Research Clinic Project Contract No. NO1-HV-1-2159-L of the National Heart and Lung Institute.

increasing utilization of coronary cineangiography has been accompanied by improved accuracy and safety of this procedure, but it is still formidable in comparison with the exercise ECG and is less amenable to periodic repetition for long-term evaluation. More important, the exercise ECG and the coronary angiogram are complementary rather than competitive, one supplying physiologic information and the other delineating anatomy. In terms of patient safety, availability and accuracy the exercise ECG is the logical procedure to follow history, physical examination and baseline tests on the subject with chest pain. Following a brief reference to the origins of stress electrocardiography, this chapter will deal with the physiologic basis for exercise testing, methods by which the exercise stress is administered, electrocardiographic data acquisition, interpretation and implications and patient selection and safety.

Clinical exercise electrocardiography for diagnostic purposes was introduced by Wood, Wolferth and Livezey, who had a patient induce chest pain by climbing nearby stairs, immediately returning for a postexercise ECG that demonstrated exertional ST segment depression.[7] Scherf and Schaffer successfully employed postexercise ECG records in the diagnosis of angina pectoris, tailoring the stress used according to each patient's individual precipitating factors.[8] Master and Jaffe, however, aiming to standardize the procedure rather than making it an individual one, added ECG recording to the step test of cardiovascular fitness.[9] In the Master test all details of ECG recording and interpretation were specified, and tables for the two-step test specified the precise amount of work to be performed during the fixed work interval. This degree of standardization made the test amenable to performance by technicians or other physician assistants under the (sometimes remote) supervision of a physician. Although an indisputable relationship was shown by Robb and Marks between two-step test results and subsequent mortality rates for large groups of life insurance clients, the accuracy of individual test results was found to be variable.[10] False positive results were reported by Friedberg and colleagues in 8% of their nonangina patients, and there were 43% false negative results in angina pectoris patients when the two-step test was used.[11] Our group evaluated the two-step test and found 35% false negative responses but did not encounter false positive responses.[12] As realization spread that low sensitivity was a principal source of weakness in the two-step test, the present era of high performance testing evolved. Contemporary exercise electrocardiography embodies three basic concepts: an understanding of the pathophysiology of angina pectoris in relation to exercise, a commitment to the acquisition of high-quality electrocardiographic data and attainment of statistically valid interpretation of the acquired information.

PATHOPHYSIOLOGY OF ANGINA PECTORIS: BASIS FOR EXERCISE TESTING

It is important to bear in mind that atherosclerotic coronary artery disease, al-though by far the most frequent cause of exertional angina and concomitant ST segment deviation, is not the only cause of angina. Localized coronary arterial spasm, found in some cases of Prinzmetal's angina, extreme ventricular overload, such as caused by aortic valve stenosis, and other unexplained instances of convincing anginal syndromes in the presence of apparently normal coronary angiograms are occasionally encountered.[13] The exercise electrocardiogram can only indicate transient myocardial ischemia; the step from this finding to a diagnosis of coronary atherosclerosis is a clinical inference based on additional clinical information and statistical probability. Regardless of the basic etiology, transient myocardial ischemia with its frequently accompanying chest discomfort and ST segment deviation is always, so far as we know, due to a disparity between myocardial oxygen requirement and oxygen availability.

The causes of excessive myocardial oxygen requirement are readily identifiable and rarely present a diagnostic problem except when two or more different causes coexist, such as aortic valve stenosis and coronary atherosclerosis. In patients with uncomplicated angina pectoris the myocardial oxygen requirement can be expected to be normal, implying that it varies in direct proportion to the work of the heart. In these patients, attacks of ischemia are typically produced when the heart performs a higher than average work load, whether this is due to exercise, the stimulus of emotion or other factors. In such conditions the myocardial oxygen requirement progressively and appropriately increases, but because of narrowed coronary arterial lumens the perfusion of one or more regions of the heart does not increase sufficiently to maintain proportion with the perfusion requirement. Inasmuch as myocardial oxygen extraction from the blood is nearly maximal at all times, increases in oxygen delivery must be accomplished almost entirely by proportional increases in coronary blood flow rate. Intense exercise can increase the myocardial oxygen requirement approximately fourfold.[14] If obstructive coronary disease permits only a twofold increase in regional myocardial perfusion, a disparity between requirement and supply will occur that immediately degrades contractile performance and electrical behavior and may induce chest discomfort (Fig. 4-1). This disparity will be rectified as soon as cardiac work is reduced below the level for which existing perfusion is adequate.

It is apparent therefore that the function of a stress test is to induce a large increase in myocardial oxygen requirement in order to uncover a significant degree of coronary obstruction that might not make itself apparent at rest. This reasoning shows also that the sensitivity of the test for detecting coronary disease is related to the degree of stress applied: In the example given above, if the stress had resulted

only in doubling the myocardial oxygen requirement a perfusion disparity would not have resulted, and the test would have been interpreted as normal.

The means by which exercise stress increases myocardial oxygen requirement are by now reasonably well known (Fig. 4-2). The working skeletal muscles require a great increase in oxygen, requiring a great increase in cardiac output; even though peripheral resistance drops to a remarkable extent an increased perfusion pressure is still required in order to circulate this increased output. The heart, in meeting the demand for increased output, achieves a slight increase in stroke volume, but the principal adjustment to this need is a progressive increase in the number of strokes per minute. This increase in rate and an appropriate increase in peak systolic pressure serve to increase the rate of tension development in each myocardial fiber. Since the oxygen requirement per minute is the product of the oxygen cost per beat

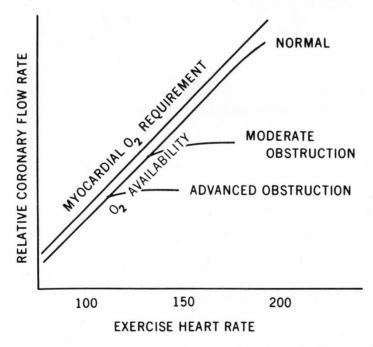

Figure 4-1. Basis for the relationship between degree of coronary obstruction and amount of exercise required to induce myocardial ischemia: The lower the exercise heart rate at which O₂ disparity develops, the more severe the expected degree of occlusion.

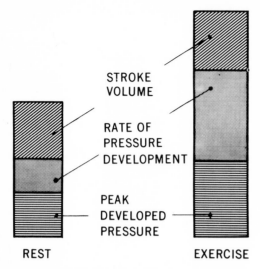

STROKE VOLUME

RATE OF PRESSURE DEVELOPMENT

PEAK DEVELOPED PRESSURE

REST   EXERCISE

Figure 4-2. Principal determinants of myocard-ial O_2 requirement per contraction. Not con-sidered are the small costs for cell maintenance and for excitation.

and the heart rate, the readily measurable quantity *heart rate* is an excellent indicator of increasing myocardial oxygen require-ment during exercise (Fig. 4-3). The value of heart rate measurement is enhanced by virtue of the fact that although the oxygen

cost per contraction changes with progres-sive exercise the changes are in the same direction as the change in heart rate.

In the normal individual maximal steady-state aerobic exercise is not limited by the coronary circulation but in most cases is limited by the perfusion of the working skeletal muscles. Therefore, nor-mally, with progressively increasing exer-cise up to near-maximal intensity, there is no significant disparity between myocardial oxygen requirement and supply. A subject who exercises to maximal or near-maximal intensity without exhibiting any evidence of insufficient myocardial perfusion will have by inference demonstrated that he or she can circulate a normal or nearly nor-mal flow of blood through the coronary vasculature. An individual with significant obstructive coronary disease, on the other hand, in the course of progressively exer-cising toward a high-intensity work load, would at some point reach a cardiac work level at which the blood flow requirement was not satisfied by the diseased coronary arteries. At this point, evidence of ischemia

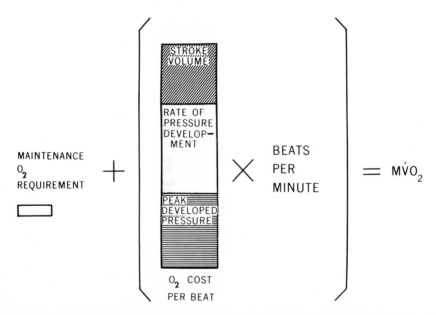

MAINTENANCE O_2 REQUIREMENT

STROKE VOLUME

RATE OF PRESSURE DEVELOP-MENT

PEAK DEVELOPED PRESSURE

O_2 COST PER BEAT

BEATS PER MINUTE

$= M\dot{V}O_2$

Figure 4-3. Myocardial O_2 requirement per minute, and hence coronary blood flow requirement, is shown to be determined mainly by the O_2 cost per beat multiplied by the heart rate. Thus the response of the heart rate to exercise is an excellent index of changing $M\dot{V}O_2$.

would be expected, and the level of work and the level of tachycardia at which ischemia began to develop may be thought of as an inverse approximation of the degree of coronary arterial obstruction (Fig. 4-1).

It is plain from the preceding discussion that any exercise test that involves only mild or moderate stress will fail to detect a significant number of subjects with moderately advanced coronary atherosclerosis. This explains why the two-step test has been found to have low sensitivity, since for a selected individual it will involve 430 kilopound-meters per minute work rate, whereas the same individual would develop a work level of 1267 kilopound-meters per minute in performing the graded exercise test (GXT), a near-maximal test (Fig. 4-4).

There are two obvious approaches to the definition of the level of stress to which

each subject will be subjected in testing for obstructive coronary disease. Each has its theoretic drawbacks, yet in use each is remarkably effective.

The first approach is to employ maximal exercise on the premise that this approach will yield the highest degree of sensitivity that can be attained by stress testing. In putting this decision into practice, however, one is faced with the question of verifying that maximal aerobic exercise has occurred. Researchers in work physiology accomplish this by performing multiple exercises at different intensities, all the while measuring oxygen consumption at each steady-state. When the O_2 consumption ceases to increase with increase in work rate, the immediately preceding work rate is proved to be the maximal aerobic exercise intensity.

Inasmuch as it is manifestly impractical

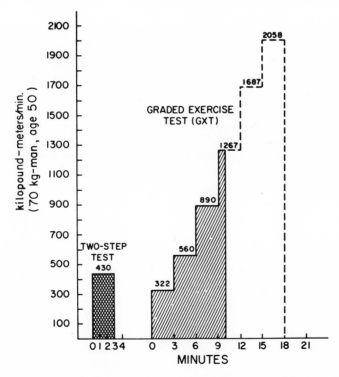

Figure 4-4. Energy cost of two-step test (*left*) and graded exercise test (*right*) for a 50-year-old 70-kg. man. Graded exercise test contrasted with a single level exercise test. Note the low work rate at the beginning of GXT and progressive increase to nearly three times the work rate of the two-step test.

to adopt the oxygen uptake–proven maximum exercise test for clinical purposes, an obvious alternative would be employment of a subjective maximal test. Such a test would involve exercise with progressive increases so gradual that the participating subject would remain near steady-state throughout the procedure by virtue of the work increments lying within the range of the normal body's homeostatic mechanisms. The subject would continue this progressive exercise as long as able to do so. Exercise would terminate in the normal individual at the point of sheer inability to develop a further increase or continuation of existing work output. The subject with exertional angina pectoris would terminate his stress test when chest discomfort developed and progressed to the point beyond which he was unwilling to endure. Results of such a test, while not identical with the oxygen consumption–proved maximum work capacity, provide a good approximation of it in the cooperative, well-motivated subject who is familiar with strenuous exercise. A theoretic weakness of the subjective maximal test is that it is indeed subjective and therefore perturbed by individual variations in motivation, spirit of cooperation and willingness to tolerate without alarm the sensory barrage originating within a body exercising at maximal capacity. Therefore, part of the interpretation of any subjective maximal exercise test is judgment by the test supervisor whether the subject made a convincing effort to perform maximally. The physician-test supervisor thus contributes his subjective element to the overall result, since some will accept as technically satisfactory degrees of subject cooperation that others would not. Clearly the experience and sophistication of the physician-test supervisor play a large role in maintaining the technical quality of subjective maximal exercise tests.

In an effort to provide objective criteria for high-performance exercise tests, our group and others have turned to heart rate response as a gauge of the actual stress of exercise. Robinson in 1938 established the basis for this approach when his study of normal men over a wide age range indicated that age was the only strong predictor of maximum exercise heart rate.[15] He found that maximum-exercise heart rate declines predictably with advancing age, and other factors such as height, weight and athletic training have little or no effect on this relationship. This relationship of maximum heart rate to age seemed such an important means of evaluating the effort of exercise that we repeated Robinson's experiments and not only confirmed the surprisingly high maximum heart rates he found in older men (about 170 beats per minute at age 60) but found the maximum heart rates in our older volunteers to be slightly higher than his[16] (Fig. 4-5). While confirming the lack of effect of other body variables upon maximum heart rate, our study showed the slight but again significant effect of athletic training upon heart rate, those who engaged in strenuous exercise at least three times weekly having maximum heart rates that averaged 7 beats per minute lower than physically untrained individuals at any age.

These maximum heart rate findings permitted construction of tables of percentages of maximum heart rate in relation to age and physical training (Table 4-1). Realizing that the sensitivity of a stress test is inseparably related to the degree of stress employed, we sought by experiment to find the highest percentage of heart rate stress that was acceptable to nearly all subjects, as well as being attainable by nearly all individuals. We found that 90% of predicted maximal heart rate represented the best criterion of high-performance exercise in the normal individual, and this level, 85 or 90% of maximal, has been favored by others as well.[17,18,19]

The test heart rate selected for each subject undergoing the graded exercise test is termed the target heart rate since it is the

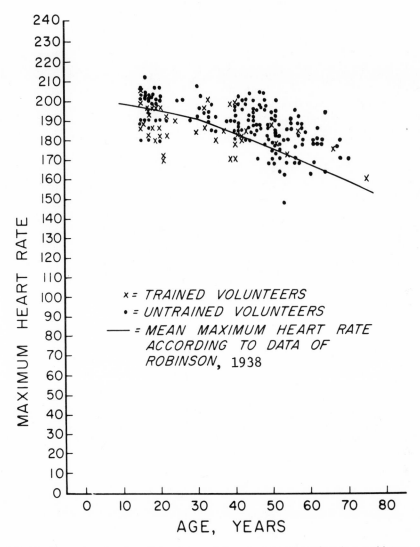

Figure 4-5. Maximum heart rate attained in relation to age in performing multistage treadmill exercise test to exhaustion.

TABLE 4-1

Exercise Heart Rate As A Function of Age and Training

	Age	20	25	30	35	40	45	50	55	60	65	70	75	80	85	90
	Max. H.R. (%)															
	100	190	188	186	184	182	180	177	175	173	171	169	167	165	163	161
Trained	90 (GXT)	171	169	167	166	164	162	159	158	156	154	152	150	149	147	145
Subjects	75	143	141	140	138	137	135	133	131	130	128	127	125	124	122	121
	60	114	113	112	110	109	108	106	105	104	103	101	100	99	98	97
	Max. H.R. (%)															
	100	197	195	193	191	189	187	184	182	180	178	176	174	172	170	168
Untrained	90 (GXT)	177	175	173	172	170	168	166	164	162	160	158	157	155	153	151
Subjects	75	148	146	144	143	142	140	138	137	135	134	132	131	129	128	126
	60	118	117	115	114	113	112	110	109	108	107	106	104	103	102	101

heart rate that is aimed for in the course of the test if a normal interpretation is to result. (In a small fraction, less than 5% of subjects, target heart rate is attained and at the same time angina or ST segment abnormality develops so that the subject has an indication of ischemic heart disease even though having reached target heart rate.) Subjects with significant coronary artery disease will develop exertional myocardial ischemia at much lower than near-maximal or maximal work levels, and when the evidence of ischemia is established by definite ST segment deviation, progressive substernal chest discomfort or both, the exercise is terminated. At this point the diagnostic information has been discovered and recorded, and there is neither need nor justification for prolonging the exercise stress beyond this point. In particular it should be understood that the target heart rate concept applies only to the thus-far-normal individual and never to the subject who has just demonstrated evidence of ischemic heart disease or any other cause of abnormal effort intolerance.

Prediction of maximum-exercise heart rate on the basis of age and physical training is not exact; standard deviation from the predicted rate is plus or minus 8 beats per minute and, allowing 2 standard deviations for approximately 95% confidence, yields a normal range that may be 16 beats per minute lower than the nominal predicted value. This degree of variation is expected in virtually any physiologic variable, and there is need to appreciate its significance so proper allowance for it can be made.

Allowance for normal maximal heart rate variance is made in either of two ways: First, if fatigue, breathlessness or any other normal consequence of peak physical effort results in termination of the exercise test when the heart rate has reached within 8 beats per minute of the normal heart rate, the test shall be accepted as technically satisfactory even though the target rate was not attained. Second, the principle of the well-motivated subjective maximal test is fully accepted within the framework of the GXT, and any test stopped below GXT target heart rate that is marked by a convincing degree of motivation will be accepted. These valid exercise challenges will nearly always have been marked by a period of sweating followed by the development of cool clammy skin, rapid labored breathing and inability to maintain a position near the front of the treadmill platform.

EXERCISE ELECTROCARDIOGRAPHY

Contemporary exercise electrocardiography, as contrasted with postexercise electrocardiography, which characterized first-generation exercise testing, is distinguished by the continuous acquisition of at least one and usually several ECG leads. This acquisition, beginning prior to exercise in the control period and extending through exercise and throughout the postexercise observation, is used for continuous display on a conveniently large monitor oscilloscope, for the activation of a cardiotachometer, and for recording selected lead samples periodically during all phases of the test. Only the availability of this continuous monitoring of the electrocardiogram, in conjunction with continuous observation of other aspects of the subject, has made clinicians willing to subject potentially diseased individuals to high-performance testing. It was previously thought unnecessary to employ rigorous monitoring techniques for less stressful procedures such as the two-step test. However, many patients develop ischemia before exceeding the stress level characteristic of mild exercise tests. This convinced us and many others of the need for high-quality monitoring whenever potentially diseased subjects are stressed in any way. The rare complications of exercise testing may occur at any level of exercise, and the need to detect these at the earliest possible moment is always with us.

The principal developments that make contemporary exercise electrocardiography feasible are (1) effective preparation of the skin followed by application of fluid contact electrodes, (2) development of light, flexible, low-noise patient cables and (3) the evolution of high-quality ECG amplifiers that possess the qualities of low inherent noise, high impedance input and high common mode rejection.

Making electrical contact with biologic tissue has always been a frustration to the electronics engineer and a challenge to the clinical investigator. With no convenient metallic snap-on connectors extending from the body, we are faced with the requirement of conveying the electrical potentials on the surfaces of living cell membranes to the metallic components of artificial electronic systems. Einthoven originally employed a virtually ideal arrangement to accomplish this when he immersed the limbs of his subjects into vessels containing salt solution, which were connected by wires to the recording apparatus. The great electrochemical disparity between cutaneous tissue cells and solid metal was mediated by interposition of a solution of electrolyte having an electrochemical potential intermediate between the source and recipient components of the system. As the reader who has seen reproductions of Einthoven's records will recall, the clarity of inscription, frequency response and registration of fine details within the QRS complex and freedom from artifactual noise content result in an overall signal quality not surpassed by direct recording electrocardiographs in routine use today.

With the advent of electron-tube ECG amplifiers, the fluid contact electrode principle was discarded in favor of directly contacting plate electrodes aided by electrolyte paste or cream. With this arrangement it was necessary for the subject to remain very still during recording, for any slippage of the electrode plates or variation in the resistance of electrode contact caused excessive baseline shift or other interference in the recorded tracing.

The fluid contact electrode principle was reintroduced to clinical electrocardiography with the report by Abarquez and colleagues of an exercise ECG system suitable for employment with a conventional electrocardiographic recorder.[20] Nonmetallic cups having a recessed metallic electrode are filled with electrolyte paste that makes the actual electrical contact with the skin when the rim of the cup is attached to the selected site, which has been previously carefully cleansed, rubbed to remove dead epithelial scales and from which skin oils have been removed by an application of acetone. With this procedure they were able to obtain stable, relatively low noise ECG recordings at medium and high levels of exercise. The unique advantages of this recording method were gradually adopted with what now seems surprising slowness. The fluid contact electrodes were tedious to prepare and unavailable commercially. Then Mason and Likar reported a simplified version of the fluid contact electrode taking advantage of new plastics and other materials that had become available.[21] These electrodes were easier to make and could be prepared in quantity. Only after the added superiority of the Mason-Likar electrodes was appreciated did equivalent factory-made electrodes appear (Fig. 4-6). These are now readily available, and in variety. The main choices are whether to adopt single-use disposable electrodes or reusable ones, involving a trade-off between convenience and expense. The other choice is between silver–silver chloride electrodes and electrodes made from some other material such as stainless steel. Silver–silver chloride electrodes have definite advantages for some types of recording because of their lower contact potential and lower susceptibility to long-term drift;

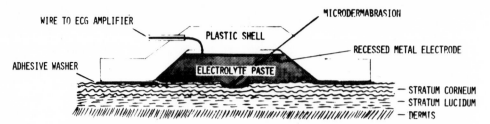

Figure 4-6. Typical fluid contact electrode illustrating the recessed metallic portion separated from skin contact by electrolyte paste. The skin has been cleaned and defatted with acetone, and a small circle of cornified epithelial scales has been removed by microdermabrasion. A plastic film washer, adhesive on both sides, holds the electrode securely on the skin. (Actual outside diameter of electrode is 2 to 2.5 cm.)

neither of these qualities is germane to the subject of exercise electrocardiography, however, and expert opinion varies with respect to whether silver–silver chloride electrodes yield superior exercise ECG records. The skill with which the skin is prepared and the electrodes applied is more important in exercise studies than the composition of the electrode material (Fig. 4-7).

The manufacture of an ECG patient cable tailored to the needs of exercise testing would seem to be a trivial challenge to the medical instrumentation manufac-

turer, yet the commercial cables presently available leave much to be desired. They should not only be light in weight and highly compliant and flexible but should also generate only a negligible amount of electrical noise when flexed or shifted. Present cables are relatively thick, heavy, bulky and noisy, yet the feasibility of constructing optimized patient cables has been demonstrated by Grais and associates.[22] High-quality cables containing up to ten conductors are fabricated by hand according to the methods of Grais and coworkers and are now available for purchase

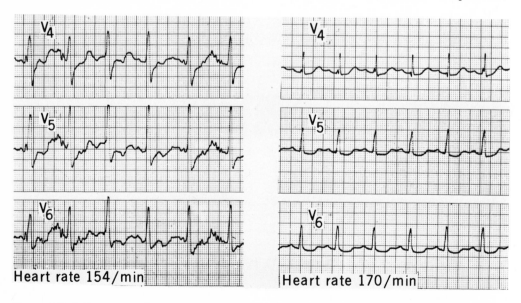

Figure 4-7. Left, poor quality exercise ECG record that appears abnormal but would not qualify for quantitative interpretation. *Right,* a high-quality exercise resulting from meticulous adherence to good skin preparation and electrode application technique. Paper speed 50 mm. per second; treadmill 3.4 miles per hour, 14% slope.

(James Development Co.). This development should provide a stimulus for large-scale manufacturers to provide a similar product.

The third major development in the evolution of high-quality exercise electrocardiography has been the ECG amplifiers themselves. Earlier amplifiers had three significant shortcomings when applied to this field: They introduced a certain measurable amount of distortion or noise, independent of the patient source, that originated in (1) the relatively large temperature-sensitive resistance elements, (2) the noise of spurious electron flights within vacuum tubes or (3) in relatively unsophisticated transistors. Improvements in materials and transistor-fabricating technique have reduced intrinsic noise nearly tenfold.

With the introduction of field-effect transistors it became practical to design ECG preamplifiers with input impedances in the 100-million-ohm range, instead of the 100-thousand-ohm range that prevailed in earlier amplifiers. This permits almost complete immunity from the kind of wave-form distortion introduced when different electrodes have different contact resistances on the skin. High-input impedance also makes negligible the earlier problem of ECG signal attenuation by the input stage, since input attenuation is determined by the ratio of source impedance to input impedance. The use of contemporary fluid contact electrodes and field-effect transistor amplifiers reduces this attenuation factor to substantially less than 1%. Finally, advances in the theory of amplifier design have made it possible to increase the common-mode rejection factor of amplifiers to 100-fold or greater. The effect of this development is to reject 60 Hz line interference and other modes of interference that are common to both leads of any input path to the extent that under ordinary circumstances this interference becomes negligible (Fig. 4-8). The incorporation of the above developments into the armamentarium of exercise electrocardiography is attributable in large part to the gradually increasing spirit of cooperation between clinicians and engineers and the small but growing breed of individuals, originally qualified in one

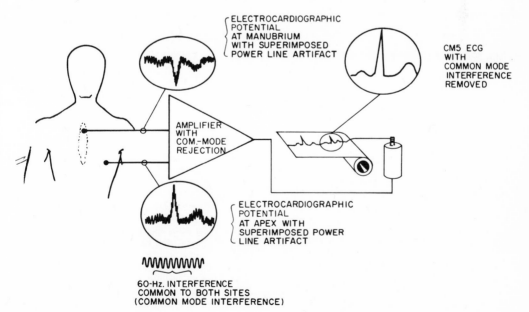

Figure 4-8. The effect of *common mode rejection* in reducing power line artifact in the ECG record.

discipline or the other, who have taken the time and trouble to become conversant in the basic principles and terminology of their colleagues in the other camp.

LEAD SYSTEMS

Clinicians have grown up with the realization that electrocardiographic phenomena exist in three-dimensional space within the body, and only an array of ECG leads providing multiple different "viewpoints" suffices to detect most of the characteristics of the EGG that have been recognized as clinically useful. That being the case, it would be surprising if all instances of myocardial ischemia such as provoked by exercise testing could be detected by a single ECG lead. Fortunately as well as surprisingly, most instances of ischemia are indeed reflected in a single lead: Blackburn and colleagues have found that about 89% of ST segment depressions present in any of the 12 conventional leads were detectable in lead V_5.[23] They found the next most sensitive leads were those located close to V_5, namely V_3, V_4 and V_6. The combination of these precordial leads and limb leads II and aVF detected all of their recognized examples of ST segment depression. Now that very rapid and efficient means of preparing the skin and attaching electrodes are available, those who maintain a no-compromise approach to exercise electrocardiography will find this combination of six leads their best choice. These leads have the advantage of familiarity throughout the field of medicine, and because of their long use, they have been subjected to the most extensive documentation. After initial registration during the resting control period, permanent records can be made at the end of each minute or at the end of each stage of exercise, the group repeated if possible, a few seconds before termination of exercise if this can be anticipated, and again immediately after cessation of exercise. The lead group is usually repeated at 2-minute intervals until the end of postexercise observation, typically 6 minutes if the ECG is stable.

Bipolar leads have come into extensive use for exercise test purposes (Table 4-2). By definition these leads consist of the potential difference between two electrodes, such as the Einthoven limb leads I, II and III as opposed to the other conventional leads that make use of the Wilson central terminal,[24] an electrical average of two or

TABLE 4-2

Some Bipolar Leads Used for Stress Electrocardiography

Lead	Proximal Electrode Location	Reference Electrode Location	Comments
CM5*	V_5 position	Manubrium	A sensitive bipolar lead for detecting ST changes
CH5	V_5 position	Forehead	Frequently used in Sweden for bicycle tests
CS5	V_5 position	Right infraclavicular fossa	Yields somewhat more muscle artifact than CM-5
CC5	V_5 position	V_6R position	This lead bears a closer resemblance to V_5 than most other bipolar leads
CB5	V_5 position	Low right scapula	Closely resembles V_5 but has more muscle artifact than most other bipolar leads
CR5	V_5 position	Right arm	Favored in northern Europe and Russia for pre-exercise and postexercise records, usually with 4 to 6 chest lead positions. High muscle artifact level during exercise

* The number 5 refers to the position on the chest of a corresponding V lead such as V_5. Thus the positive electrode could be located in any numbered V lead position. Ordinarily the position yielding the largest R wave is preferred if only one lead is to be recorded.

more leads whose aim is to create an electrically neutral reference point against which the active or exploring electrode is graphically compared. Before the field-effect transistor era, when the simplest means of avoiding interference problems involved the use of radiotelemetry, ECG telemetry transmitters could accommodate only bipolar leads, and therefore these leads were used extensively.

Optimal location of the electrodes that comprise a bipolar lead is very important and is strongly influenced by the use to which the resultant signal is to be put. For example, in monitoring the heart rate responses of competition swimmers, the electrodes are located over the upper and lower portions of the sternum in order to minimize interference from the hard-working skeletal muscles of the thorax. For cardiac rhythm monitoring, one electrode over the midprecordium and one at the upper sternum provide good P wave registration as well as clear registration of ventricular premature complexes. For exercise electrocardiography, where the main consideration is sensitive detection of ST segment shifts due to ischemia, the "active" or positive electrode is always located at or near the V_5 location, usually where the R wave is greatest. Opinion differs as to the ideal location of the reference electrode, recommended sites including upper and lower sternum, right infraclavicular fossa, right lateral chest (V_6R), right arm, right scapula and even locations on the head such as ear lobe or forehead.

One question concerning the use of bipolar leads for detection of myocardial ischemia is the relative susceptibility of these leads to ST segment depression due to nonischemic causes such as hyperventilation or changes in body position. Blackburn and colleagues, in comparing merits and disadvantages of bipolar leads, found that the lead from the V_5 position to the manubrium sterni (CM5) was the bipolar lead of choice for detecting ST segment displacement and had about the same sensitivity as conventional lead V_5 or perhaps a trifle more.[25] Thus the use of the CM5 bipolar lead for electrocardiography during and after exercise (but not substituting for the complete 12-lead rest and control tracing) is justifiable when practical considerations rule out the use of the six conventional leads.

The vectorcardiographic leads of Frank[26] have seen limited use in the field of exercise electrocardiography, mainly in clinical research projects, especially those oriented toward developing computer interpretation of the resulting records.[27] As in the case of the resting ECG the attraction of Frank leads lies in the theoretic economy of recording all or most of the characteristics of the ECG via three mutually perpendicular ECG leads.[28] Although the dipole theory of classical vectorcardiography has been disproved,[29] these leads have been found diagnostically useful in practice. Exercise electrocardiography strives to detect abnormal ST segment displacement occurring in any direction, not only from left to right, as reflected in V_5 and V_6, but also in the head-foot direction or the front-back direction. Whether the added complexity of these corrected leads will confer increased sensitivity, specificity or both to the stress test has not yet been determined. Initial experience, especially with transverse lead X, suggests that ST segment displacements are lower in this lead than in conventional leads and require compensating modifications and interpretation criteria.[25]

The application of topographic electrocardiography, mapping the thorax with electrodes over every few centimeters of the surface, has not yet spread to exercise electrocardiography, but there seems to be no good reason why it should not. Holt and colleagues have utilized arrays of 120 or more ECG electrodes in order to calculate the electrical signal strength emanating from different regions of the ventricles,[30] and Kornreich, utilizing Holt's ECG data, has claimed that a subset of only nine leads is sufficient to reproduce all the diagnostic information contained in the original set.[31] It is possible that a similar approach to the exercise electrocardiogram would be equally rewarding.

EXERCISE ECG INTERPRETATION

The time course of exercise ECG findings is as important as the individual findings themselves. Deviation of the ST segment is the only ECG finding that has been proved specific for myocardial ischemia, but this is true only if the ST segment deviation, usually depression but occasionally ST elevation, is temporally related to circumstances likely to provoke ischemia. The typical ischemic type of reaction to exercise stress would begin with an isoelectric and normal-appearing ST segment in the resting control period, and this would prevail through the initial period of light exercise and on until a critical ischemic threshold was reached and gradual ST segment depression developed. The concomitant development of characteristic chest discomfort would be likely, and ST segment depression in progressively greater degree

would occur until the test was interrupted. With termination of exercise stress the circulatory disparity would be abolished and ST segments would promptly become isoelectric again along with the disappearance of any other type of pathophysiologic manifestations of ischemia (Fig. 4-9). Thus, episodic or reversible periods of myocardial ischemia characteristic of angina pectoris involve *transient* rather than chronic deviation of the ST segment. Chronic ST segment abnormality may be the result of diverse causes such as healed myocardial infarction, ventricular overload with or without hypertrophy, electrolyte disorders, drug effects, hyperventilation and even changes in body position.

The effect of assimilation of a carbohydrate-rich meal upon serum potassium concentration is known to cause an increase in borderline and false positive exercise ECG responses,[32] and for that reason stress tests should not be conducted during the postprandial period but rather should be timed at least 2 hours after a light meal or longer after a heavier one (Table 4-3). If there is any reason to doubt the normality of the serum potassium concentration, such as known renal disease, or diuretic

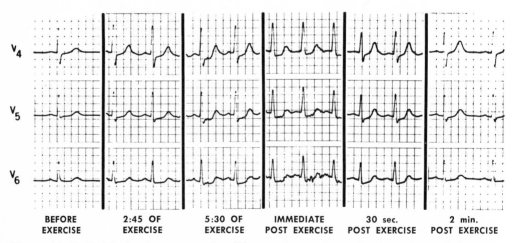

| BEFORE EXERCISE | 2:45 OF EXERCISE | 5:30 OF EXERCISE | IMMEDIATE POST EXERCISE | 30 sec. POST EXERCISE | 2 min. POST EXERCISE |

Figure 4-9. Typical ischemic response in mild to moderate obstructive disease: ST displacement is seen beginning at time 2:45, progressing with increased work rate at 5:30, definitely abnormal *immediate post exercise* but no longer fulfilling criteria of abnormality by *30 sec post exercise*. By *2 min post exercise* the record is entirely normal.

therapy, the potassium level should be checked on the day of testing and normality confirmed.

Digitalis therapy is known to cause false positive exercise ECG responses, and it is desirable that effects of digitalis glycoside be allowed to wear off at least 10 days prior to exercise ECG testing. Indeed, one should reconsider whether stress testing is indicated at all in a person who is being appropriately treated with digitalis, for in most such cases the response to the stress test will not result in a significant alteration in the management of the patient.

Antianginal agents when employed in effective dosage are known to prolong the amount of exercise tolerated prior to development of myocardial ischemia, and stress testing is highly useful in evaluating the beneficial effects of such drugs. Uncommonly, if ever, will these agents entirely prevent the development of myocardial ischemia at the most severe level of exercise encountered during stress testing, so the antianginal agents are not a significant source of false negative results. It is important, however, to be aware if they are being taken, so that their effects can be considered in evaluation of the anginal threshold that the test demonstrates.

It has recently been reported that tranquilizers and other psychotropic drugs may cause false negative exercise ECG results and, less commonly, false positive results as well.[33] Further confirmation of these findings is needed, for at present neither the mechanism of action for producing this effect nor the basis for predicting which way the false change will go has been satisfactorily explained.

Disorders of intraventricular conduction are known to affect the ST segment, and in the presence of left bundle branch block the effects of ischemia cannot be specifically identified. Right bundle branch block distorts the ST segment and T wave in the anteroposterior direction, affecting leads V_1, V_2 and perhaps V_3; however, this effect

TABLE 4-3

Equivocating Factors In Exercise ECG Interpretation

1. Left ventricular hypertrophy or overload
2. Abnormal ST-T at rest
3. Abnormal QRS: LBBB, other IVCD
4. Digitalis glycosides
5. Glucose or other carbohydrate load
6. Electrolyte imbalance
7. Coronary vasodilators
8. Adrenergic blocking agents, quinidine, procainamide
9. Tricyclics, other psychotropic drugs
10. Insufficient exercise tachycardia

is not ordinarily seen in the lateral leads, and it is generally accepted that ST segment deviations in leads V_4–V_6 can be interpreted in the usual way with only slight if any reduction in the accuracy of the result. Finally, Ellestad and Wan have recently confirmed what I would have intuitively predicted; namely, that the survivor of myocardial infarction has a better prognosis if he does not demonstrate ST segment depression on exercise testing than if such depression is manifested.[34] In other words, stress test results are important even in patients known to have advanced coronary artery disease. If previous infarction has caused great distortion of the QRS contour and direction of the main R wave vector, one may assume that left ventricular activation has been disturbed also. In such cases ST deviation may not always represent myocardial ischemia, and in particular, transient ST elevation may be due to aneurysmal bulges or local dyskinesia rather than simple hypoxia of otherwise normal healthy myocardium.[35]

In order to realize precision and reproducibility of test results, quantitative criteria of ST segment changes are employed. It has been found that when interpretation is made by inspection alone or by nonstandard criteria, there is a wide variation among physicians in the interpretation of exercise ECG.[36] The criterion that has been used by most clinicians for the longest time requires that the previously normal resting ST segment must become depressed with flat or down-sloping contour extending at least 80 msec. past the QRS-ST junction. This depression must be at least 0.1 mV. (1 mm.) in amplitude. It is not usually stated just where along the ST segment this amplitude measurement will be performed; if the ST segment is flat this is unimportant, but if it is down sloping then some specific point of measurement, such as "40 msec. after the J point," is necessary in order for the measurement criterion to have quantitative meaning. This is important because T wave inversion alone can cause 0.1 mV. of ST-T depression 80 msec. after the J point even when there is no significant depression of the J point itself. T wave inversion without J point depression is not a specific indicator of ischemia,[37] and ST segment criteria should be selected so as not to include isolated T wave inversion. The criteria advocated here have two advantages: Interpretations based on them correspond well with those based on other different but well-accepted criteria, and they are quantitatively precise, their results comparing well with clinical course and angiographic findings for a positive, isch-

emic type of ECG response: There must be deviation of the QRS-ST junction (J point) of at least 0.1 mV. from the baseline, and the first 80 msec. of the ST segment must (a) be flat with respect to the baseline; (b) slope away from the baseline (down sloping, for depressed J point, up sloping for elevated J point); (c) slope at a rate of less than 1 mV. per second if the slope is toward the baseline (steeper ST segment slopes are classified as normal). At recommended paper recording speed of 50 mm. per second, a 1 mV. per second slope represents an angle of 11.3 degrees or 20% grade. An example of an abnormal response meeting the combined J point deviation and ST segment slope criteria is shown in Figure 4-10. To assure that baseline quality is satisfactory for interpretation a straight line should be drawn through three successive QRS onsets. These criteria may be applied to other leads than the traditionally employed V_5 lead, but in the anterior chest leads such as V_1–V_3, ST segment elevation is a normal phenomenon and should not be construed to represent ischemia. ST segment depression in these leads is indicative of ischemia, as it is in lateral leads. In Figure 4-11 for example, all three monitor leads have become criti-

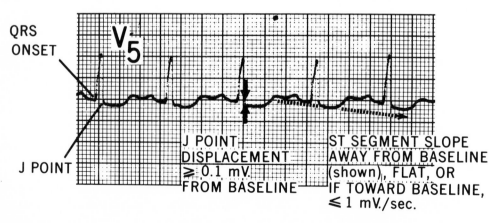

Figure 4-10. Application of quantitative criteria of abnormal ST segments. The baseline must be straight, with at least three successive QRS onsets lying on the same horizontal line. The J point is displaced from this baseline at least 1 mm. (*arrows*). A line is constructed tangential to the first 80 msec. of the ST segment. If abnormal it will not slope back toward the baseline as steeply as 1 mV./sec. (a 1:5 slope at 50 mm. per second chart speed).

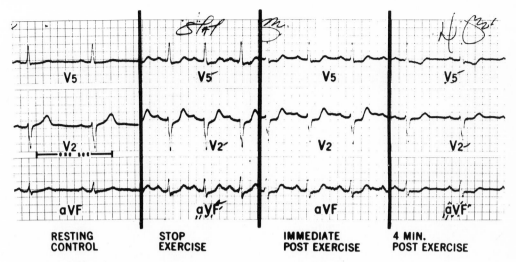

Figure 4-11. Highly abnormal response in patient with proved advanced coronary disease. At *stop exercise,* only V₅ is abnormal, but *immediately post exercise* all three leads are abnormal. Delayed normalization of ST is shown in V₅ *4 min post exercise.*

cally abnormal in the Immediate Post Exercise record.

Other ECG abnormalities may be encountered in the course of stress testing, and indeed stress tests are frequently conducted specifically to search for some of them, e.g., atrial and ventricular arrhythmias, to evaluate the efficacy of antiarrhythmic therapy. In the absence of ST segment deviation, however, no other abnormalities should be used to diagnose the presence of exertional ischemia.

PROGNOSTIC SIGNIFICANCE OF EXERCISE ECG RESULTS

Robb and Marks, reviewing the survival data of insured patients who had undergone two-step tests, found that a sixteen-fold increase in mortality rate attended those who showed pronounced ST segment depression.[10] It is reasonable that profound ischemia in response to relatively mild stress would be related to an advanced degree of coronary obstructive disease. Only slightly less astonishing is the finding by Doyle and Kinch that following conversion to an ischemic type treadmill test response there is an 85% incidence of coronary events in the ensuing 5 years.[38]

This compares with only about 5% incidence of coronary events among negative responders. Ellestad and Wan, employing an even more strenuous stress test, found an incidence of 9.5% new coronary events per year among positive responders as compared with 1.7% among negative responders.[34] These findings give more than ample justification of the effectiveness of stress electrocardiography in aiding the diagnosis of ischemic heart disease. No other non-invasive procedure except the patient, skillful review of the medical history rivals the sensitivity and specificity of the stress electrocardiogram, and indeed a sizable fraction of the population can be identified by stress testing as suffering from coronary atherosclerosis even though prior to testing these individuals have been asymptomatic and their condition therefore undetectable by questioning.

CLINICAL OBSERVATIONS

The exercise test offers a unique opportunity for the physician to observe many facets of a patient's personality, including whatever emotional component may be associated with exercise-induced symptoms, the location and time course of these symptoms as they are actually experienced and the relationship between symptoms and objective data such as ST segment changes or rhythm and conduction disturbances. For this reason, even apart from safety considerations, it is well worthwhile for patients to be observed by a physician during exercise tests. However, this reasoning may not necessarily apply to stress tests performed on asymptomatic volunteers who are part of population screening projects or participating in physiologic research projects.

Patient Safety. Although patients who are free of heart disease are not significantly endangered by the exercise involved in a properly performed GXT, patients with coronary artery disease, always at some risk of infarction or cardiac arrest, are subjected to a slight and temporary increase of this risk by taking an exercise test. Knowing this, physicians are obligated to make every effort to minimize the risk of the individuals tested, and this can be accomplished by scrupulous attention to the three principal components of patient treatment.

Prevention implies that each candidate for stress testing will be interviewed, examined and have a 12-lead resting ECG interpreted prior to initiation of exercise stress. Of greatest importance is recognition and elimination from testing of any individual with acute or unhealed myocardial infarction. Such infarctions have been known to occur between the time that an exercise test was appropriately requested for evaluation of a chest pain problem and the time that the patient actually arrived at the testing facility.

There is increased hazard of myocardial infarction in patients with chest pain that fulfills certain criteria such as original onset of pain less than 4 weeks ago, chest pain that in the last 4 weeks has become progressively more severe, prolonged or easier to provoke, or chest pain that occurs at rest and without obvious precipitating cause.

Such patients should probably be treated on the assumption that the chest pain is ischemic in origin and testing postponed until chest pain is stable for 4 weeks or longer. Patients with uncontrolled atrial or ventricular arrhythmias should have testing deferred until these are brought under satisfactory regulation. Patients with mild to moderate aortic valve stenosis may be exercised if aerobic capacity estimation is desired to aid in patient treatment and counseling, but blood pressure must be monitored carefully in these individuals and exercise terminated upon any suggestion of abnormal blood pressure response. Individuals with moderate to severe aortic stenosis should not be subjected to stress testing because of the known risk of mortality associated with exercise in these patients. Other possible contraindications to stress testing are listed in Table 4-4.

Recognition refers to effective monitoring of the test subject so that any abnormality is detected and interpreted properly with a minimum of delay. It is an appropriate challenge to the clinician to acquire as much information as possible about his subject with the facilities at hand: These may include advanced electrocardiographic equipment but will also include skillful use of the clinician's own eyes, ears and touch. The ECG equipment not only permits continuous evaluation of the ST segment but also serves for monitoring heart rhythm and the course of heart rate with respect

TABLE 4-4

Contraindications to Exercise Testing

1. Myocardial infarction—impending, acute or healing
2. Unstable angina pectoris
3. Severe aortic stenosis
4. Congestive heart failure
5. Severe hypertension
6. Uncontrolled cardiac arrhythmias
7. Intracardiac conduction block greater than first degree
8. Acute systemic illness
9. Unwillingness to give informed consent

to work rate. It is common policy to interrupt exercise if ventricular premature beats become so frequent that more than one VPB is visible on the oscilloscope at one time, or if the VPBs exhibit multiform contour. Two or more consecutive VPBs represent an indication to terminate exercise, as does the development of any degree of intracardiac block or any recognized shift in pacemaker focus (Table 4-5).

Heart rate response to exercise gives useful clues for patient evaluation. Rapid heart rate immediately on beginning exercise is usually a result of anxiety and typically becomes normal during the first 3 minutes of exercise. Inappropriately high heart rates that persist beyond 3 minutes usually indicate physical deconditioning and poor aerobic capacity. A leveling off of a previously normal heart rate response indicates that the subject has begun performing what is for him maximal or near-maximal exercise. A very much lower than average heart rate response may be a normal variant in a small percentage of subjects but is most likely the result of intensive athletic training or in the elderly subject may be due to degenerative disease of the sinoatrial node. Propranolol or other beta-adrenergic blocking agent will of course reduce the resting and exercise heart rate regardless of the age of the subject, and it is essential to be aware of this drug effect if it is present. When the effect of this drug is present, target heart rates will not be attained, and subjects will terminate exercise according to one of the indications for stopping exercise other than heart rate (Table 4-5).

Indirect brachial blood pressure should be measured before exercise and at least once in each stage of exercise (Fig. 4-12). It is checked again immediately post exercise and periodically, e.g., every 2 minutes, during the postexercise period. Patients with uncontrolled systemic hypertension should be eliminated from exercise testing until satisfactory therapy is achieved. Dur-

TABLE 4-5

GXT Indications for Terminating Exercise

1. Attainment of GXT target heart rate and maintaining it for 1 minute, or to the end of a treadmill stage, or until heart rate exceeds target rate by eight beats per minute
2. Angina-like pain that is progressive during exercise
3. Diagnostic degree of ischemic type of ST depression or elevation during exercise
4. Ectopic supraventricular tachycardia, regular or irregular
5. Ventricular premature beats aggravated by exercise or precipitated by exercise, over 25% of beats
6. ECG consistent with ventricular tachycardia
7. *Any* recognized type of intracardiac block precipitated by exercise
8. Signs of peripheral circulatory insufficiency (pallor, diminished pulse, clammy skin, exhaustion)
9. Drop in systolic blood pressure during exercise
10. Excessive fatigue or dyspnea
11. Failure of ECG monitoring system
12. Subject wishes to stop exercise

ing exercise the procedure is interrupted if blood pressure becomes "dangerously" high, for example, 260/120 mm. of mercury, although any such cutoff point is arbitrary since I am unaware of any hypertensive complication of exercise testing. On the other hand, a drop in systolic blood pressure or failure to increase systolic pressure with increasing work load represents a clear hazard and calls for exercise termination as soon as the presence of this phenomenon has been confirmed by a repeat reading. The possibility of this occurrence in the presence of aortic valve stenosis has been mentioned; the other principal cause is coronary artery disease, and it has recently been reported that patients manifesting such reactions have very far advanced disease involving two or more major coronary vessels.[39]

Other aspects of clinical monitoring include frequent questioning of the patient regarding the development of chest pain, in which case the quality, location and subsequent time course are noted. We termi-

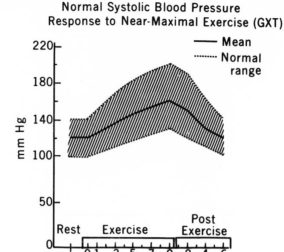

Figure 4-12. All normal subjects demonstrate a progressive rise in systollic blood pressure when performing the GXT. Mean and normal range blood pressure response in our laboratories is shown. Diastolic blood pressure normally changes very little (usually not over 10 mm. Hg) during the test.

nate exercise if chest discomfort consistent with angina pectoris develops and progresses in intensity during exercise. The gait of the exercising subject can yield useful information about musculoskeletal defects and coordination. Deterioration of gait may be the first sign of exercise intolerance. Periodic palpation of the skin of the torso or forehead allows one to estimate the degree of stress that the current work rate represents to the exercising subject. Mild stress will cause little or no change, moderate stress will result in increased skin warmth, moderately severe stress is marked by warmth and sweating, and near-maximal to maximal stress is associated with the development of cool, clammy skin. This comes about as cutaneous vasoconstriction aids in conserving the cardiac output for the brain, heart and working muscles.

Treatment begins with the appropriate termination of exercise upon recognition of any danger signal and proper management of the subject in the postexercise period. If the subject develops a precipitous drop in heart rate or blood pressure, the recumbent position with legs elevated should be employed, and an intravenous infusion begun without delay to facilitate drug therapy. If, however, the hoped-for salutary normalization of rate and pressure occurs promptly, the procedure of establishing an infusion may be as promptly abandoned. Ordinarily, after near-maximal or maximal exercise the sitting position is more comfortable than lying down. Ventricular arrhythmias nearly always cease spontaneously upon termination of exercise, but one should be prepared to administer an intravenous bolus of lidocaine if the arrhythmia persists or is poorly tolerated. Proper planning and practice should make it possible to administer countershock within a few seconds after the need for it is recognized. Patients being countershocked for ventricular fibrillation or very rapid ventricular tachycardia should be hospitalized and monitored at least over night. Likewise, patients with prolonged or very severe angina pectoris precipitated during exercise testing should be considered suffering from intermediate coronary syndrome and hospitalized. Prearrangements should be made to permit the immediate transfer of a patient to the nearest coronary care unit if evidence of myocardial infarction develops. Fortunately, complications of exercise testing are quite uncommon.[40] In order to maintain and even improve the current safety record enjoyed by stress testing it is necessary to maintain constant vigilance for contraindications to testing, reasons for stopping exercise and effective means of minimizing the severity of complications.

SUMMARY

The high-performance exercise ECG test is the most useful non-invasive laboratory aid for the diagnosis of coronary artery disease. Reflecting the physiology of the stressed myocardium, it bears a complementary relationship to the coronary angiogram, which reveals arterial anatomy. The foundation of the stress test is the fact that arterial narrowing usually restricts coronary blood flow only at high levels of myocardial perfusion requirement, while allowing appropriate coronary flow when the demands are modest. Heart rate is a sensitive indicator of the increasing myocardial O_2 requirement during exercise, so while an abnormal response may occur at virtually any heart rate, a normal response is meaningful only if a high heart rate was achieved during exercise.

Greatest sensitivty for detecting coronary artery disease is attained with the greatest cardiac work and highest heart rate. For this reason, maximal exercise has been proposed as the standard stress. As clinically employed, maximal exercise is a subjective determination. Others, favoring an objective criterion of satisfactory performance, recommend 90% of predicted maximum heart rate as the end point for normal responders.

Exercise electrocardiography has evolved in low-noise patient electrodes and cables, sophisticated ECG amplifiers and improved writing galvanometers that permit ECG acquisition and recording all during exercise as well as afterward. In-exercise ECG monitoring has contributed to

the safety of high-performance testing and is now considered essential for all patients. Leads used for monitoring and diagnosis include simple bipolar (two electrode) leads like CM5 as well as the conventional unipolar chest leads and some limb leads.

Interpretation of the exercise ECG requires high-quality records as well as standardized criteria. In addition, the numerous sources of erroneous results must be recognized or excluded. When this is done, exercise ECG results have strong prognostic significance, identifying patients with at least ten times greater than average risk of suffering a coronary event. The usefulness of the stress test is increased by the clinical observations available during exercise in addition to the ECG. This constant observation of the patient throughout the stress test contributes to the excellent safety record enjoyed by stress test laboratories.

ACKNOWLEDGMENT

It is a pleasure to acknowledge the assistance given me by my colleague, David Roitman, M.D. Thanks are also due to Mrs. Myrnie Driskill and Mrs. Juanita Brasher for their assistance in preparing this manuscript.

REFERENCES

1. Lown, B., and Wolf, M.: Approaches to sudden death from coronary heart disease. Circulation 44:130, 1971.
2. Bruce, R. A., Blackmon, J. R., Jones, J. W., and Strait, G.: Exercising testing in adult normal subjects and cardiac patients. Pediatrics 32:742, 1963.
3. Hilsenrath, J., Hamby, R. I., and Hoffman, I.: Pitfalls in the prediction of coronary artery disease from the electrocardiogram or vectorcardiogram. J. Electrocardiol. 6:291, 1973.
4. Aronow, W. S., Bowyer, A. F., and Kaplan, M. A.: External isovolumic contraction times and left ventricular ejection time/external isovolumic contraction time ratios at rest and after exercise in coronary heart disease. Circulation 43:59, 1971.
5. Craige, E.: Apexcardiography. *In* Noninvasive Cardiology, edited by A. M. Weissler. New York, Grune & Stratton, 1974, pp. 1–38.
6. Feigenbaum, H.: Coronary artery disease. *In* Echocardiography, edited by H. Feigenbaum. Philadelphia, Lea & Febiger, 1972, pp. 199–211.
7. Wood, F. C., Wolferth, C. C., and Livezey, M. M.: Angina pectoris. Arch. Intern. Med. 47: 339, 1931.
8. Scherf, D., and Schaffer, A. I.: The electrocar-

diographic exercise test. Am. Heart J. 43:927, 1952.

9. Master, A. M., and Jaffe, H. L.: Electrocardiographic changes after exercise in angina pectoris. J. Mount Sinai Hosp. N.Y. 7:629, 1941.

10. Robb, G. P., and Marks, H. H.: Latent coronary artery disease: Determination of its presence and severity by the exercise electrocardiogram. Am. J. Cardiol. 13:603, 1964.

11. Friedberg, C. K., Jaffe, H. L., Pordy, L., and Chesky, K.: The two-step exercise electrocardiogram. A double-blind evaluation of its use in the diagnosis of angina pectoris. Circulation 26:1254, 1963.

12. Sheffield, L. T., and Reeves, T. J.: Graded exercise in the diagnosis of angina pectoris. Mod. Concepts Cardiovasc. Dis. 34:1, 1965.

13. Prinzmetal, M., et al.: Angina pectoris. A variant form of angina pectoris. Am. J. Med. 27:375, 1959.

14. Kitamura, K., et al.: Hemodynamic correlates of myocardial oxygen consumption during upright exercise. J. Appl. Physiol. 32:516, 1972.

15. Robinson, S.: Experimental studies of physical fitness in relation to age. Arbeitsphysiol. 10:251, 1938.

16. Lester, F., Trammell, P., Reeves, T. J., and Sheffield, L. T.: Effect of age and athletic training on maximal heart rate during treadmill exercise. Clin. Res. 15:28, 1967.

17. Ascoop, C. A., Simoons, M. L., Egmond, W. G., and Bruschke, A. V. G.: Exercise test, history, and serum lipid levels in patients with chest pain and normal electrocardiogram at rest: Comparison to findings at coronary arteriography. Am. Heart J. 82:609, 1971.

18. Ellestad, M. H., Allen, W., Wan, M. C. K., and Kemp, G. L.: Maximal treadmill stress testing for cardiovascular evaluation. Circulation 39:517, 1969.

19. Mason, R. E., and Likar, I.: A new approach to stress tests in the diagnosis of myocardial ischemia. Trans. Am. Clin. Climatol. Assoc. 76:40, 1964.

20. Abarquez, R. F., Freiman, A. H., Reichel, F., and LaDue, J. S.: The precordial electrocardiogram during exercise. Circulation 22:1060, 1960.

21. Mason, R. B., and Likar, I.: A new system of multiple-lead exercise electrocardiography. Am. Heart J. 71:196, 1966.

22. Grais, I. M., Campbell, D. E., and Adolph, R. J.: A 12-lead patient cable for electrocardiographic exercise testing. Am. Heart J. 87:203, 1974.

23. Blackburn, H., Katigbak, R., Mitchell, P., and Imbimbo, B.: What electrocardiographic leads to take after exercise? Am. Heart J. 67:184, 1964.

24. Wilson, F. N., Johnston, F. C., Macleod, A. G., and Barker, P. S.: Electrocardiograms that represent the potential variations of a single electrode. Am. Heart J. 9:447, 1934.

25. Blackburn, H., et al.: Standardization of the exercise electrocardiogram. A systematic comparison of chest lead configurations employed for monitoring during exercise. In Physical Activity and the Heart, edited by M. J. Karvonen and A. Barry. Springfield, Ill., Charles C Thomas, 1967, pp. 101–133.

26. Frank, E.: An accurate, clinically practical system for spatial vectorcardiography. Circulation 13:737, 1956.

27. Blomqvist, G.: The Frank lead exercise electrocardiogram. A quantitative study based on averaging technic and digital computer analysis. Acta Med. Scand. 178 (Suppl. 440): 5, 1965.

28. Hu, K. C., Francis, D. B., Gau, G. T., and Smith, R. E.: Development and performance of Mayo-IBM electrocardiographic computer analysis programs (V70). Mayo Clin. Proc. 48:260, 1973.

29. Flowers, N. C., Horan, L. G., and Brody, D. A.: Evaluation of multipolar effects in the high-fidelity standard electrocardiogram by means of factor analysis. Circulation 32:273, 1965.

30. Holt, J. H., Barnard, A. C. L., Lynn, M. S., and Svendsen, P.: A study of the human heart as a multiple dipole electrical source. Circulation 40:687, 1969.

31. Kornreich, F.: The missing waveform information in the orthogonal electrocardiogram (Frank leads). Circulation 48:984, 1973.

32. Riley, C. P., Oberman, A., and Sheffield, L. T.: Electrocardiographic effects of glucose ingestion. Arch. Intern. Med. 130:703, 1972.

33. Laws, J. G., Satinsky, J. D., and Linhart, J. W.: Treadmill exercise test in female patients. Circulation 50 (suppl. 3): 8, 1974.

34. Ellestad, M. H., and Wan, M. K. C.: Predictive implications of stress testing. Follow-up of 2700 subjects after maximum treadmill stress testing. Circulation 51:363, 1975.

35. Chahine, R. A., Mathur, V. S., Raizner, A. E., and Luchi, R. J.: Significance of the exercise induced ST segment elevation. Circulation 50 (suppl. 3): 9, 1974.

36. Blackburn, H., et al.: The exercise electrocardiogram: Differences in interpretation. Report of a technical group on exercise electrocardiography. Am. J. Cardiol. 21:871, 1968.

37. Sheffield, L. T., et al.: On-line analysis of the exercise electrocardiogram. Circulation 40: 935, 1959.

38. Doyle, J. T., and Kinch, S. H.: The prognosis of an abnormal electrocardiographic stress test. Circulation 41:545, 1970.

39. Thomson, P. D., and Kelemen, M. H.: A reliable and easily elicited sign of critical coronary artery narrowing. Circulation 50 (suppl. 3): 9, 1974.

40. Rochmis, P., and Blackburn, H.: Exercise tests. A survey of procedures, safety and litigation experience in approximately 170,000 tests. J.A.M.A. 217:1061, 1971.

Chapter 5

Holter Monitor Electrocardiography

CALVIN L. WEISBERGER AND EDWARD K. CHUNG

When a physician wishes to evaluate a patient's cardiac rhythm during his usual daily activities, he can utilize the technique of Holter monitoring. The Holter technique utilizes a precordial lead system that is connected to a portable electrocardiographic monitor. The ECG signal is recorded on magnetic tape, which may record 10, 12 or 24 hours of electrocardiogram. The Holter technique has the sensitivity to detect not only various cardiac arrhythmias but also changes in conduction pattern and the S-T segment and T wave abnormalities.[1-4]

The tape from the Holter recorder is played back on a scanner. A trained technician with this equipment can scan a 10-hour tape recording in about 20 minutes. The 12- and 24-hour recordings require a proportionally longer time for scan. This rapid scanning is performed by utilizing four basic aids to the recognition of cardiac rhythm and conduction abnormalities.

The ECG wave forms are rapidly superimposed upon each other on an oscilloscope. The scanning technician can readily recognize alteration in wave form and play back representative strips of ECG. Besides the wave-form superimposition, the scanner has an audible tone built in that varies with changes in heart rate and wave form. By sensing the tone change the technician can be alerted to recognize the ECG changes. Another visual tool is a line display of rate and beat-to-beat interval spacing changes that also serves to alert the scanner to record representative strips. A most important part of the Holter monitor system is the patient's diary. The patient keeps a record of his activities, the time of these activities and the presence and timing of symptoms (Fig. 5-1). The time the monitor is turned on is recorded, and the tape runs at constant speed for 10 hours, 12 hours or 24 hours, depending upon the capacity of the equipment. Therefore, it is possible to correlate the ECG rhythm strips with the time of symptoms by using a clock synchronized to the monitor. When the actual electrocardiogram is reproduced from recorded tape, the physician can interpret the detailed rhythm and wave form to correlate with his patient's activities during the monitored period.

Some of the various indications for Holter recording are included in Table 5-1. In short, the technique can be used to obtain a diagnosis such as paroxysmal tachyarrhythmias, bradyarrhythmias or atrioventricular block.[5] The recorder may identify

TIME	ACTIVITY	SYMPTOMS
10:00AM	START RECORDING	
10:30 AM	Walking in STREET	fluttering feeling in chest
11:00 AM	Resting on BENCH	none
noon	Eating lunch	"indigestion"
1:15 Pm	Walking Steps to office	Short of BREATH
1:30 Pm	Sitting in office	shortness of breath relieved
2:30 Pm	Business meeting, ARgument	chest pain and shortness of breath
2:45 Pm	After nitroglycerin	feeling better
4:00 Pm	Driving home	anxiety
5:45 Pm	Eating dinner	Feel O.K.
7:00 Pm	Watching television	
8:30 Pm	Got up to go to bathroom	lightHEADED
8:45 Pm	Resting-feel	feel better
9:30 Pm	IN BED	Feel O.K.
10:00 pm	Monitor off	

Figure 5-1. Patient's diary card for the Holter monitor.

episodes of angina or anginal equivalent by the S-T segment and T wave alteration.[3] The recorder can also be used to evaluate the incidence of extrasystoles and whether they occur as group beats or with the R-on-T phenomenon.[6] Another important use of Holter monitoring is in the evaluation of antiarrhythmic therapy.[7] By determining whether the incidence of arrhythmia is decreased or abolished by a given dosage of drug the physician is able to assess the efficacy of his therapy. During digitalis therapy, the Holter monitor can identify digitalis-induced arrhythmias and also give an indication of rate control, especially in atrial fibrillation during various activities. In patients with artificial pacemakers the technique can evaluate the status of pacemaker function. It can also give an indication of the time that a demand pacemaker is actually pacing. This can predict the lifespan of the pacemaker.

Early stages of malfunction of the pacemaker can be detected by the Holter monitor.

INSTRUCTION TO THE PATIENT

The patient is first instructed in the nature of the examination. He is advised what activities to include and to exclude during the monitoring period. In general, the patient must be advised not to get the electrodes or the recorder wet. He must also be advised not to finger the electrodes during the recording period as this may produce artifacts in the recording. The patient is advised how to remove the electrodes at the end of the recording period. The patient should be presented with a diary and instructed to keep a careful record of activities, symptoms and their time of occurrence. He should be reminded not to forget to return the diary when he returns the recorder. The patient should be given a list of types of activities to record such as exercise, walking stairs, emotional upsets, arguments, smoking, bowel movements, urination, meals, sexual intercourse, medicines and sleep periods (Fig. 5-1). More than usual daily activity should be clearly indicated in the diary.

PROCEDURE FOR LEAD PLACEMENT

The Holter monitor system utilizes a bipolar electrode system.[8] This consists of three electrodes: the exploring (usually colored red), indifferent (colored white) and ground electrodes (green). Two basic electrode positioning systems are used, although any suitable modification is acceptable. The general application is a bipolar modification of lead V_4 or V_5. This usually gives a good way of analyzing P waves, QRS complexes, S-T segment and T wave abnormalities. The QRS complex is usually upright when this lead placement is used. In this system, the exploring electrode is placed over the fifth rib in the left midclavicular line. The indifferent electrode is placed high over the sternum, and the ground is placed over the fifth rib in the right midclavicular line (Fig. 5-2A). The placement over the bone is to minimize muscle-motion artifact. The other basic lead placement is a modified V_1 lead, which is used primarily for cardiac rhythm analysis with less concern with the S-T and T wave changes (Figure 5-2B). The lead V_1 position usually records a prominent P wave and also facilitates differentiation between right and left bundle branch block configurations. This position consists of the exploring electrode over the lower sternum, the indifferent over the upper sternum and the ground over the fifth rib in the right midclavicular line (Fig. 5-2B). Before the electrodes are attached the skin should be shaved and defatted, with acetone, and antiperspirant should be applied and allowed to dry. After the leads are securely applied, loops of the connecting wire from each

Table 5-1

Clinical Uses of Holter Electrocardiogram

Diagnosis of Arrhythmias
    Premature contractions (extrasystoles)
    Tachyarrhythmias
    Bradyarrhythmias
    Brady-tachyarrhythmia syndrome
    Conduction disturbances
    Wolff-Parkinson-White syndrome
Diagnosis of Myocardial Ischemia
    Classical angina
    Atypical angina
    Nocturnal angina
    Prinzmetal's angina
    Asymptomatic ischemic ECG change
Evaluation of Antiarrhythmic Drug Therapy
    Efficacy of drug
    Toxicity of drug
Evaluation of Artificial Pacemaker Function
    Missed capture
    Inadequate sensing function
    Runaway pacemaker
    Cardiac arrhythmias related to or induced by pacemaker
Miscellaneous
    Follow-up of myocardial infarction
    Rhythm response to daily activities
    Ischemic response to daily activities
    Evaluation of various drugs
    Evaluation of ill-defined symptoms (such as dizziness, fainting, palpitation)

lead should be taped to the patient's skin to prevent sudden tension on the wire from disconnecting a lead. The lead system should then be connected to a conventional ECG to verify the utility of the lead morphology and baseline steadiness. Control recordings should be made in the supine, sitting and standing positions as the configuration of the P wave, QRS complex and S-T,T waves may change depending upon the patient's position. The lead system is then connected to the monitor, which should be prechecked to confirm whether the unit contains a fresh battery supply and a blank magnetic tape. The time the monitor is activated is recorded on the patient's diary, and the patient can be dismissed. The monitor may be carried over the shoulder or connected to a belt, depending on the make and model of the instrument.

The monitoring period should almost

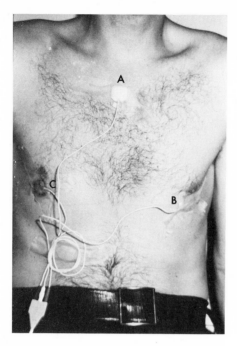
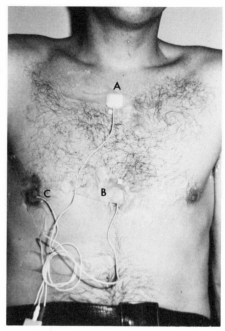

Figure 5-2. Lead placement: *Left,* General electrode position; *right,* P wave specific position. *A,* indifferent electrode (white); *B,* exploring electrode (red); *C,* ground electrode (green).

never be less than 10 hours. Lown and his associates demonstrated the need for monitoring at least for 10-hour periods. The tape with 24-hour capability allows one to monitor the patient through both his active daytime activities and his inactive evening and sleeping periods with one recording.[9,10]

When the recorder and tape are returned the tape should be scanned as soon as possible. At present, this is done either at the recording institution (physician's private office or heart station of the hospital), if a scanner and trained technician are present, or at a processing laboratory where the tape is sent for scanning, with the diary.

The report usually consists of representative ECG rhythm strips of the recording that show cardiac arrhythmias and abnormalities in the QRS complex, S-T and T waves, in addition to the rhythm strips recorded during the periods when symptoms were noted by the patient in the diary. Various techniques have been employed for the quantitation of phenomena in the re-

cording. Trend records can be reported that show the variation in heart rate throughout the period correlated with time and diary notes. A technique for quantitating events is to print out random 1-minute strips during each hour of recording, quantitate events on these and extrapolate to the total period. This is called the serial rhythm strip method and is, of course, only a coarse estimate of the actual frequency of ECG abnormalities. Another technique for quantitating events is by constructing a histogram using the R-R interval indicator.[11] Utilizing this technique, one can quantitate the occurrence of the predominant (for example, sinus rhythm) R-R interval and all other R-R intervals within the recording period. At present, this technique is available through very few laboratories, but it does give one excellent accurate quantitation data.

ILLUSTRATIVE CASE STUDIES

Ten illustrative cases showing the most common and clinically important electrocardiographic abnormalities have been selected for this chapter.

Case 1. The monitor rhythm strip in Figure 5-3 belongs to a 58-year-old man with a past history of diaphragmatic (inferior) myocardial infarction. He had complained of nocturnal dyspnea for several weeks. These episodes were associated with a sensation of extreme heaviness in the chest. There was, however, no history of palpitation, chest pain, nausea, diaphoresis or weakness. There was no evidence of congestive heart failure. An exercise electrocardiogram was positive, being stopped because of chest pain at a 5-met exercise level. A Holter monitor recording was obtained in order to document the ischemic event during his usual activity, including his sleeping period. As can be seen in the recording, during the night when the patient was in bed, his S-T segment became markedly depressed. The patient awoke with the sensation of heaviness in the chest and shortness of breath. It was assumed that the findings represented nocturnal left ventricular ischemia, probably produced by the increased venous return associated with the supine position. The patient received digoxin 0.25 mg. daily, and by the sixth day of therapy the nocturnal symptoms had disappeared. The Holter recordings obtained later showed no S-T segment depression through the night, and the above-mentioned symptoms had subsided.

Case 2. The Holter rhythm strips in Figure 5-4 are those of a 34-year-old man who complained of sudden episodes of jumping sensations in his neck. These were associated with a feeling of irregular heart beats. There was, however, no history of chest pain, dyspnea, dizziness or weakness. He was not taking any drugs. The physical examination was within normal limits, as was the 12-lead electrocardiogram. There was no clinical or laboratory evidence of thyroid disease or anemia. A 10-hour Holter monitor was obtained. One can readily see the occurrence of paroxysmal atrial flutter-fibrillation. The dominant rhythm throughout was sinus, however. Since no cause could be found for the ectopic rhythm the patient was treated with quinidine sulfate orally. Following quinidine therapy the paroxysmal atrial flutter-fibrillation was abolished completely.

Case 3. The strips in Figure 5-5 are examples of those of a 45-year-old man 3 months after recovery from diaphragmatic (inferior) myocardial infarction. There had been a problem with frequent ventricular premature contractions during his hospitalization, and he had been treated with procainamide (Pronestyl). The drug had been discontinued 2 months after the patient's discharge from the hospital. Soon after discharge, he began to experience episodic dizzy spells associated with palpitation. A routine ECG in the physician's office showed the evidence of old diaphragmatic myocardial infarction but no

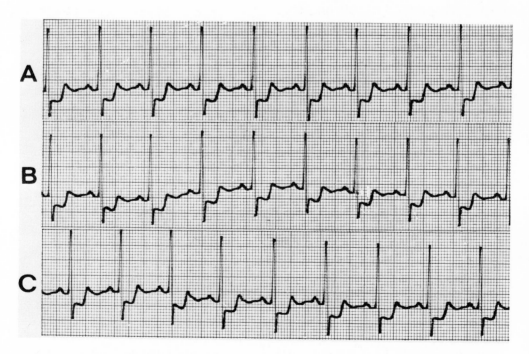

Figure 5-3. Marked S-T segment depression during myocardial ischemic event. Rhythm strips A, B and C are not continuous.

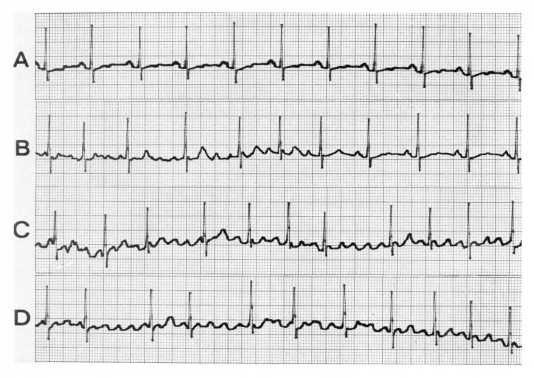

Figure 5-4. Sinus rhythm with paroxysmal atrial flutter-fibrillation. Rhythm strips A,B,C and D are not continuous.

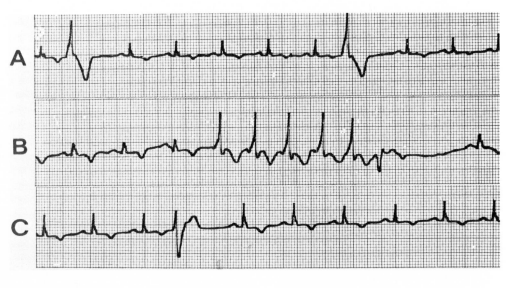

Figure 5-5. Sinus rhythm with frequent multifocal ventricular premature beats and an area (strip B) of paroxysmal ventricular tachycardia followed by a long pause. Rhythm strips A,B and C are not continuous.

evidence of any cardiac arrhythmia. The Holter monitor ECG shows ventricular premature contractions from two foci and a short episode of ventricular tachycardia (Fig. 5-5). The fifth beat of this series (rhythm strip B) is followed by a different QRS complex that may represent a ventricular fusion beat with another ventricular premature focus, followed by a long pause until sinus rhythm is restored. The patient was treated with quinidine sulfate orally. Another Holter monitor recording documented decreased frequency of ventricular premature contractions. There was also symptomatic improvement with respect to dizziness and palpitation.

Case 4. The Holter monitor recording in Figure 5-6 belongs to a 72-year-old man who had experienced several episodes of syncope. These were not associated with chest pain or shortness of breath. The syncopal episodes were not precipitated by exercise, neck position change or straining at voiding or defacation. Their occurrence appeared to be entirely unpredictable. Physical examination did not reveal any specific findings suggestive of an etiology for the syncope. The 12-lead ECG showed sinus arrhythmia and no other significant ECG abnormalities. The Holter monitor recording demonstrates the occurrence of Mobitz type II A-V block. The patient received a permanent transvenous demand pacemaker, and no further episode of syncope was observed.

Case 5. The Holter monitor recording (Fig. 5-7) obtained from a 40-year-old woman with type A Wolff-Parkinson-White syndrome demonstrates three group beats with "normal" QRS morphology during sinus rhythm with anomalous (W-P-W) A-V conduction. The implication was that the group beats with normal QRS contour represent re-entry beats that conduct in retrograde fashion through the bypass tract and antegradely through the A-V junction. The P waves are not clearly seen in group beats, however. In this patient, recurrent tachyarrhythmias were treated with propranolol (Inderal). Propranolol has been shown to be the drug of choice in the treatment and prevention of regular tachycardia associated with Wolff-Parkinson-White syndrome.[12]

Case 6. The Holter recording in Figure 5-8 belongs to a 45-year-old woman with a history of an intermittent pounding sensation in the chest associated with a feeling of extreme warmth. She denied a prior history of cardiac disease, dyspnea on exertion, chest pain, paroxysmal nocturnal dyspnea or pedal edema. The episodes were precipitated by emotional excitement or physical exercise, and they would last several minutes to

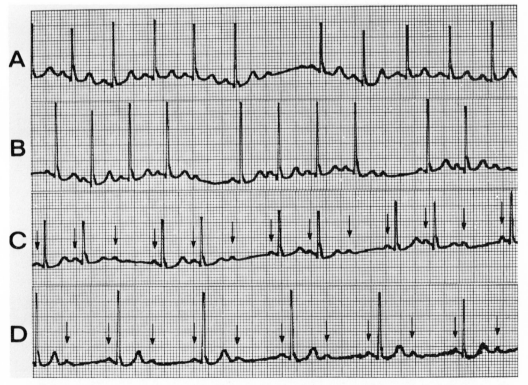

Figure 5-6. Sinus P waves (*arrows*). The rhythm is sinus with Mobitz type II A-V block with varying A-V ratios. Strip D reveals 2:1 A-V block. Rhythm strips A,B,C and D are not continuous.

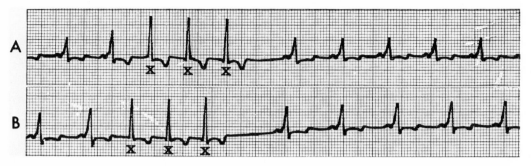

Figure 5-7. Wolff-Parkinson-White syndrome with short episodes of paroxysmal supraventricular tachycardia and normal QRS complex (*X*). Rhythm strips A and B are not continuous.

an hour or more. The patient had never had an electrocardiogram during her symptomatic episodes. As part of her diagnostic work-up, the Holter monitor recording was obtained. The palpitations occurred during the recording period and subsequently were identified as paroxysmal atrial tachycardia. The patient was found to have hyperthyroidism, and treatment with propranolol (Inderal) abolished the episodes while antithyroid therapy was initiated.

Case 7. The Holter monitor recording in Figure 5-9 is that of a 48-year-old woman with a diagnosis of rheumatic heart disease. The pri-

mary lesion was mitral stenosis. She has had atrial fibrillation and has been taking digoxin for several years. Prior to the Holter monitor recording the patient began to have episodes of severe shortness of breath associated with pounding in the chest. The shortness of breath would be relieved soon after the pounding in the chest ceased. Physical examination revealed no change from her many previous visits. The office ECG documented atrial fibrillation with well-controlled ventricular response and was suggestive of right ventricular hypertrophy. The Holter monitor recording demonstrates nonparoxysmal A-V junctional tachycardia in the presence of

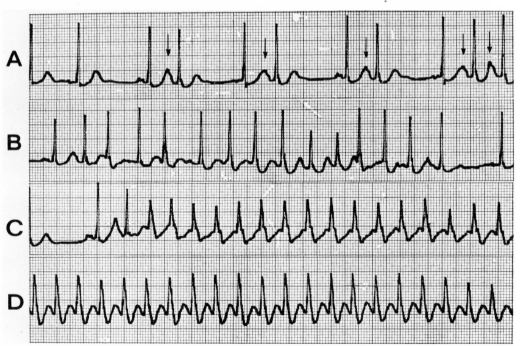

Figure 5-8. Sinus rhythm with frequent atrial premature contractions (*arrows*) and paroxysmal atrial tachycardia (rate 175 beats per minute). Note that the QRS complexes during the paroxysmal atrial tachycardia are bizarre because of aberrant ventricular conduction. Rhythm strips A,B,C and D are not continuous.

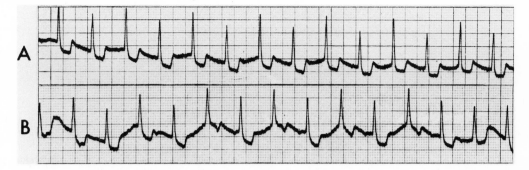

Figure 5-9. Nonparoxysmal A-V junctional tachycardia (rate 106 beats per minute), due to digitalis intoxication, in the presence of atrial fibrillation, producing complete A-V dissociation. In addition, 2:1 electrical alternans is present. Rhythm strips A and B are not continuous.

atrial fibrillation, producing complete A-V dissociation. It is well known that nonparoxysmal A-V junctional tachycardia, especially in the presence of atrial fibrillation, is one of the most common digitalis–induced cardiac arrhythmias.[13] There was improvement with withdrawal of the drug.

Case 8. The recording in Figure 5-10 is that of a 75-year-old man with congestive heart fail-

ure. The symptoms and physical signs were well controlled with 0.25 mg. digoxin a day and hydrochlorothiazide 50 mg. every other day. He had not complained of palpitation during therapy, nor had any arrhythmia been detected. On a follow-up visit to his physician, occasional ectopic beats were noted on the routine ECG recording. The 10-hour Holter monitor recording reveals ventricular parasystole in the presence of sinus rhythm. Initially, digitalis toxicity had been

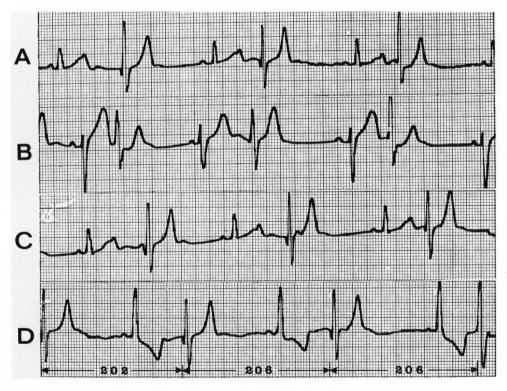

Figure 5-10. Sinus rhythm with ventricular parasystole. Note varying coupling intervals with constant interectopic intervals. The numbers represent hundredths of a second. Rhythm strips A,B,C and D are not continuous.

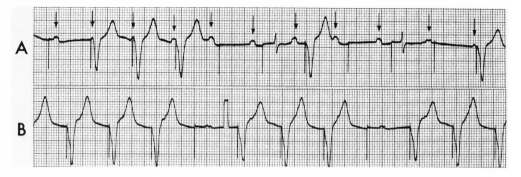

Figure 5-11. Sinus P waves (*arrows*). The basic rhythm is sinus with complete A-V block (ventricular rate 42 beats per minute) and intermittent ventricular pacemaker rhythm. Note occasional failure of the ventricular capture by the artificial pacemaker. Rhythm strips A and B are not continuous.

considered a possibility because of the ventricular ectopic beats. However, confirmation of the ventricular parasystole by a Holter monitor recording excludes the possibility of digitalis intoxication. It has been shown that parasystole is *not* a digitalis-induced arrhythmia.[13] Quinidine therapy was instituted, and the parasystolic beats decreased in frequency.

Case 9. The Holter monitor tracing in Figure 5-11 belongs to a 64-year-old woman with a ventricular demand pacemaker in place for 18

months. She was having a slow pulse rate from time to time. The Holter monitor recording was obtained to evaluate the function of the pacemaker and to document the episodes of slow pulse rate. The natural slow cardiac rhythm appears intermittently because the pacemaker spikes often fail to capture the ventricles. Obviously the patient's underlying complete A-V block is shown intermittently during failure of the ventricular capture. The pacemaker electrode in this patient had shifted to a wrong position. Repositioning the electrode resulted in restora-

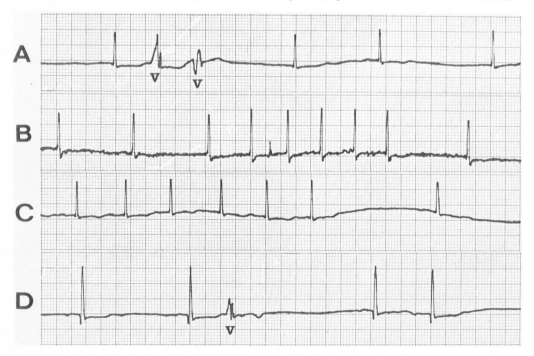

Figure 5-12. Brady-tachyarrhythmia syndrome. The basic rhythm is most likely marked sinus bradycardia and arrhythmia with frequent ventricular premature contractions (*V*) and paroxysmal atrial tachycardia. Rhythm strips A,B,C and D are not continuous.

tion of the consecutive ventricular capture by the artificial pacemaker. The possibility of other forms of malfunctioning artificial pacemaker is excluded.

Case 10. The Holter monitor recording in Figure 5-12 belongs to a 70-year-old woman with a history of intermittent syncopal episodes. As part of a complete medical work-up a 10-hour Holter monitor recording of her cardiac rhythm was obtained. The illustration shows that she has areas of both severe bradyarrhythmia and tachyarrhythmia. This ECG finding is termed bradytachyarrhythmia syndrome.[12] An artificial pacemaker with a slightly overdriving pacing rate was successful in the treatment of the bradytachyarrhythmia syndrome.

SUMMARY

At the present time the Holter monitor electrocardiogram is one of the most important non-invasive diagnositc tests in our daily practice. The primary purpose of the Holter monitor ECG is to diagnose various cardiac arrhythmias with accuracy, especially when the routine 12-lead electrocardiogram fails to record the arrhythmia because of its transient and episodic nature. The precise cause of a dizzy spell or a fainting episode can be confirmed by the Holter monitor ECG when the symptoms are directly related to either tachyarrhythmias or bradyarrhythmias.

The secondary purpose of the Holter monitor ECG is to document ischemic events by recognizing the S-T segment, T wave abnormalities or both, especially at rest or during sleep. This is particularly valuable when the chest pain is atypical and when the exercise electrocardiogram is equivocal. It is common experience to find that the patient's complaint may be totally unrelated to the actual ischemic event or any cardiac arrhythmias. For instance, the electrocardiographic findings, including those of the Holter monitor, may be completely normal or negative even when the patient definitely experiences a true sensation of palpitation. The Holter monitor then is of great value for reassurance purpose.

In addition, artificial pacemaker function can be assessed by the Holter monitor ECG. Many other clinical applications of the Holter monitor ECG are listed in Table 5-1.

REFERENCES

1. Stein, S., and Tzivoni, D.: The reliability of the Holter-Avionics system in reproducing the ST-T segment. Am. Heart J. 84:427, 1972.
2. Hinkle, L. E., Jr., Carver, S. T., and Stevens, M.: The frequency of asymptomatic disturbances of cardiac rhythm and conduction in middle-aged men. Am. J. Cardiol. 24:629, 1969.
3. Stern, S., and Tzivoni, D.: Dynamic changes in the ST-T segment during sleep in ischemic heart disease. Am. J. Cardiol. 32:17, 1973.
4. Iyenfar, R., Castellanos, A., and Spence, M.: Continuous monitoring of ambulatory patients with coronary disease. Prog. Cardiovasc. Dis. 13:392, 1971.
5. Bleifer, S. B., Bleifer, D. J., Hansmann, D., and Sheppard, J. J.: Diagnosis of occult arrhythmias by Holter electrocardiography. Prog. Cardiovasc. Dis. 16:569, 1974.
6. Bleifer, S. B., Karpman, H. L., Sheppard, J. J., and Bleifer, D. J.: Relation between premature ventricular complexes and development of ventricular tachycardia. Am. J. Cardiol. 31:400, 1973.
7. Koch-Weser, J.: Antiarrhythmic prophylaxis of ambulatory patients with coronary heart disease. Arch. Intern Med. 129:763, 1972.
8. Kossman, C. E., et al.: Report of Committee on Electrocardiography, American Heart Association. Recommendations for standardization of leads and specifications for instruments in electrocardiography and vectorcardiography. Circulation 35:583, 1967.
9. Stern, S., and Tzivoni, D.: Early detection of silent ischemic heart disease by 24-hour electrocardiographic monitoring of acute subjects. Br. Heart J. 36:481, 1974.
10. Lown, B., Tykocinski, M., Garfeiu, A., and Brooks, P.: Sleep and ventricular premature beats. Circulation 48:691, 1973.
11. Simborg, D. W., Ross, R. S., Lewis, K. B., and Shepard, R. H.: The R-R interval histogram. A technique for the study of cardiac rhythms. J.A.M.A. 197:145, 1966.
12. Chung, E. K.: Electrocardiography: Practical Applications with Vectorial Principles. Hagerstown, Md., Harper & Row, 1974.
13. Chung, E. K.: Digitalis Intoxication. Amsterdam, Excerpta Medica, 1969.

Chapter 6

Computer Electrocardiography

CESAR AUGUSTO CACERES

Electrocardiogram analysis by computer has begun to pass from the research phase to a validated, standardized, cost-effective technique with defined quality of interpretations. The automatic capability is now readily available to physicians in many parts of the world. In dealing with automated electrocardiographic analysis, there is a need to consider the concept of a "system" from data acquisition to storage and retrieval, with the central point being the stability of the software. Several ECG computer programs have been or are in development by many groups. Several hardware system components for ECG analysis have been developed and made commercially available. The U.S. Public Health Service's former Medical Systems Development Laboratory coordinated early efforts of many concerns and fitted them into the first model of an overall integrated system design of both software (computer programs) and hardware to show the inherent advantages of automatic analysis.[1,2] A number of other programs and systems now exists for both standard and other lead systems.[3]

Each community and each user have specific requirements for ECG analysis that may require modification and extension of the basic system's design. Additionally, data input from various classes of ECGs (stress, resting diagnostic, screening or resting), comparison needs and long-term storage requirements are modifiers that have to be taken into consideration. The geographic location of physicians is pertinent to criteria utilization and can further affect system operations. An optimum system can service both individual physicians and hospital-based services at the requisite cost and quality standards by a variety of hardware/software combinations now commercially available, if needs have been established by careful analysis.

The original design must be oriented for changes to avoid obsolescence and, most importantly, to allow for volume increments projected in both number and kind of electrocardiograms. Throughout a period of service, however, an automated system requires quality control. The system must continuously be evaluated for repeatability, signal fidelity, noise and equipment stability. Quality control techniques require careful methodologic documentation. Education of users is also a continuing process.

BASICS

A system for resting diagnostic or screening, stress and monitoring electrocardiography will generally encompass the following basic subsystems:

Signal acquisition
Transmission
Preprocessing
Processing
Display
Storage and retrieval
Accounting

In the original design of a system, general considerations are: quality (meeting specifications), compatibility with neighboring systems for back-up needs, maintenance requirements and operational costs. The system should have several attributes:

Assurance of patient and lead identification
Uniform calibration of the signal throughout telephone transmission or tape acquisition
Assurance of technical quality of the signal
Methodology to use redundancy when technician cannot record the full leads usually processed
Flexibility for criteria changes when necessary

The automated product should be superior to manual methods in quality. Additionally, the design of the components of an ECG system must be with full recognition that specially trained electrocardiographic personnel are, and can be expected to remain, in short supply. From technician operator through to physician, the components of any system must be studied to conserve manpower and diminish overhead costs.

Signal Acquisition. Conventional paper recordings are now best obtained by several newly designed, commerically available, three-channel ECG machines. Many of these new models can also serve as input to computer systems through telephone linkage. No one should purchase a three-channel unit without at least future adaptability to computer use. Commerical acquisition units now available either transmit an analog signal by telephone or record the ECG signal on analog magnetic tape for playback to a computer. Both types are generally mobile units. The acquisition units that produce tape for "batch processing" produce economies in certain instances. The choice depends on individual site considerations, "turn-around" time requirements and volume of ECGs. Rapid turn-around time (i.e., real time) is a desirable goal but not required in some applications like screening, although it is useful for technician operations.

Transmission by Telephone to a Computer. The first telephone trials were from offices in situations similar to those of current community physician needs. ECGs transmitted with portable ECG machines taken to patients' homes have also been investigated in feasibility trials, and that experience (good and bad) has been helpful in research, development and trials. Experiences have included local telephone transmission and long-distance transmission via private and public lines from many points in the United States and by various other facilities such as satellite from France and Tokyo and radio link to South America. The problems discovered laid the foundation for now readily available transmission units. Transmissions have been successful and have included long-term, routine day-to-day operations in emergency rooms, special screening systems, etc.

Processing. The major sections of an ECG processing software (program) package are (1) pattern recognition, (2) interpretation, (3) editing or other record-keeping purposes and (4) internal controls for the system itself. The pattern recognition portion of the software usually contains logic for condensation and combination of measurement data. The interpretation software allows for interaction of criteria and measurement data. The design of the software should be oriented for modifications based on future evaluations and on new research.

Generality incorporated in the pattern analysis program can permit it to be used as the basis for all types of ECG work: standard 12 lead, monitoring and stress. Such generality could, for example, allow for use of both vectorcardiographic and standard leads with one program. However, such generality is not currently readily available. A program may perform selective "averaging" to select appropriate complexes, do rhythm analysis, locate and measure the wave amplitude and durations, format and print these measures, compute axis, determine the interpretation to be made and classify the ECG as normal, borderline, atypical or abnormal or into other desired categorizations. The computer program must have been designed so that provisions can be made for bad data and rejection of bad data. Redundancy checks should have been added to compensate for rejected data.

Display. An acceptable report from an automated system requires time and effort in design *and* education of the user. If it is not in a format acceptable and understandable to the clinician, its use is limited. Much time has been spent in developing report outputs acceptable for routine clinical use, but educational methodology must be included during installation of systems to achieve optimum use.

The display subsystem should provide a format suitable for both clinician and record-room use. Additionally, if it is to be used in a research institution, other formats may be needed. The display should allow for:

Hard copies of the ECG report for use by the submitting physician, hospital house staff and heart station, i.e., copies as needed
A reproduction of the tracing for quality control of the processing and data acquisition system
A computer storable form (such as digital tape or disk) for retrieval and comparison purposes

In the future there is the possibility of a computer-generated voice report.

Storage and Retrieval. Many methods exist, ranging from very mundane indexing storage and retrieval systems to large "online" sophisticated systems. Economics and statistics are both significant to the overall effort. Raw data, measurements or interpretive codes or both can be stored on appropriate media within a computer system. Software specifications for cost-effective record retrieval at a specific site can be developed only after full consideration by physician groups and record-room personnel of the needs and uses at the specific institution.

The precise biologic and technical variation of the ECG signal over a short term is a problem in retrieval. These phenomena must be studied further for development of optimal guidelines for the appropriateness of data to be retrieved in a judicious manner for comparisons.

Computer-generated statistical studies from stored data may shed significant light on the natural history of disease so that indicators of each stage in an individual might be predictive. This implies the design of statistical subsystems to allow for the storage and retrieval of ECG information that is useful for clinical service as well as for research.

Billing and accounting must also be incorporated as a practical subsystem within the storage and retrieval capabilities of the system.

Economic Considerations. Clinics and hospitals require that operational costs be low in order to justify using an automated system. There is no question that the value of any system to the user must be greater than its cost. In all cases of use of automation, the projected costs must be less than manual methods, but, by-product benefits must be considered in these calculations. Savings in the record room or in the administrative area should not be forgotten.

Labor and overhead reductions are possible and increase as system capacity is reached. ECG processing system costs cannot be based on computer speed. For example, a "slower" computer may fulfill all medical needs for speed and be extremely economical.

Minimum cost is rarely a suitable factor upon which purchase of a system should be based. Some features of a system may result in such operational convenience that they will be considered worth the price. In this regard one must study real needs to each specific institution. There are also many acceptable methods of measuring and estimating costs. Importantly, the selection of method will influence results of the analysis.

OPERATIONS

Practicality. The utmost economy is achieved when electrocardiograms are taken in one central area on admission to a clinic, ward or hospital. Depending upon the average age of a hospital population and the number of patients who go to elective surgery, for example, it might be a reasonable procedure to exclude patients from electrocardiography, on order of the physician, rather than to ask him to make a special request. This is said in view of the fact that it might be possible to provide the patient in general with better service and lower costs if volume is obtained at a single site. It often happens that the ECG required is ordered after admission. The difference in hospital operational costs is appreciable. Centralization makes it possible to schedule technicians better and to use them more productively throughout the entire day rather than in many locations for portions of a day. Prior study shows that, on an average, an ECG on the wards takes 15 minutes or more of technician time as opposed to 5 to 10 minutes in a central location.

It has long been considered by some that an ECG interpretation should be available in preliminary form for use immediately after the tracing is taken. Since it is not feasible to have 24-hour 7-day a week cardiologist interpretation, a computer is the next best and can be quite suitable. This requires that computer limitations be well known. There are, of course, some areas in which, as opposed to the cardiologist, the computer is weak. The areas are primarily in the area of arrhythmia subclassification, but the computer does usually tell well enough whether an arrhythmia is present or not and so allows the intern, resident or practitioner to make a decision regarding immediate action or consultations.

A central issue for automation is how it can provide more expeditious and efficient service. Appropriate training of technicians is necessary to achieve this. It is inherent in any computer operation that those most immediately concerned, the technicians, become responsible for good system results. Responsibility for proper scheduling, quality control, supervision and training of technicians must be considered for best results of computer operations. Those, other than ECG technicians, in various areas of the hospital, who might be needed to take electrocardiograms during emergency hours should also be trained.

There are ancillary savings, if billing can be facilitated or multiple ECG copies are available at insignificant cost, if mounting of tracings can be diminished and if such improvements assist the record room. All of this amounts to saving in secretarial and clerical time, which administratively is significant.

Criteria for Computer ECG. Electrocardiographic criteria have evolved in the last 50 to 70 years as a result of the physician's empiric association of wave forms to disease. But we have become increasingly aware that there are many problems due to observer variability or error in the usage of those criteria. It is in part to solve these problems that automation has been introduced. Automation forces us to consider standardization and requires us to better define our empiric criteria. Automation forces us to objectively review our performance as well.

Usage of computerized ECGs has brought about a significant number of comments and studies indicating the errors and problems in computer quality. Many studies clearly and objectively define: (a) lack of computer criteria, (b) machine error and (c) programming omission faults. More importantly, these have forced us to review the manual system and its evaluation. The basic question is whether the computer product has less quality, overall, than the manual system. To answer this implies that the physician's level of quality needs to be defined before a fiducial quality point can be applied to automation.

Years of usage usually lead us away from daily cognizance of the details in the criteria that we use in diagnosis. Automation of any type is forced to rigidly adhere at all times to precisely defined criteria. Because of this, when the computer fails, we can evaluate the problem objectively. We cannot do the same for the manual system. A point for computers is that their level of quality is readily definable and as such can be studied, checked and, after planning, predetermined.

The disadvantage of computers in the 1970s is that existent physician criteria are not yet fully defined. Further, the physician changes the criteria he uses on the basis of certain factors not always in a textbook, i.e., the patient's type of work, a body de-

formity and a host of other factors, without, quite often, realizing he has changed the ground rules. That is artistry that we cannot economically incorporate into the computers of today. This implies that logically a computer should be used first, and in series with a physician, in order to leave the factors that require personal judgment up to the individual physician.

Observer Variability. A comparison between a physician's interpretation and a computer's interpretation of a tracing will differ with the physician, depending upon his criteria and his variability. The varying normal range for a wave's amplitude or axis cited in standard texts begins to show why we must expect interphysician variability. Physician variability is based more on human factors. If the computer follows author A, B or C and we disagree, we can always correct the result as it refers to our patient, when we find it necessary, but we know the criteria were used consistently, and this is an advantage.

A review by any physician of any group of tracings on two occasions some weeks apart, so that he cannot recognize the tracings, will quickly show that agreement with oneself or with one's peers is difficult and that there is variance 30% or more of the time. Even in the area of normality, it is not certain that two groups of cardiologists will agree, even though they may generally agree on criteria. For example, two groups of well-qualified university electrocardiographers read the same group of ECGs; 9% disagreed on what was normal, and a higher percentage disagreed on abnormality (Table 6-1). The data suggest the level of observer variability that must be expected in such a complex human action as ECG reading. Variability on the part of the human is a significant part of the case against computer electrocardiographic automation. It means that each physician can differ from the computer as he differs from every other human.

The incidence of computer false positive

TABLE 6-1

Percentage Agreement between Two
Cardiology Groups in Reading
561 ECGs

	Normality Categorization (%)	Abnormality Categorization (%)
Agreement	17.6	42.1
Disagreement	8.9	31.4

interpretations of ECGs has been reported as anywhere from 2 to 30%, depending on the program. The incidence of false negative interpretations has usually been reported as 5% or slightly more. The computer's clinical accuracy is thus a problem. In part, the false positives are due to the computer's following of defined criteria that we do not always follow. The false negatives are in part due to lack of criteria in our empiric system. Thus, these two areas show where there is need of further clinical research.

In any event the computer ECG certainly does not provide a diagnosis. The physician alone can do that on the basis not only of the ECG but of input from other sources. The computer ECG does describe better one of the factors that has to be placed into context with other factors.

Computer Drawbacks. While observer variation is reduced, the computer-interpreted ECG has not yet competed in several areas with ECGs read by conventional methods. Arrhythmias are a good example. Computers easily pick up the very common ones, but there is still need for a physician's direct interpretation for the unusual arrhythmia in most instances. Although the incidence of these arrhythmias is high in intensive care areas, they are evident on less than 1% of the total ECGs taken. For the most part, mechanical reasons, cost of computer memory, etc., have been the main drawbacks to arrhythmia analysis by

computer. These problems are being rapidly overcome. Comparison of ECGs is another area where the costs may currently be higher than the results are worth.

Machine error of 4 or 5% is common with any machine *system*. We can expect to have this with a computer electrocardiographic system as well since it incorporates many mechanical and electronic components. The lack of computer programs to accurately measure certain variables, e.g., termination of the QRS complex and waves of diminutive amplitude, or to differentiate artifacts may also be drawbacks in specific classes of ECGs. But automation is an area of rapid change. Some of the statements regarding drawbacks do not represent facts of the 1970s but obstacles that existed in the developmental machine systems in the late 1960s. Whatever the percentage error in the computer system, it should be properly contrasted to 30% human variability.

The various programs available must still be considered to be in a developmental stage. All diagnoses made require subsequent confirmation by a physician to varying degrees, and that will always be the case. The purpose of the computerized ECG is, of course, to assist—not supplant—the physician.

In one study in which approximately 10,000 ECGs were taken on Civil Service workers in the early 1960s, the important finding was that although the computer was initially said to have had too many false positive results, on reevaluation of the subjects years later the conclusion was that perhaps the physicians had had false negatives. In that study, the incidence of heart disease morbidity was high in the group picked out as positive by the computer, really only rigidly following the cardiologists criteria.[4] The cardiologist, however, cannot adhere to his own criteria as rigidly.

Problem Areas in Programming and Design. It cannot be emphasized too strongly that introduction of any new component into any machine system can measurably alter the final product. New programming, new data terminals, etc., when installed mean repetition of all tests as required for a new system.

Uniform calibration of the signal and noise elimination throughout telephone transmission requires adaptive reprogramming. Although several successful nationwide telephone services now exist, noise is still a problem for acquisition of stress electrocardiography and monitoring.

The area of tape recording still has problems of repeatability. These must be carefully monitored if tape is to be used. These, like noise in telephone transmission, can affect the diagnostic output.

The development of suitable quality-control procedures for fidelity, resolution and accuracy documentation needs emphasis. An automated electrocardiographic system is an amalgamation of various subsystems into one operating system configuration suitable to meet specific needs, usually for dedicated ECG computers.[5] An operating network of processing computers should be considered to eliminate downtime problems that will occur in any system.

Time Saving. It is often stated that automated electrocardiographic interpretation will relieve the physician of a time-consuming task, allowing him additional time for more critical functions. Others have suggested that only when computer-ECG programs are fully automated will this assertion be valid. Some providers of automated ECGs have said that physician supervision should no longer be required. The continuing need for overview will obviously never be eliminated in any health or medical care system, although certain computer-interpreted categories are gradually allowing great confidence. Currently the convenience of having a computer prescreen ECGs at, for example, 2:00 A.M., may save considerable time, and that type of advantage should be seriously considered.

The objective automatic measurement of intervals and durations by the computer does save time but not always for the physician only. The time and cost savings for the student, technician or other paramedical persons should also be considered. The studies done by Dobrow and associates in Hartford show at least a fivefold improvement in reading service tracings.[6] Certainly physician time is valuable, but if we save technician time too, that is no loss to the physician, and it is a gain to the patient. Computer feedback by telephone directly to the technician immediately after taking the tracing, for example, helps many acquisition problems, and this is reflected in diminished record-room and mounting problems.

The complexity of the computer can also create some personnel problems, but alternative approaches to computer use, such as technician review, require a high degree of motivation and excessive training for personnel who may not remain long on the job. We can consider use of technicians, paramedical personnel, etc., but from the point of view of speed of obtainment of results, diagnostic accuracy, accessibility and cost, they are satisfactory only in unique circumstances. The cost of installing a computerized program is less than the costs of installing a noncomputerized detection program when one considers training time, turnover of personnel and all related logistic problems.

Surprisingly, community physicians have found fewer obstacles to computer ECG use than university practitioners. Those in research have particularly emphasized the faults even as the community physician has begun to supply overall timesaving service for his patient through automation.

Research and Service. Collection of electrocardiographic signals from several populations must begin in order to better define various subpopulation groups by signal parameters. The initial impressions, after processing of several hundred thousand electrocardiograms, are that at present we have barely begun to utilize the full capability of the electrocardiogram. Programs for the display of the percentile distribution of amplitudes, durations and axes commonly used in electrocardiographic interpretation have been developed. Applicability of these and other statistical techniques to research needs to be reviewed.

The purpose of computer-generated statistical studies must primarily be to describe the natural history of possible disease so that the indicators of each stage in an individual can be predictive. We must obtain numerical values for thresholds all along the line of possible disease detection. With every change in subject status, we should raise the question of where to set predictive thresholds. The design of a statistical subsystem to allow for the storage and retrieval of ECG information that is useful for research is a first step.[7] Significant areas of clinical diagnosis have been studied, and potential for new criteria have become evident.[8]

CLINICAL IMPLICATIONS

The central issue is, of course, how physicians can provide more expeditious and efficient service. A publication by the American Medical Association states: "It is reasonable to expect that government and industry will make broader commitments to develop further the applicability of the computer to medical practice. The ultimate responsibility for the effective utilization of computers, however, will lie within the medical community."[9] Correctly, it is up to physicians to assure that efforts are successful. The physician has to learn three items in order to use automated ECGs. The first involves understanding the display given by the computer. One is presented and explained in Figure 6-1. The second is the method by which criteria function in a computer. One set of computer criteria is presented and described in

Table 6-2. The third item refers to overall understanding of the integration of the basis of electrocardiography and the purpose of computers in any field.

A headline recently warned of the risks of malpractice by physicians and hospitals should computers set the accepted medical standard where "the computer could have cured, minimized or prevented medical problems." In the Journal of the American Medical Association, a letter described the first case of "computerogenic heart disease." A physician had received a computer's interpretation of his six-lead screening electrocardiogram. First-degree heart block and S_1, S_2, S_3 syndrome were "diagnosed." The author of the letter stated that, "In this case the computer diagnosis did not save time and effort of physicians. The apprehensive patient underwent thorough studies of pulmonary function and consulted so far two specialists who declared him to be healthy."

A clear dilemma exists for the physician. Nonuse as well as use of computers will present problems. In considering the dilemma we should bear in mind two points. The first is that it will always be up to the physician to diagnose the meaning of an interpretation in a particular patient. The computer interpretation will simply be an aid in assuring that we overlook no data in assessing the patient's status. The second point is that in the computer era medical education implies acquisition of knowledge that relates to new techniques that promote an improvement in diagnosis as well as how to intersperse those new techniques with the existing body of knowledge.

What Is an ECG Interpretation? A clinical electrocardiographic interpretation depends on use of classifications tailored by the physician to suit his own clinical practice. These classifications are built up from the correlations of multiple combinations of electrocardiographic parameters and their measurements to clinical entities.

TABLE 6-2

*Computer Criteria**

Code		Objective Statement	Interpretive Statement: Infarct Anterior and Anterolateral
320	ATY	SLOW R PROGRESSION V LEADS RA .15 MV or less	
317	ATY	R .10 MV OR LESS V2 AND V3	FIBROSIS OR INFARCT: ANTERIOR
321	B	Q/S OR SMALL R V2-3 Ra less than or equal to .07 MV	FIBROSIS OR INFARCT: ANTERIOR
322	B	QR V2-V4	FIBROSIS OR INFARCT: ANTERIOR
323	B	SMALL OR ABSENT R V2-5 Ra .01 to .10 MV	FIBROSIS OR INFARCT: ANTERIOR
327	B	Q/QS .04 SEC. 1, AVL, V4-6† Q of .04 sec. and .09 MV *and* more than $\frac{1}{4}$ Ra	INFARCT: ANTEROLATERAL
324	AB	SMALL OR ABSENT R V2-5† Ra .10 MV or less	INFARCT: ANTERIOR
330	AB	Q/QS .04 SEC. 1, AVL V4-6† Q of .04 sec. and .09 MV *and* more than $\frac{1}{4}$ Ra	INFARCT: ANTEROLATERAL
325	AB	Q OR QS, NEGATIVE T, V2-V5† Criteria 323 or 324 and Ta or T'a − .10 or more neg. or STe .08 MV or more positive Ta-STe .05 MV or smaller	INFARCT: ANTERIOR, ? AGE
331	AB	Q/QS AND NEG. T'S 1, AVL, V4-V6 Criteria 327 or 330 and Ta or T'a − .10 MV or more neg.	INFARCT: ANTEROLATERAL, ? AGE
326	AB	Q OR QS, ELEVATED ST, V2-V5 Criteria 323 or 324 and STo and STm .15 MV or more positive	INFARCT: ANTERIOR, ACUTE
332	AB	Q/QS, ST-T CHANGES 1, AVL, V4-V6 Criteria 327 or 330 and STo and STe .07 MV or more positive	INFARCT: ANTEROLATERAL, ACUTE

* The simplified listing indicates what in general the computer used to interpret the tracing in Figure 1 diagnosis of anterior infarct. It looked at the table of values in Figure 1 B and reviewed precordial R waves. The finding of small (.15 mv. or less) waves in any precordial lead will trigger consideration of at least one of the diagnoses listed. In this instance, diagnosis 324 was the best fit.

It is at this stage that the general categorization of the ECG is made. Some of the diagnoses on the listing are atypical (*ATY*), others borderline (*B*), and in this instance abnormal·(*AB*). Differences in opinion about what makes an anterior infarct, if not resolvable on a consensus basis, can through listings such as this be handled on an individual site basis.

† When multiple Q/QS mentioned in criteria, Qs need be present in two leads only.

If the clinical electrocardiogram or any other clinically used "electromedical" signal is to be examined by a computer, the specialist in the subject matter must develop a step-by-step organization and detailed logic of the material. With this available the "computer specialist" is able to properly detail the procedures that the computer will follow to perform the desired service for the practicing physician.

Clinical definitions of electrocardiographic parameters and electrocardiographic interpretations have been developed during the past half-century from study of graphic recordings made on instrumentation constructed without the benefit of basic knowledge of the signal actually generated in the heart. Current methods of recording are based on string galvanometers patterned after those of the

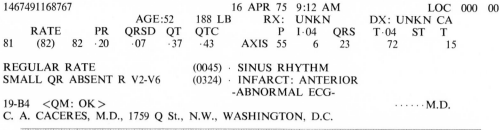

1467491168767   16 APR 75 9:12 AM   LOC 000 00
                    AGE:52   188 LB   RX: UNKN   DX: UNKN CA

RATE		PR	QRSD	QT	QTC		P	I·04	QRS	T·04	ST	T
81	(82)	82	·20	·07	·37	·43	AXIS 55	6	23	72		15

REGULAR RATE   (0045) · SINUS RHYTHM
SMALL QR ABSENT R V2-V6   (0324) · INFARCT: ANTERIOR
                                        -ABNORMAL ECG-

19-B4 <QM: OK>   ·····M.D.
C. A. CACERES, M.D., 1759 Q St., N.W., WASHINGTON, D.C.

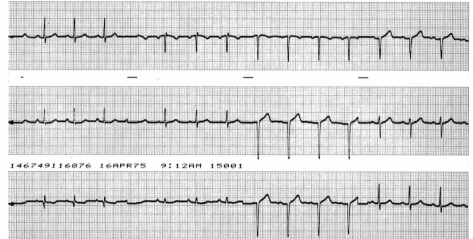

Figure 6-1. A, A simultaneous three-channel display is shown. Leads were recorded in approximately 2.8-second time blocks. Date and time of processing are shown. (If batch-processed, it will still be processed time. If from tape, there is still no commercial terminal that inserts the time of actual recording). A location number (000-00) is seen at the upper right hand corner of the interpretation. A patient-identifying number of 13 digits was used and is seen at the upper left hand corner. Some patient data can be input into the system. This can be used in diagnosis if desired. (Calibration scales for each channel are used to adjust values as presented in *B.* The computer will correct all data in each lead.)

The heart rate is derived from the RR intervals in each lead strip. The lowest rate, the mean, in parentheses, and the highest rate are printed. PR interval, QRS duration (QRSD), QT, and corrected QT values (QTC) are given. The computer uses the QTC for its interpretations. The frontal axis for the P wave, the initial .04 of a second (I.04), the QRS, and the terminal .04 of a second (T.04) are given based on areas under the curve. ST and T vectors, if computed, are based on amplitude alone. In this example, no significant ST was present.

The interpretation is divided into two parts. These are separated by numbers in parentheses at the center of the report. They are codes for each interpretation made.) The essence of the criteria for the statement on the right is given on the left. In this particular program, a new user-oriented one, designed by some who developed the MSDL Public Health Service Program, and Hewlett Packard personnel, it is possible to change the statements based on user preferences. The final interpretative line gives, if desired, a categorization such as Normal, Atypical, Borderline, and Abnormal[10] Designation of program number and a quality monitor (QM) code is seen at the lower left hand corner above the responsible physician's or clinic's name and address. The computer can store physician and clinic listings so that each report is individualized for each user, even though the computer may be handling several accounts. Space for the physician's signature is at the lower right hand corner. Only after a signature can a computer data report be considered valid medical information.

1467491168767 < T   16 APR 75   9:12:24 AM   LOC 000 00

I	II	III	AVR	AVL	AVF		V1	V2	V3	V4	V5	V6
·08	·13	·04	−·09	·03	·11	(PA)	−·06	·03	·07	·07	·08	·08
·10	·15	·09	·12	·06	·13	(PD)	·09	·05	·11	·11	·15	·12
	−·04	−·29				(Q/SA)	−1·38	−2·62	−2·11	−1·23		
	·02	·04				(Q/SD)	·05	·08	·06	·06		
1·04	·72	·41	·02	·70	·17	(RA)					·23	1·05
·04	·03	·02	·01	·04	·04	(RD)					·04	·04
−·33	−·17		−·91	−·28		(SA)					−·81	−·32
·02	·02		·03	·02		(SD)					·03	·02
				·20		(RPA)						
				·02		(RPD)						
						(STO)	−·09	·07				
						(STM)		·13	·06	·07		
						(STE)		·20	·13	·13	·06	
·16	·14	−·08	−·19	·14	·09	(TA)	−·12	·48	·48	·41	·31	·23
·19	·18	·17	·21	·16	·20	(PR)	·17	·20	·20	·21	·21	·21
·06	·07	·06	·06	·06	·04	(QRS)	·05	·08	·06	·06	·07	·06
·37	·37	·33	·35	·35	·53	(QT)	·35	·37	·37	·36	·39	·39
81	82	81	82	82	82	(RATE)	82	81	81	81	82	82
2	2	2	2	2	2	(CODE)	2	2	2	N2	2	2

Figure 6-1B. For research and statistical or quality control, it may be helpful to view the measurements the computer used to derive the interpretations. These are given for the 12 standard leads, and for each wave there is an amplitude and duration value, e.g., *PA, PD.* S-T onset (*STO*), S-T midpoint (*STM*) and S-T end (*STE*) are given. No duration is presented for the T since it is not always possible to know where it actually begins.

P-R, QRS and Q-T summations are given along with heart rate. A code line indicates which complex in a lead strip was measured by the computer. In general, it will select the same complex for each three-lead set. Selection is based on baseline noise, proximity to onset and end of lead strip and number of complexes present. It may thus select different complexes if there is a need.

In this program, the 12 leads are used for their redundancy value. The program does not aim to make each measurement with the highest precision but rather to provide sufficient cost-effective data so that the criteria program can select to provide an accurate answer. Thus, the computer can cope with technician errors or missing leads at least some of the time.

early 20th century. They are not the best, or even an accurate, way of recording components of the wave forms that give electrocardiograms their basic characteristics. However, a methodology of interpretation, based on tracings produced by that type of instrumentation, has been developed, and the wave forms in those tracings have been correlated to pathologic findings. Although the instrumentation and recording characteristics are empiric, a vast amount of useful clinical material is correlated to the existing system. The imprecise recording does not destroy the value of clinicopathologic associations that have been made and are in current use.

With this background, it is evident why the wave forms of the clinical electrocardiogram can be read automatically only when the computer's program is based on the definitions that the wave forms have in clinical medicine. Thus, the primary task in automation has fallen on the physician. He has had to supply the proper input to a computer programmer to assure desired computer output.

Programming requires a knowledge of detail. It must be emphasized that there is no clinical need for strict objectivity in electrocardiography under current practices. A physician may say, for example, that he interprets "patterns" of curves. In actuality, he means that he performs, mentally, several different functions:

1. He recognizes the curves by their slope, amplitude, duration and sequence
2. He identifies and names each curve by arbitrary criteria established by Einthoven in the 1900s.
3. He subjectively contrasts the amplitude, duration and slope of each curve with values and patterns that are blends of "standards" in the literature and in his specific practice.
4. He picks out those values that are outside the range that he associates with normal.
5. He groups these "abnormals" according to a set of rules or criteria that he has established to categorize electrocardiograms in a classification scheme that he considers suited to his practice.

Computers have been programmed to do the same. They differ from the human in the objectivity of each step performed.

Any criteria set for a computer-aided electrocardiographic system is usually in a concise and easy format. The evaluation that must be made after computer processing is actually if these criteria have relationship to clinical data. There is no way of ascertaining, for example, whether an orthogonal-lead system is better or worse than the 12-lead system simply by comparing computer outputs. Since the criteria come from a variety of sources, one must further note that the validity of 12-lead or orthogonal-lead systems is based on the specific selected criteria in a specified lead system. Computer use is relevant to any ECG lead system as a tool. An evaluation of the diagnostic worth of specific criteria used in electrocardiographic analysis is what is actually needed. This additionally suggests that the computer is of secondary and not primary importance (the criteria are of primary importance) in electrocardiographic use.

It might be, for example, that one could suggest that a specific set of criteria applied in an orthogonal-lead and another set of criteria applied in a 12-lead system would yield the proper clinical diagnosis. However, one could not by testing one criterion from one lead system and another criterion from another lead system conclude that one or the other lead system is better or worse. The evaluation of a lead system is basically an engineering consideration. Can the lead system reproduce signals on the surface that are precisely or accurately reflective of what is going on at the generator site? One needs, in effect, engineering, mathematic or other similar data to be appreciative of the differences.

What Must the Physician Do? As we begin the computer era of electrocardiography the physician's educational responsibility is perhaps somewhat more complex than in the past. The computer can do certain repetitive things better than we can ourselves. It can help us establish a performance standard for ourselves. It can also cause us to make mistakes if we rely on it too heavily. If the physician is going to go into an area where electrocardiography is used, training in electrocardiography is still necessary. But further, the physician must learn how to use computer output in order to improve his use of electrocardiography in patient care.

We hope eventually to see medical information systems consisting of large computers performing centralized data storage, retrieval and statistical analysis functions, receiving data from a system of small or minicomputers whose function is to perform data collection, analysis and interpretation. The advantages of such systems will be felt when small "terminals" such as for ECG can be installed anywhere—in the physician's office, outpatient clinic, coronary care unit, or hospital screening center.

During several public symposium sessions, electrocardiographic experts have matched themselves against computer-interpreted electrocardiograms. It was obvious that no one lost. The computer generally found everything that the experts independently and collectively interpreted. However, there are still problems in the field of electrocardiography specifically highlighted by the entrance of computers into the field of medicine. The lack of good criteria for human or computer use for children's electrocardiograms is a problem, and there is a need to study exercise and stress results on the electrocardiogram to see if computer monitoring can identify coronary-prone individuals. On the clinical side the remarkable incidence of questionable electrocardiograms in outpatient populations that usually are denied electrocardiographic health screening has been noted. The study of Neufeld and associates is an example.[4]

The Prediction and Prevention of Disease—A Possibility. We are admittedly just beginning to document the advantages that technology offers in a concrete sense. By the early 1960s we knew what the answers had to be but it takes a long time to get data verified and published. The report by Neufeld and colleagues about computer ECGs typifies the issue.[4] The report is the first study that definitively answers the question regarding the advantage of a computer in reading ECGs. Analogously it tells us that the implementation of technology in other medical data areas can similarly produce quantum improvements.[4]

Analysis in relation to electrocardiographic findings, apart from arrhythmias (dysrhythmias), showed the presence of evidence of any of the following abnormalities in a resting electrocardiogram recorded in 1963 to be associated with a significant increase in incidence of myocardial infarction: left axis deviation, nonspecific T wave changes, ischemic changes, conduction disorder (right or left bundle-branch block), left ventricular hypertrophy.

Another finding in regard to the electrocardiographic examinations is extremely interesting. The five year incidence of myocardial infarction was significantly higher among those subjects whose electrocardiograms were computer-interpreted in 1963 as giving evidence of possible or probable infarct, but in whose paper tracings the cardiologists found no signs of infarct, than among subjects not so shown by computer.

This report took 10 years to appear. But, we should not wait 10 years to obtain an analogous answer from other medical areas before we act.

Continuing Education. One aspect of computer use that should not be forgotten is its capability to act as a passive educator. If the display is properly planned it serves to identify interpretations and as the basis for their having been made. Although useful to all grades of practitioners as a constant mentor, it is extremely helpful in training of students at all levels. With sufficient use there is a continuing passive learning experience with consistent logic.

CONCLUSIONS AND SUMMARY

We can now use many studies as models for medical signals and data and act accordingly. What was philosophy in the past should now, with the proof given, be considered methodology. We emphasize and stress the computer advantage. If the physician uses the computer interpretation as a baseline level, a quality enhancement of the physician's health service can result. We can postulate that if a computer allows detection of possible disease earlier than simply by routine observation, physiologic signal monitoring by computer in intensive care areas could in fact show patient trends and earlier detection of hazardous stages.

The up slope of the curve of computer electrocardiographic interpretation usage has increased. An estimate is that 3 to 4% of 80,000,000 ECGs made annually in the United States are done by computers. It should be parenthetically said that no one has lost his practice to a computer as a result of the increasing use. There are those who argue that the computer will not improve their reading of electrocardiograms, that the computer will not increase their productivity and that it will add to costs. These statements are true only for unique environments. The ideal ECG computer system is, of course, not yet available for every environment, but with the increasing availability of such systems, the physician must consider how the computer can improve his diagnostic services, no matter where he practices the art of ECG interpretation. Several good systems have been designed. It is now up to the physician to transfer the meaning of computerized ECG interpretations to patients.

The computer is not, however, just a tool for the physician. It is a tool for the technician and paramedical person. When used in conjunction with them, the computer becomes part of a system in which diminished physician manpower can outperform the most generous physician staffing pattern. This point is essential in health planning for the future. Through technology, performance improvement can be expected in technician and paramedical efforts with end results evident in enhanced physician quality. This must be documented more definitively, but we already have vivid demonstrations. Unit cost reductions can also result and can be proven by controlled productivity studies.

REFERENCES

1. Schmitt, O., and Caceres, C. A.: Computer Assisted Studies of Biomedical Problems. Springfield, Ill., Charles C Thomas, 1964.
2. Caceres, C. A., and Rikli, A. E.: Diagnostic computers. Springfield, Ill., Charles C Thomas, 1969.
3. Caceres, C. A., and Dreifus, L. S.: Clinical Electrocardiography and Computers, New York, Academic Press, 1970.
4. Neufeld, H. N., Medalie, J. H., Riss, E., and Goldbourdt, U.: Selected findings of the Israeli ischemic heart disease study. Geriatrics 134 (Feb.) 1973.
5. Caceres, C. A.: Large vs small, single vs multiple computers. Comput. Biomed. Res. 3:445, 1970.
6. Dobrow, J. R., Calatayud, J. B., Abraham, S., and Caceres, C. A.: A study of physician variation in heart-sound interpretation. Med. Ann. D.C. 33:305, 1964.
7. Abraham, S., and Caceres, C. A.: Statistical computer methods for diagnosis. *In* Data Acquisition and Processing in Biology and Medicine, edited by K. Enslein. New York, Pergamon Press, 1964, vol. 3, pp. 277–288.
8. Cornfield, J., Dunn, R. A., Batchlor, C. D., and Pipberger, H. V.: Multigroup diagnosis of electrocardiograms, Comput. Biomed. Res. 6:97, 1973.
9. Ryan, G. A., and Monroe, K. E.: Computer Assisted Medical Practice, the AMA's Role. A. M. A. Publication OP-377, Chicago, 1971.
10. American Heart Association Risk Factor Screening Guide, 1971.

Chapter 7

Vectorcardiography

EDWARD K. CHUNG

GENERAL CONSIDERATIONS

Definition of Vectorcardiogram.[1-8] Vectorcardiogram is defined as the recording of the electrical activity generated by the heart and presented in loop form in spatial representation, from three-dimensional views. The three-dimensional views are the horizontal (transverse), frontal (anterior-posterior) and left sagittal (lateral) planes.

The P sÊ loop, QRS sÊ loop and T sÊ loop are formed during atrial depolarization, ventricular depolarization and ventricular repolarization respectively. The major axis of the QRS sÊ loop is normally directed posteriorly, inferiorly and to the left. The major axes of the P sÊ loop as well as the T sÊ loop are almost parallel to that of the QRS sÊ loop in a normal heart. In addition, the beginning point and the end point of the QRS sÊ loop usually coincide, namely, the loop is closed. When the QRS sÊ loop is not closed an S-T vector is said to be present. The S-T vector is the distance from the beginning point to the end point of the QRS sÊ loop when the loop is open.

Spatial QRS sÊ Loop. The spatial QRS sÊ loop includes three-dimensional views, namely, horizontal, frontal and left sagittal

planes, of the QRS sÊ loop (Fig. 7-1).[2,3,6-8] The QRS loop of each view is as if the shadow of the spatial QRS sÊ loop is recorded. Arrows indicate the direction of the QRS loop (A, anterior; P, posterior; S, superior; I, inferior; L, left; R, right).

Relationship between ECG Complexes and VCG Loop. There is a close relationship between the electrocardiographic QRS complexes in the precordial leads (Fig. 7-2B) and the vectorcardiographic QRS loop in the horizontal plane (Fig. 7-2A).[1,7] When the fundamental principles of electrocardiography and vectorcardiography are understood, construction of the vectorcardiographic loop from the electrocardiographic complexes and vice versa is easily accomplished (Fig. 7-2).

Standard Leads and VCG Loop. Similarly there is a close relationship between the electrocardiographic QRS complexes in the standard extremity leads and the QRS loop in the frontal plane if Einthoven's triangle (Fig. 7-3A) and a hexaxial reference frame (Fig. 7-3B) are utilized.[1,7] Again construction of the vectorcardiographic QRS loop from the electrocardiographic QRS complexes and vice versa can be accomplished without much difficulty if the

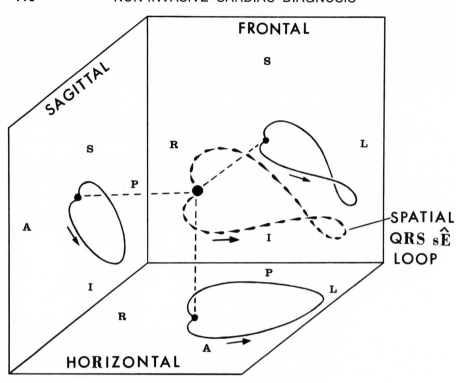

Figure 7-1. Spatial QRS sÊ loop.

principles of vectorcardiography and elec-trocardiography are well understood (Fig. 7-3).

Three-Dimensional Views.   Three-di-mensional views of the vectorcardiogram include horizontal plane (transverse or superior-inferior view), frontal plane (anterior-posterior view) and left sagittal plane (left lateral view).[2,3,6-8] The hori-zontal view in the vectorcardiogram cor-responds to the precordial (chest) leads of the electrocardiogram, whereas the fron-tal plane in the vectorcardiogram corre-sponds to the extremity (limb) leads of the electrocardiogram.

Among three-dimensional views, the horizontal plane offers more information than any of the others in most of clinical situations, including anterior myocardial infarction, posterior myocardial infarction, chamber enlargement, bundle branch block and Wolff-Parkinson-White syndrome. The horizontal plane is *not* altered in diaphrag-matic (inferior) myocardial infarction, however.

Components of Vectorcardiogram. There are three major components of the vector-cardiogram—direction, magnitude and in-scription.[2,3,6-8] The most important one is the direction, and next in importance is the inscription. The magnitude probably offers the least information for vectorcardio-graphic analysis.

For example, the earliest alteration in right ventricular hypertrophy is the right-ward and anterior shift of the QRS axis, and the next change will be the alteration of the inscription. The magnitude may or may not be altered significantly. Another example is left ventricular hypertrophy in which the first alteration will be the left-ward and posterior shift of the QRS axis. The actual magnitude of change is not as important as the altered direction of the major QRS axis in the diagnosis of left ventricular hypertrophy.

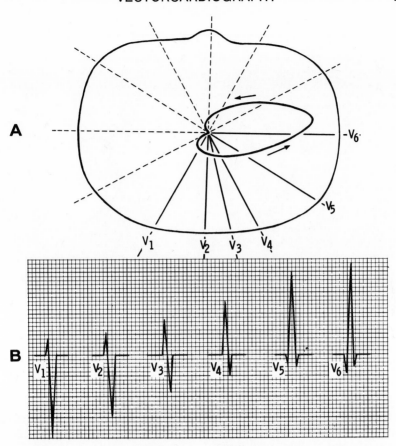

Figure 7-2. Relationship between VCG loop (*A*) and ECG complexes (*B*).

Frank Lead System. A total of seven electrodes is used in the Frank lead system (Fig. 7-4).[2,3,7] Five electrodes are located at the level of the fifth intercostal space (ICS) around the circumference of the chest. Electrodes A and I are placed in the left and right midaxillary lines (LMAL and RMAL) respectively and electrodes E and M are situated in the midline, anteriorly and posteriorly (AML and PML) over the sternum and thoracic spine respectively. Electrode C is located halfway between electrodes A and E so that the angle between the transverse lines drawn from zero point to electrodes A and C will be approximately 45 degrees. Electrode H is placed over the back of the neck, and electrode F is placed on the left leg.

The X lead is directed from right to left (extension of the horizontal line connecting electrodes I and A), and the Z lead is directed anteriorly (extension of the horizontal line connecting electrodes M and E). The Y lead is directed vertically from head to leg.

The Frank lead system is most commonly used for vectorcardiographic analysis at most medical institutions at the present time.

X,Y,Z Leads.[1] As described above (see Fig. 7-4), the X lead is analogous to lead I, whereas the Y lead is analogous to lead aVF of the conventional electrocardiogram.[1] The Z lead is a posteroanterior lead that is analogous to an upside-down pattern of lead V_1 or V_2 of the conventional electrocardiogram.

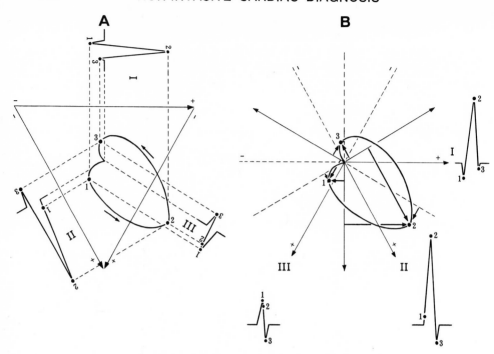

Figure 7-3. Diagram of standard leads and VCG loop.

Various Vectors in The QRS and T Loop. Each dot in the vectorcardiogram is calculated to be 0.0025 second in duration. A series of instantaneous 0.01-, 0.02-, 0.03-, 0.04-, 0.05-, 0.06-, 0.07- and 0.08-second vectors is shown during a cardiac cycle (Fig. 7-5). The QRS or T loop connects the individual instantaneous vectors in sequence during a cardiac cycle.[2,3,6-8]

The 0.04-second vectors are usually considered to be the maximum QRS vectors. The efferent limb implies the first half of the loop from the beginning point (E) to the longest distance from the E point, whereas the afferent limb signifies the last half of the loop (Fig. 7-5).

TABLE 7-1

Dots of the QRS Loop*

4 dots	0.01 second	28 dots	0.07 second
8 dots	0.02 second	32 dots	0.08 second
12 dots	0.03 second	36 dots	0.09 second
16 dots	0.04 second	40 dots	0.10 second
20 dots	0.05 second	44 dots	0.11 second
24 dots	0.06 second	48 dots	0.12 second

* Each dot = 0.0025 second

In myocardial infarction the initial 0.02- to 0.04-second vectors are most commonly altered. Right bundle branch block characteristically produces the conduction delay involving the last 0.04-second vectors, whereas Wolff-Parkinson-White syndrome causes the conduction delay involving the initial 0.02- to 0.04-second vectors. The conduction delay is easily recognized by the closely spaced dots in sequence.

The dot has a teardrop appearance, and the blunt end indicates the direction of the vector loop (Fig. 7-5).

In a normal heart the major axes of the QRS and T sÊ loop are almost parallel to each other so that the angle between the two axes should be less than 60 degrees. If the angle is more than 60 degrees, the T sÊ loop is said to be discordant to the QRS sÊ loop, and the term wide QRS-T angle may be used.

Dots of the QRS Loop. Table 7-1 shows dots of the QRS loop in relation to the different timing in sequence: Four dots indicate 0.01-second vectors; eight dots,

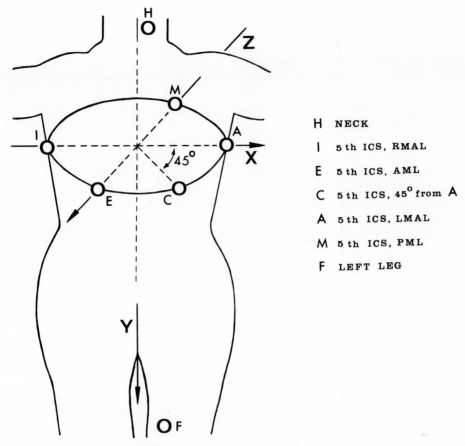

Figure 7-4. Frank lead system. *ICS,* intercostal space; *RMAL,* right midaxillary line; *AML,* anterior midline; *LMAL,* left midaxillary line; *PML,* posterior midline.

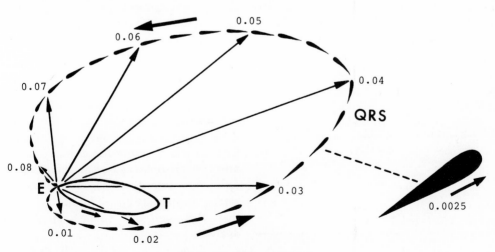

Figure 7-5. QRS and T loop.

0.02-second vectors.[2,3,6-8] It should be remembered that each dot represents 0.0025 second.

When any form of intraventricular conduction disturbance occurs, a larger number of dots of the QRS loop will be recorded. In general, the QRS loop contains more dots for children than adults.

Direction of Inscription.[2,3,6-8] Table 7-2 reveals the direction of the inscription. In a normal heart the inscription is counterclockwise in the horizontal as well as the left sagittal planes. This applies to the P, QRS and T sÊ loops. In fact, the P sÊ loop shows a counterclockwise inscription in all three planes. The inscription of the QRS loop in the frontal plane varies according to the direction of the major vector (axis); namely, the inscription is counterclockwise when the axis is less than +45 degrees and clockwise when the axis is more than +45 degrees. The inscription of the T loop also varies.

Order of VCG Interpretation. Following is the order for vectorcardiographic interpretation.[1-8]

1. QRS Loop. As can be expected, the QRS loop has the greatest importance in routine VCG analysis, particularly in the horizontal plane. The initial vector should be carefully analyzed first. Alteration of the initial QRS sÊ vector may be due to anteroseptal myocardial infarction, left bundle branch block, Wolff-Parkinson-White syndrome and, less commonly, right ventricular hypertrophy. Following analysis of the initial vector, the 0.01-, 0.02-,

0.04-, 0.06- and 0.08-second vectors will be analyzed in sequence. When there is an intraventricular conduction disturbance, 0.10-, 0.12- and even 0.14- or 0.16- second vectors will be present. The conduction delay is manifested by the closely spaced dots in sequence in the involved area. Lastly, any other abnormality should be mentioned if present.

2. T Loop. An approach similar to that described in the analysis of the QRS loop should be applied in T loop analysis. In particular, the concordance or discordance of the T loop with the QRS loop should be mentioned. Left ventricular hypertrophy or left bundle branch block characteristically produces 180 degrees discordance between the T and QRS sÊ loops because of the secondary T loop abnormality. In addition, the T loop configuration in the secondary T loop abnormality tends to be thin and long, whereas in the primary T loop abnormality as seen in myocardial ischemia it is round.

3. S-T Vector. When the QRS loop remains open the S-T vector is said to be present. In the majority of normal individuals, no significant S-T vector is noted. However, not uncommonly, a slight to moderate S-T vector may be present in young healthy adults, particularly in blacks. S-T vectors may be observed in many abnormal conditions, including acute myocardial infarction, left or right ventricular hypertrophy, left or right bundle branch block, pericarditis and various drug effects.

4. P Loop. Analysis of the P loop is often difficult because of its small size and its superimposition on the T loop. Left atrial hypertrophy produces an increased leftward and posterior force, whereas right atrial hypertrophy causes an increased inferior and anterior force. In general, the same principles described in the analysis of the QRS loop are applied in P loop analysis.

5. Conclusions. After each item de-

TABLE 7-2

Direction of Inscription

	P Loop	QRS Loop	T Loop
H	C.C.	C.C.	C.C.
LS	C.C.	C.C.	C.C.
F	C.C.	C.C. (Less than +45°)	C.C. or C.
		C. (More than +45°)	

H, Horizontal; LS, left sagittal; F, frontal; C.C., counterclockwise; C., clockwise

scribed above is analyzed, a normal vector-cardiogram or abnormal vectorcardiogram is diagnosed. If the vectorcardiogram is abnormal, a specific abnormality such as acute myocardial infarction or right bundle branch block should be described.

Value of the Vectorcardiogram. The most important role of the vectorcardio-gram is to assist in better understanding of the electrocardiogram.[1-11] In fact, it is the best teaching tool for this purpose. With-out knowing the vector concept, it is im-possible to understand various electro-physiologic events. It should be emphasized that the vectorcardiogram is not a re-placement for the electrocardiogram, but it often provides valuable diagnostic infor-mation that may not be obtained from the conventional electrocardiogram. The elec-trocardiographic diagnosis is frequently confirmed by the vectorcardiographic diag-nosis. For example, a poor progression of R waves in leads V_{1-3} on the ECG may be due to a normal variant (Fig. 7-6A and B), but it could be due to left ventricular hypertrophy (Fig. 7-7A and B), lung dis-ease (Fig. 7-8A and B), left bundle branch block (Fig. 7-9A and B), anteroseptal or anterior myocardial infarction (Fig. 7-10A and B) and Wolff-Parkinson-White (W-P-W) syndrome type B. In these cir-cumstances, the vectorcardiogram often clarifies the diagnosis. Another example is a tall R wave in lead V_1 on the ECG that may be due to a normal variant (Fig. 7-11A and B), right ventricular hyper-trophy (Fig. 7-12A and B), posterior myocardial infarction (Fig. 7-13A and B), right bundle branch block (Fig. 7-14A and B), W-P-W syndrome type A (Fig. 7-15A and B) and idiopathic hypertrophic sub-aortic stenosis. The vectorcardiogram often differentiates these possibilities.

In addition, more accurate diagnosis can be made in the following conditions by VCG analysis: diaphragmatic (inferior) myocardial infarction, posterior myocar-dial infarction, multiple myocardial infarc-tion, myocardial infarction associated with bundle branch block, right ventricular hypertrophy, biventricular hypertrophy and W-P-W syndrome.

Various QRS Loops—RSR′ Pattern (Right Bundle Branch Block Pattern) in Lead V_1.[1-11] Four different mechanisms may produce a similar, if not identical, electrocardiographic finding in lead V_1 (Fig. 7-16). Not uncommonly, normal in-dividuals may show a right bundle branch block (RBBB) *pattern* (RSR′) in lead V_1 that is a normal variant (A). Otherwise, an RSR′ pattern could also be due to right ventricular hypertrophy (B), true RBBB (C) or posterior myocardial infarction (D). Vectorcardiographic analysis in the horizontal plane usually differentiates these four diagnostic possibilities.

The schematic vectorcardiographic loops A,B,C and D are the horizontal representa-tion (Fig. 7-16).

CHAMBER ENLARGEMENT

Ventricular Hypertrophy. A schematic representation of left ventricular hyper-trophy (B) and right ventricular hyper-trophy (C) in comparison with normal ventricles (A) is shown in Figure 7-17. In left ventricular hypertrophy there are markedly increased posterior and leftward forces during ventricular depolarization (B), but right ventricular hypertrophy pro-duces increased forces anteriorly and to the right (C). The diagrams in Figure 7-17 are the horizontal representation.

Left Ventricular Hypertrophy: Diagnos-tic Criteria.[2,3,6-8,10] The most important diagnostic criterion is the increased QRS forces posteriorly and to the left (Fig. 7-7A and B). The loop is often enlarged, but the increased size alone is not sufficient for diagnosis of left ventricular hyper-trophy. When there is marked left ventric-ular hypertrophy the inscription of the QRS sÊ loop may be reversed or show a figure-of-eight configuration, particularly in the horizontal plane. In addition, the initial

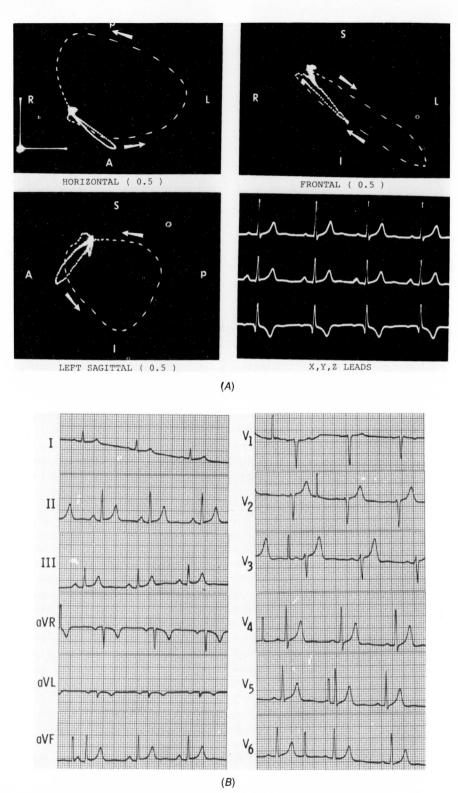

Figure 7-6. VCG (*A*) and ECG (*B*) were obtained from a 49-year-old man without demonstrable heart disease. Poor progression of R waves in leads V_{1-3} on ECG is normal variant confirmed by VCG.

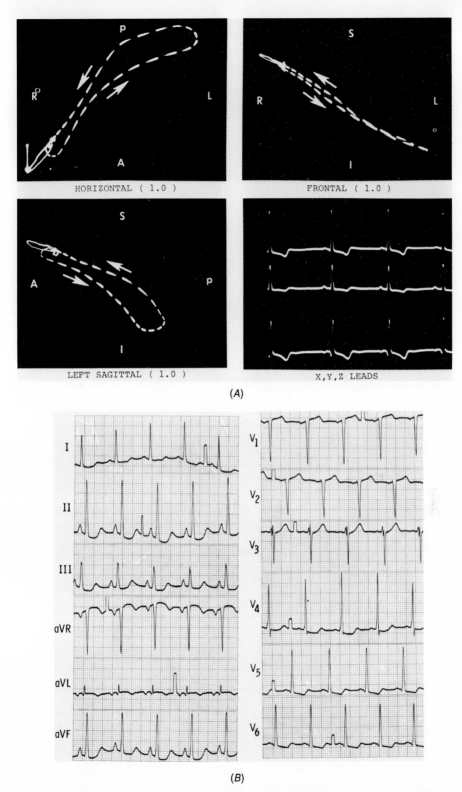

Figure 7-7. VCG (*A*) and ECG (*B*) were obtained from a 45-year-old man with congestive heart failure due to aortic stenosis. These tracings show typical left ventricular hypertrophy. Poor progression of R waves in leads V$_{1-3}$ is simply due to left ventricular hypertrophy.

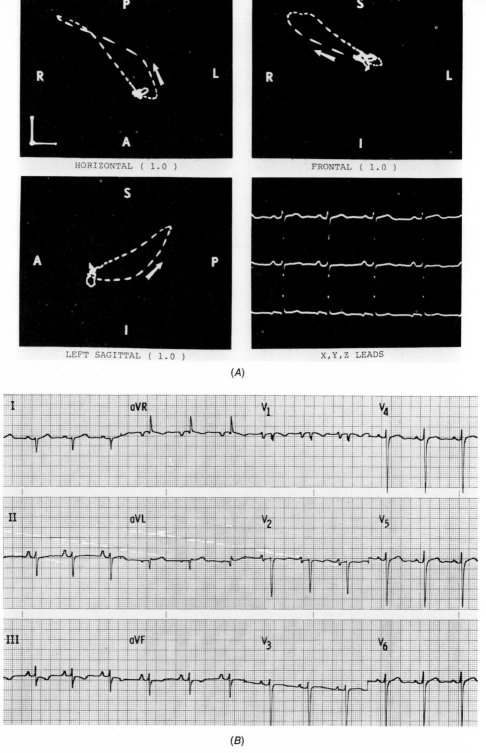

Figure 7-8. VCG (*A*) and ECG (*B*) were obtained from a 38-year-old miner with advanced chronic cor pulmonale. These tracings show right ventricular hypertrophy. Poor progression of R waves in leads V_{1-4} in this case is due to marked right ventricular hypertrophy.

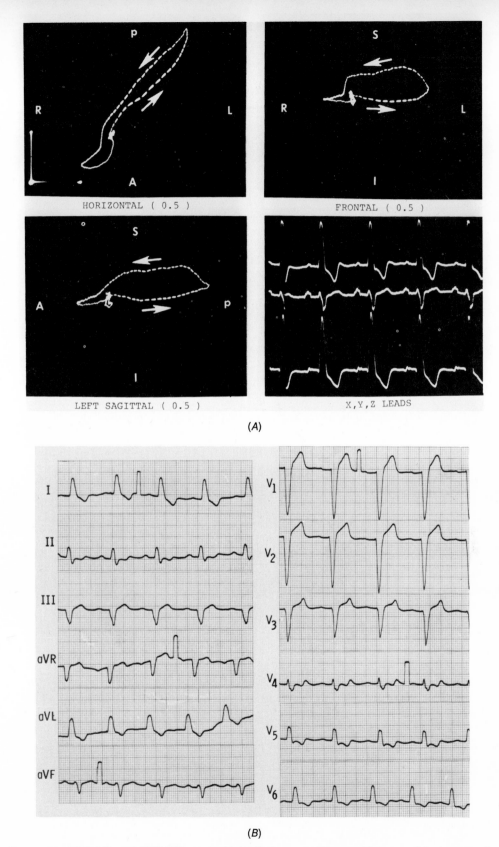

HORIZONTAL (0.5)

FRONTAL (0.5)

LEFT SAGITTAL (0.5)

X,Y,Z LEADS

(A)

(B)

Figure 7-9. VCG (*A*) and ECG (*B*) were obtained from a 73-year-old man with hypertensive heart disease. These tracings show a typical left bundle branch block.

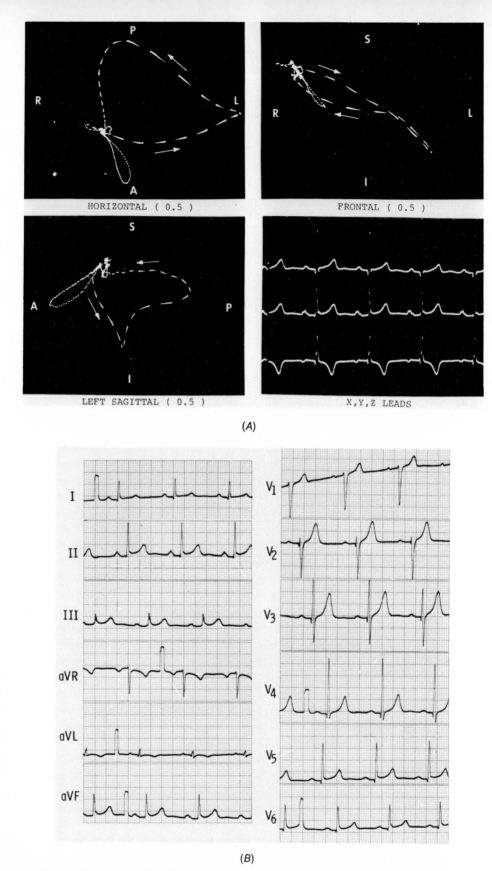

Figure 7-10. VCG (*A*) and ECG (*B*) were obtained from a 56-year-old man with coronary heart disease. These tracings reveal a localized anterior myocardial infarction. The evidence of myocardial infarction is not clear on the ECG but the finding is obvious on the VCG.

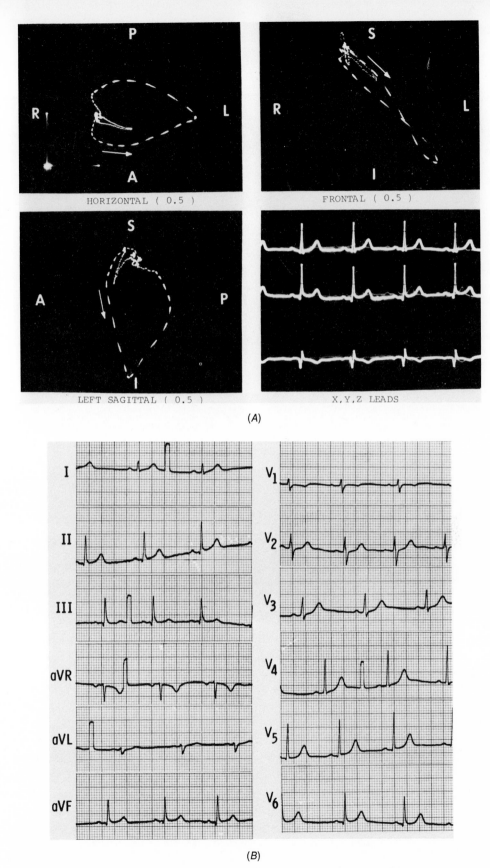

Figure 7-11. VCG (*A*) and ECG (*B*) were obtained from a 22-year-old healthy woman. Relatively tall R wave in lead V₁ on ECG is a normal variant confirmed by VCG.

127

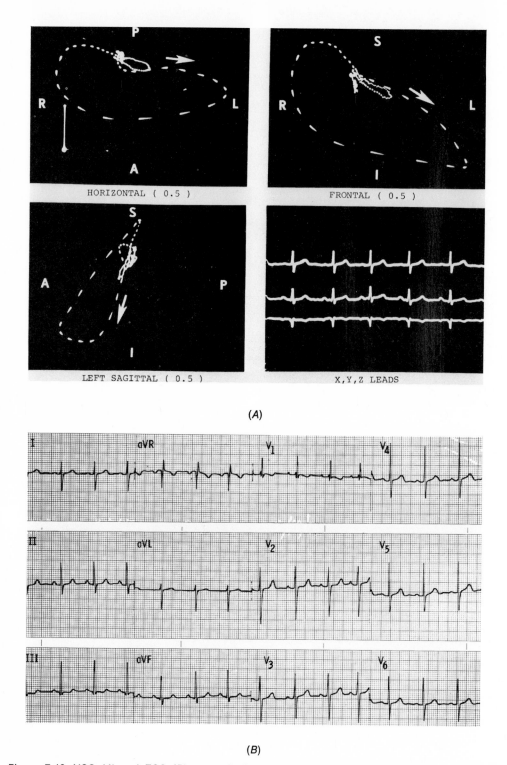

(A)

(B)

Figure 7-12. VCG (*A*) and ECG (*B*) were obtained from a 16-year-old girl with severe pulmonic stenosis associated with atrial septal defect, secundum type. These tracings show unequivocal right ventricular hypertrophy.

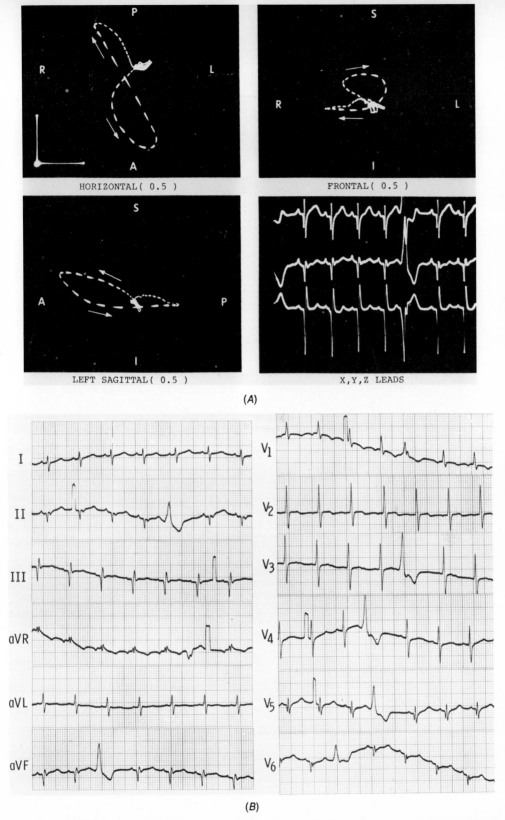

HORIZONTAL(0.5)

FRONTAL(0.5)

LEFT SAGITTAL(0.5)

X,Y,Z LEADS

(A)

I

II

III

aVR

aVL

aVF

V₁

V₂

V₃

V₄

V₅

V₆

(B)

Figure 7-13. VCG (*A*) and ECG (*B*) were obtained from a 39-year-old man with coronary heart disease. These tracings reveal diaphragmatic posterolateral myocardial infarction. Note frequent ventricular premature contractions.

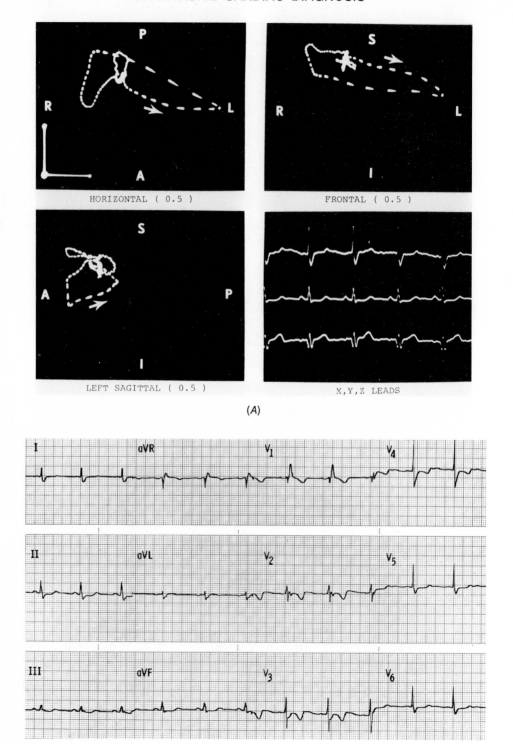

Figure 7-14. VCG (*A*) and ECG (*B*) were obtained from a 65-year-old man with coronary heart disease. These tracings show a typical right bundle branch block.

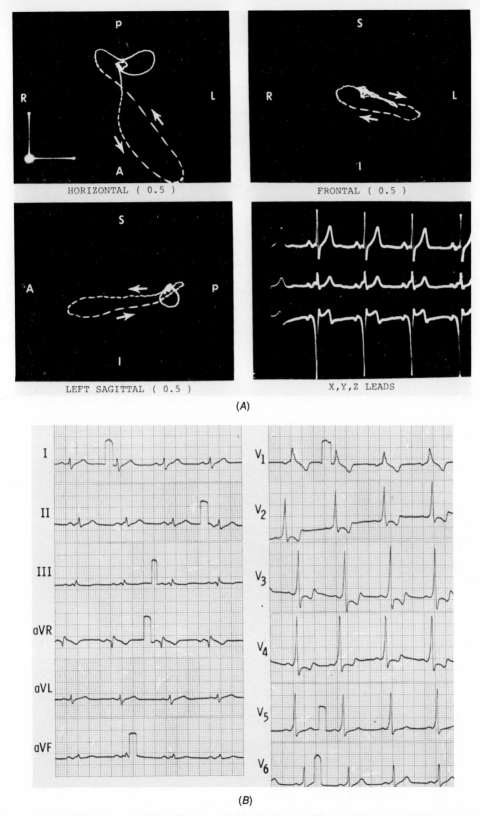

Figure 7-15. VCG (*A*) and ECG (*B*) were obtained from a 52-year-old man with frequent episodes of paroxysmal atrial fibrillation. These tracings reveal Wolff-Parkinson-White syndrome type A.

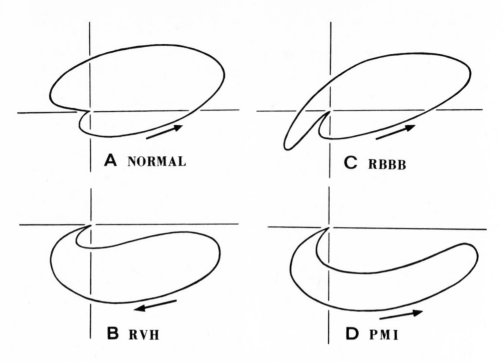

Figure 7-16. Various QRS loops—RSR′ in V₁. *RBBB,* right bundle branch block; *RVH,* right ventricular hypertrophy; *PMI,* posterior myocardial infarction.

QRS vector may show a reversed direction in severe left ventricular hypertrophy.

The T sÊ loop is usually 180 degrees discordant to the QRS sÊ loop in systolic overloading left ventricular hypertrophy (Fig. 7-7A and B). However, the T sÊ loop may be concordant or only slightly discordant to the QRS sÊ loop in diastolic overloading left ventricular hypertrophy. An S-T vector is often present in systolic overloading left ventricular hypertrophy, and it is usually directed anteriorly, superiorly and to the right.

Right Ventricular Hypertrophy: Diagnostic Criteria.[2,3,6–8,10,11] The most important diagnostic criterion is the increased QRS force anteriorly and to the right (Fig. 7-12A and B). At times there may be increased rightward force posteriorly, particularly in chronic cor pulmonale (Fig. 7-8A

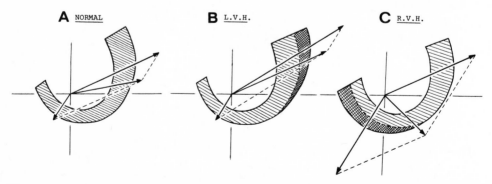

Figure 7-17. Ventricular hypertrophy. *LVH,* left ventricular hypertrophy; *RVH,* right ventricular hypertrophy.

and B) and less commonly in mitral stenosis (Fig. 7-18A and B). When the right ventricle is significantly enlarged, the inscription of the QRS sÊ loop is often reversed in one or more planes, particularly in the horizontal plane. In severe right ventricular hypertrophy, not uncommonly the initial QRS vector may be abnormal, namely, it may be directed anteriorly and to the left instead of rightward. Right axis deviation is observed in almost every case of right ventricular hypertrophy.

The T sÊ loop is often 180 degrees discordant to the QRS sÊ loop in systolic overloading right ventricular hypertrophy. The S-T vector may be present in severe systolic overloading right ventricular hypertrophy, and it is usually directed posteriorly and to the left.

BUNDLE BRANCH BLOCK: DIAGNOSTIC CRITERIA

Left Bundle Branch Block.[1-3,6-8,10] A unique vectorcardiographic finding of left bundle branch block is an abnormal initial QRS sÊ vector (Fig. 7-9A and B); that is, the initial vector in left bundle branch block may be directed anteriorly or posteriorly and to the left. Another important VCG finding is a conduction delay involving the midportion or terminal 0.04-second vectors (at times entire afferent limb) of the QRS sÊ loop (Fig. 7-9A and B). The maximum vector is usually deviated far posteriorly and to the left. The inscription of the QRS sÊ loop is often reversed in one or more planes, particularly in the horizontal plane, and a figure-of-eight configuration is not uncommon, especially in the horizontal plane. In addition, the QRS sÊ loop is often enlarged regardless of the presence or absence of coexisting left ventricular hypertrophy. Therefore, the diagnosis of left ventricular hypertrophy *cannot* be made in the presence of left bundle branch block vectorcardiographically, although many patients with left bundle branch block have anatomic evidence of left ventricular hypertrophy.

The T sÊ loop is usually 180 degrees discordant to the QRS sÊ loop in a pure left bundle branch block (Fig. 7-9A and B). In addition, a significant S-T vector is present, and it is usually directed anteriorly, superiorly and to the right.

Right Bundle Branch Block.[1-3,6-8,10,11] In right bundle branch block the initial QRS sÊ vector is normal. A characteristic VCG finding in right bundle branch block is a conduction delay involving terminal 0.04-second vectors (Fig. 7-14A and B). The terminal deflection is usually directed anteriorly and to the right. The QRS sÊ loop may reveal a figure-of-eight or, at times, a double figure-of-eight configuration in one or more planes, particularly in the horizontal or sagittal plane. The QRS sÊ loop is frequently enlarged, but this VCG finding does not indicate right ventricular hypertrophy. However, it should be noted that right bundle branch block shown in the electrocardiogram may actually represent right ventricular hypertrophy, which is confirmed by VCG analysis (Fig. 7-19A and B). Marked left or right axis deviation shown in the frontal plane in the presence of right bundle branch block often indicates coexisting left anterior or posterior hemiblock respectively (Fig. 7-20A and B).

The T sÊ loop is often 180 degrees discordant to the major axis of the QRS sÊ loop. The S-T vector may be present, but it is not as pronounced as in left bundle branch block. When the S-T vector is present, it is usually directed posteriorly and to the left.

MYOCARDIAL INFARCTION: DIAGNOSTIC CRITERIA[1-8]

Anteroseptal Myocardial Infarction. A characteristic feature of anteroseptal myocardial infarction is the abnormal initial QRS sÊ vector; namely, the initial vector

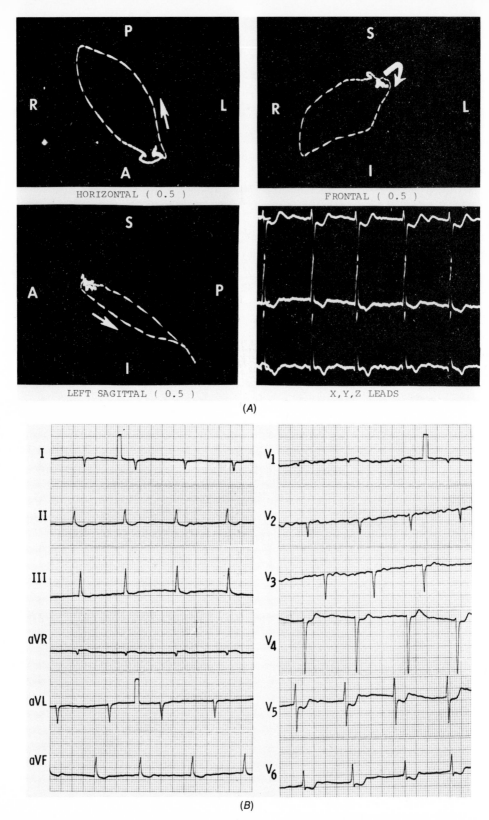

Figure 7-18. VCG (*A*) and ECG (*B*) were obtained from a 37-year-old woman with severe congestive heart failure due to mitral stenosis. These tracings show right ventricular hypertrophy compatible with mitral stenosis. The cardiac rhythm is atrial fibrillation with intermittent non-paroxysmal A-V junctional tachycardia. Pseudo anteroseptal myocardial infarction is produced as a result of severe right ventricular hypertrophy (*B*).

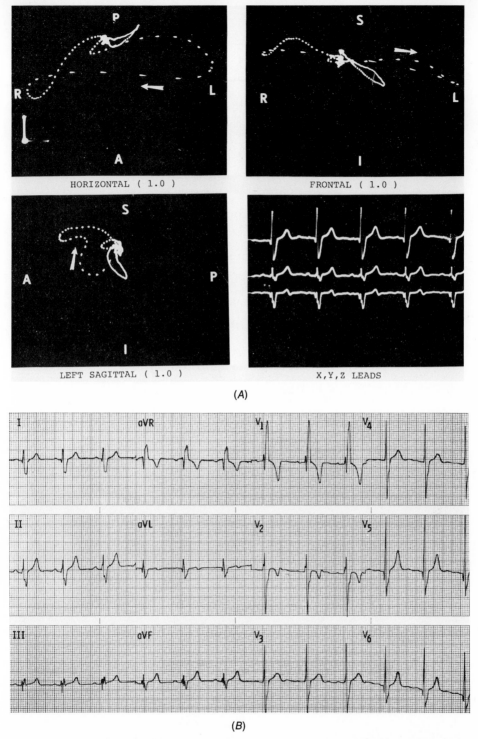

HORIZONTAL (1.0)

FRONTAL (1.0)

LEFT SAGITTAL (1.0)

X,Y,Z LEADS

(A)

(B)

Figure 7-19. VCG *(A)* and ECG *(B)* were obtained from a 17-year-old boy with tetralogy of Fallot. The basic rhythm is sinus with a rate of 65 beats per minute. The diagnosis of right bundle branch block can be made without difficulty on the basis of wide QRS complexes (QRS interval, 0.16 second) and RR' pattern in lead V_1 with deep and slurred S waves in leads. I, aVL and V_{4-6}. However, right ventricular hypertrophy *cannot* be diagnosed with certainty electrocardiographically. Only suggestive evidence for right ventricular hypertrophy is a very tall R wave in lead V_1 in the presence of right bundle branch block, but this finding is *not* a reliable criterion. Under this circumstance the vectorcardiographic diagnosis is definitely superior to the electrocardiographic diagnosis.

135

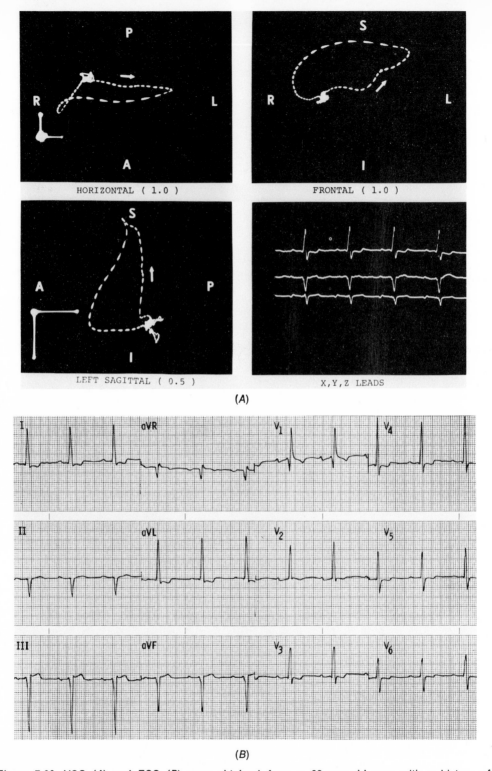

Figure 7-20. VCG (*A*) and ECG (*B*) were obtained from a 62-year-old man with a history of Adams-Stokes syndrome. The basic rhythm is sinus with a rate of 62 beats per minute and first degree A-V block (P-R interval, 0.26 second). A combination of right bundle branch block and left anterior hemiblock (QRS axis, −50 degrees) with first degree A-V block indicates trifascicular block, which is obviously a form of incomplete bilateral bundle branch block. The diagnosis of left ventricular hypertrophy can be made electrocardiographically but right ventricular hypertrophy cannot be diagnosed with certainty. In this circumstance the VCG study confirms the diagnosis of right ventricular hypertrophy. The left atrium is also enlarged.

136

is directed posteriorly and to the left (Fig. 7-21A and B) instead of rightward and anteriorly as in a normal heart. Usually, 0.01- and 0.02-second vectors are abnormally directed, and there is often posterior and rightward bowing of these vectors (Fig. 7-21A and B).

The direction of the T sÊ vector varies, depending upon the stage of myocardial infarction. In the acute stage the T sÊ vector is commonly directed posteriorly and to the left. The S-T vector is present only during the acute phase, and it is directed anteriorly and to the right. In old myocardial infarction the T sÊ loop is often normally directed, and no S-T vector is present.

Anterior Localized Myocardial Infarction. In anterior localized myocardial infarction the initial QRS sÊ vector is normal. Immediately following the initial normal vector the initial 0.02-second (at times slightly longer) vectors are abnormally directed posteriorly and to the left (Fig. 7-10A and B). There is often posterior bowing of the 0.02-second vectors. The inscription may be reversed in the horizontal or sagittal planes or both, and a figure-of-eight configuration may be produced in one or more plane (Fig. 7-10A and B).

The direction of the T sÊ loop again varies according to the phase of myocardial infarction; for example, the T sÊ loop is often deviated posteriorly and to the left (at times to the right) in the acute stage. For the same reason the S-T vector is present only in the acute stage, and it is directed anteriorly and to the right (at times to the left).

Anterolateral Myocardial Infarction. In anterolateral myocardial infarction the initial QRS sÊ vector as well as the initial 0.01-second vectors are normal. The abnormal vectors include the initial 0.02- to 0.04-second vectors, which are directed posteriorly and to the right (Fig. 7-22A and B). There is often posterior and rightward bowing of the efferent limb. The in-

scription may be reversed, and the loop may show a figure-of-eight configuration in the horizontal plane or other planes.

The direction of the T sÊ loop is determined by the stage of myocardial infarction. In acute myocardial infarction the T sÊ loop is directed posteriorly and to the right, and only acute myocardial infarction produces the S-T vector, which is directed anteriorly and to the left.

Extensive Anterior Myocardial Infarction. In a practical sense the diagnostic criteria of extensive anterior myocardial infarction include a combination of all the diagnostic criteria of anteroseptal, anterior localized and anterolateral myocardial infarction. Therefore, the entire QRS sÊ loop will be displaced far posteriorly and slightly to the left, simply as a result of loss of the entire anterior force (Fig. 7-23A and B). The inscription of the QRS sÊ loop is often reversed in the horizontal and left sagittal planes. In the acute stage of myocardial infarction the T sÊ loop is usually deviated posteriorly and slightly to the left. The S-T vector is present only during the acute stage, and it is directed anteriorly, either slightly to the left or slightly to the right.

Diaphragmatic Myocardial Infarction. The characteristic feature of diaphragmatic myocardial infarction is superior displacement of the initial 0.02- to 0.04-second vectors (usually 0 degree or more superior displacement), associated with a superior bowing of these vectors (Fig. 7-24A and B). The inscription may be reversed in the sagittal or frontal planes or both, and a figure-of-eight configuration may be observed in these planes. It is important to remember that the horizontal plane is *not* altered in pure diaphragmatic myocardial infarction.

In the acute stage of myocardial infarction the T sÊ loop is usually deviated superiorly and often to the right. The S-T vector is present only during the acute stage and it is directed inferiorly.

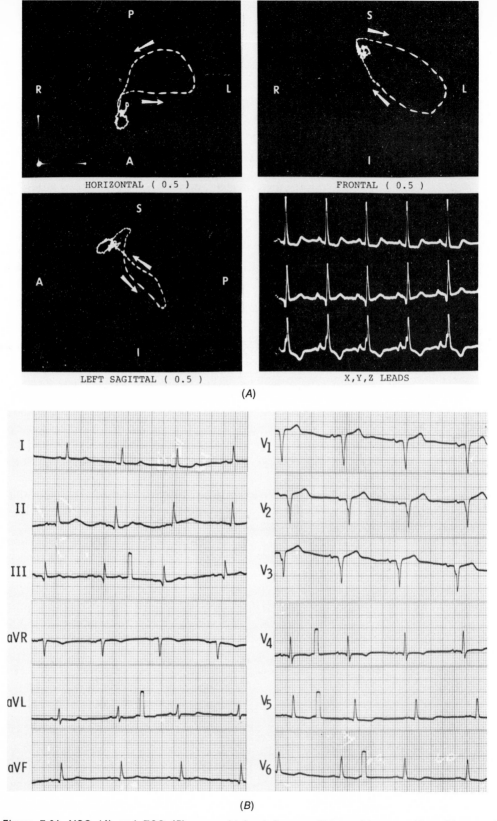

Figure 7-21. VCG (A) and ECG (B) were obtained from a 67-year-old man with a history of heart attack on two different occasions. These tracings show anteroseptal and diaphragmatic myocardial infarction.

138

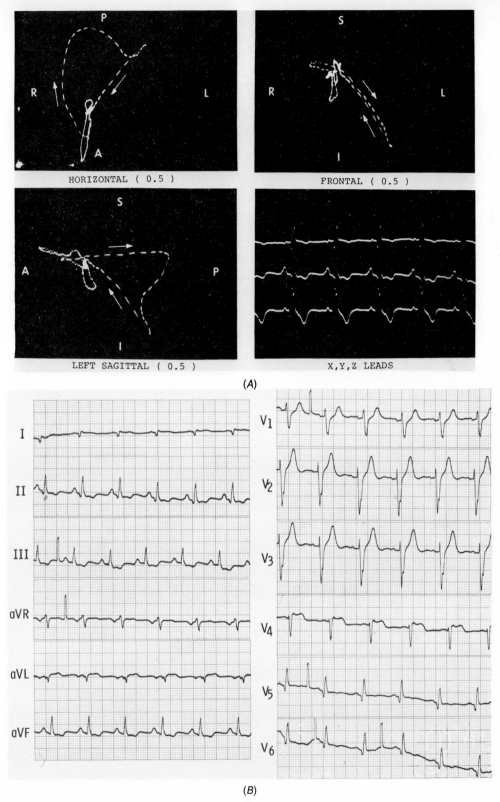

HORIZONTAL (0.5)

FRONTAL (0.5)

LEFT SAGITTAL (0.5)

X,Y,Z LEADS

(A)

Figure 7-22. VCG (*A*) and ECG (*B*) were obtained from a 58-year-old man with coronary heart disease. These tracings reveal anterolateral myocardial infarction.

139

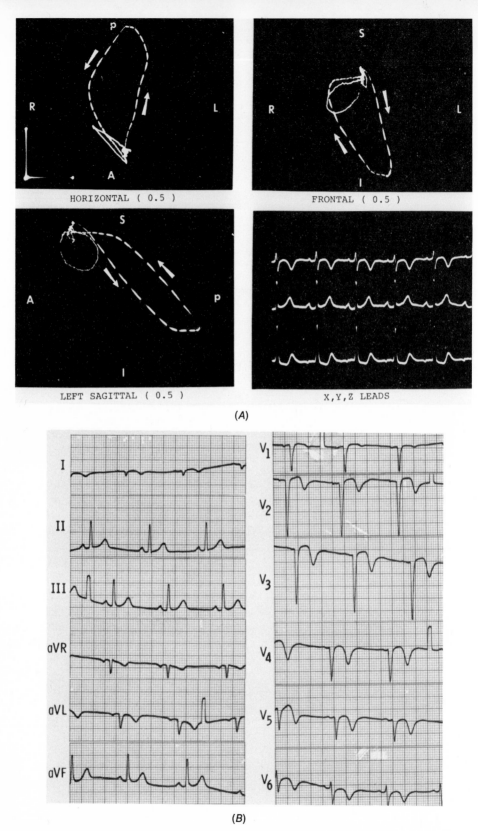

Figure 7-23. VCG (*A*) and ECG (*B*) were obtained from a 62-year-old man with coronary heart disease. These tracings show extensive anterior myocardial infarction.

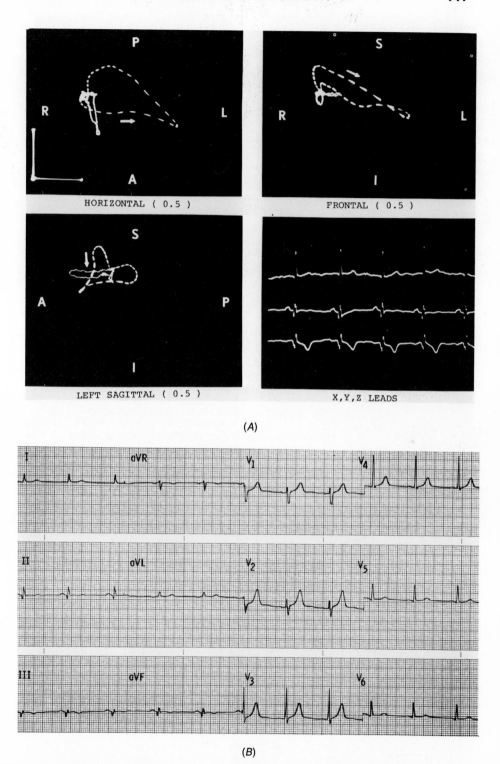

(A)

(B)

Figure 7-24. VCG (*A*) and ECG (*B*) were obtained from a 45-year-old man with coronary heart disease. These tracings reveal diaphragmatic myocardial infarction with posterior myocardial ischemia.

Posterior Myocardial Infarction. A unique feature of posterior myocardial infarction is anterior (and often rightward) displacement of 0.02- and 0.04-second vectors of the QRS sÊ loop with anterior bowing of these vectors (Fig. 7-13A and B). The inscription may be reversed in the horizontal or sagittal planes or both, and a figure-of-eight configuration may be observed in these planes. The above VCG abnormality is due to total or partial loss of posterior QRS force (Fig. 7-13A and B).

In the acute stage of posterior myocardial infarction, the T sÊ loop is often displaced far anteriorly and to the right. The S-T vector is present only during the acute stage, and it is directed posteriorly and often to the left.

It should be noted that posterior myocardial infarction is frequently associated with involvement of the diaphragmatic and lateral wall (diaphragmatic posterolateral myocardial infarction, Fig. 7-13A and B).

WOLFF-PARKINSON-WHITE SYNDROME

A unique feature of W-P-W syndrome is the conduction delay involving the initial 0.01-, 0.02-, 0.03- and, at times, 0.04-second vectors of the QRS sÊ loop (Fig. 7-15A and B). The direction of the initial vector varies markedly, depending upon the location of the anomalous conduction system. In general, the initial vector is directed anteriorly in type A W-P-W syn-drome, whereas in type B W-P-W syndrome it is directed posteriorly and leftward. The inscription may be normal, but it may be reversed in one or more planes. A figure-of-eight configuration may also be observed in one or more planes. The direction of the T sÊ loop varies markedly, but it is often 180 degrees discordant to the QRS sÊ loop, particularly in type B W-P-W syndrome. The S-T vector may or may not be present, and its direction also varies markedly according to the type of W-P-W syndrome.

REFERENCES

1. Chung, E. K.: Electrocardiography: Practical Applications with Vectorial Principles. Hagerstown, Md., Harper & Row, 1974.
2. Chou, T. C., Helm, R. A., and Kaplan, S.: Clinical Vectorcardiography, ed. 2. New York, Grune & Stratton, 1974.
3. Benchimol, A.: Vectorcardiography. Baltimore, Williams & Wilkins Co., 1973.
4. Dimond, E. G.: Electrocardiography and Vectorcardiography, ed. 4. Boston, Little, Brown & Co., 1967.
5. Hoffman, I.: Vectorcardiography. Philadelphia, J. B. Lippincott Co., 1971, vol. 2.
6. Kennedy, R. J., Varriale, P., and Alfenito, J. C.: Textbook of Vectorcardiography. Hagerstown, Md., Harper & Row, 1970.
7. Massie, E., and Walsh, T. J.: Clinical Vectorcardiography and Electrocardiography. Chicago, Year Book Medical Publishers, 1960.
8. Winsor, T.: Primer of Vectorcardiography. Philadelphia, Lea & Febiger, 1972.
9. Chung, E. K., Walsh, T. J., and Massie, E.: Wolff-Parkinson-White syndrome. Am. Heart J. 69:116, 1965.
10. Ellison, R. C., and Restieaux, N. J.: Vectorcardiography in Congenital Heart Disease. Philadelphia, W. B. Saunders Co., 1972.
11. Walsh, T. J.: The vectorcardiogram in cor pulmonale. Prog. Cardiovasc. Dis. 9:363, 1967.

Chapter 8

Echocardiography

CLAUDE R. JOYNER

Echocardiography, the pulsed reflected ultrasonic method of cardiac examination, was introduced by Edler and Hertz in 1954.[1] Since this initial report, the technique has become firmly established as a reliable and safe method of non-invasive study of a wide range of structural and functional cardiac abnormalities. Applications include the recording of abnormalities of anatomy and motion that may exist in patients with valve disease, intracardiac tumors, pericardial disease, congestive cardiomyopathy, idiopathic hypertrophic subaortic stenosis, congenital heart disease or coronary artery disease.

The principles involved in diagnostic ultrasound are well known and have been outlined in several reviews.[2-4] A single piezoelectric crystal functions as both the transmitter and the receiver of the high-frequency vibrations. Short repetitive pulses are emitted, and the echoes that are returned from acoustically reflective interfaces are detected by the receiver during the intervals between pulse transmission. Most of the instruments that are used in clinical echocardiography have a frequency of 2.0 to 2.5 mHz, and a repetition (sampling) rate between 200 and 2000 per second. The instrument used in many of our studies emits a 1-μsec. pulse of ultrasound at a repetition rate of 2000 per second. Thus, the transducer transmits during only 1/500 of each second and is in the receive mode during the remainder of the time. The laws of reflection and refraction dictate that the amplitude of the returning echoes depends upon the strength of the acoustical reflecting surface and the angle of incidence of the transmitted beam. Therefore, the strongest echoes are detected from reflecting structures that are perpendicular to the path of the ultrasonic beam. The returning echoes are amplitude modulated and displayed as spikes above the baseline of an oscilloscope (A mode). Intensity modulation of the signal converts the pattern from an amplitude spike to a dot of varying intensity. The intensity of a dot is determined by the amplitude of the echo, and the width is determined by the width of the base of the echo spike. When the intensity-modulated pattern is swept across the screen of an oscilloscope or a physiologic recorder, an M-mode presentation of moving echoes is inscribed. Figure 8-1 is a schematic representation of the A-mode and M-mode presentation of the anterior mitral leaflet. The M-mode display is calibrated in centimeters of tis-

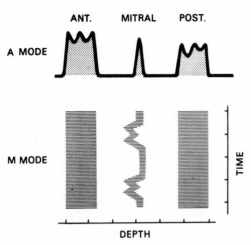

Figure 8-1. Schematic A-mode and M-mode presentation of the anterior mitral leaflet echo. M mode produces a time-distance display of movement. *ANT.,* anterior heart and mediastinal structures; *POST.,* posterior heart and lung. (Joyner, C. R.: Ultrasound and ultrasonic instrumentation. *In* Ultrasound in the Diagnosis of Cardiovascular-Pulmonary Disease. Copyright 1974 by Year Book Medical Publishers, Chicago. Used by permission.)

sue since the mean sound velocity in human tissue is known to be 1540 m. per second.[5]

RECORDING TECHNIQUE

Ultrasonic visualization of the heart and great vessels is restricteed to transducer placement and beam projections that do not traverse pulmonary tissues because lung is an extremely poor transmitter of ultrasonic energy. The distinctive pattern of the mitral valve echo is an excellent landmark within the heart. Orientation is best achieved by first locating the anterior mitral leaflet echo and proceeding from this point for confident imaging of other intracardiac structures.

Examination is customarily undertaken with the patient in the supine position. In most individuals the mitral valve is located by placing the transducer in the third or fourth left interspace 1 to 4 cm. lateral to the left sternal border, and directing the beam posteriorly and slightly medially.

However, it must be emphasized that variations in thoracic configuration and cardiac position determine the best acoustical window through which the mitral valve may be seen. In some patients this may even be the second interspace, and in others it may be the fifth or sixth interspace. Regardless of the transducer position the anterior mitral leaflet is recognized as a structure with a large amplitude of movement at a depth of 6 to 10 cm. from the transducer. Figure 8-2 illustrates the path of the ultrasound beam directed to record maximum motion of the anterior mitral leaflet. The beam traverses the right ventricle, interventricular septum and anterior mitral leaflet and usually passes through the left atrium just above the atrioventricular groove. The heart is scanned from this position by tilting the transducer to change beam direction. As the beam is directed in a more medial and cephalad projection, the aortic root, aortic cusps, and left atrial cavity are visualized. Caudad and lateral angulation from the mitral position directs the beam through the right ventricle, interventricular septum, posterior mitral leaflet and left ventricular posterior wall.

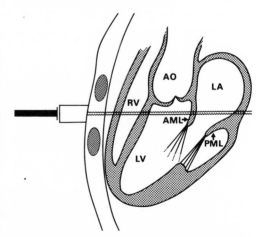

Figure 8-2. Transducer position and ultrasound beam direction to record anterior mitral leaflet motion. *RV,* right ventricle; *AO,* aorta; *LV,* left ventricle; *AML,* anterior mitral leaflet; *LA,* left atrium; *PML,* posterior mitral leaflet.

Figure 8-3 is an M-mode scan from a patient with severe coronary artery disease and chronic obstructive pulmonary disease. Moving from left to right, the scan begins with the beam directed through the aorta and left atrium. The thin aortic cusps are seen between the walls of the aorta and present a boxlike configuration during systole. The boundaries of the left atrium are the posterior aortic wall and the posterior atrial wall, which usually shows low-amplitude motion. As the transducer is tilted in a lateral and caudad direction, the anterior aortic wall becomes the interventricular septum, and the posterior aortic wall is in continuity with the anterior mitral leaflet. The relatively immobile left atrial wall merges with the thicker, actively contracting, left ventricular posterior wall. The posterior mitral leaflet, which moves in a direction opposite to that of the anterior leaflet, is seen on the right of the scan. The right ventricle of this patient is dilated because of pulmonary disease, and the septal motion is diminished because of coronary artery disease.

The tricuspid valve may be quite difficult to record from normal individuals; however, movement of this valve can be recorded from most patients with pulmonary hypertension, atrial septal defect or mitral stenosis. The tricuspid pattern is obtained by identifying the aortic valve echo and then tilting the transducer to direct the beam in a slightly medial and caudad direction. Gramiak and associates described a method that now makes possible the visualization of the pulmonary valve.[6] After the aortic root is located the transducer is moved one interspace higher and the beam angled superiorly and laterally toward the left shoulder.

Patient variability and the lack of uniformity in commercial ultrasonoscopes make it impossible to give a precise summary of the control adjustments that must be made to insure a satisfactory echocardiographic examination. The "operator factor" is critical in avoiding inconclusive or incorrect diagnoses. Instrument adjustments must be made while the pattern is observed on the oscilloscope to insure the best possible definition of structures. These skills can be acquired only by training in

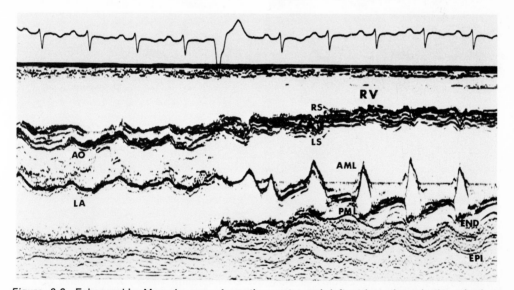

Figure 8-3. Echographic M-mode scan from the aorta and left atrium through the mitral apparatus (see text for details). *AO,* aorta; *LA,* left atrium; *RV,* right ventricle; *RS,* right side of the septum; *LS,* left side of septum; *AML,* anterior mitral leaflet; *PML,* posterior mitral leaflet; *END,* endocardium; *EPI,* epicardium.

an established laboratory or after a long period of experience and self-education.

THE MITRAL VALVE ECHOCARDIOGRAM

The Normal Mitral Pattern. Figure 8-4 is a normal pattern from the anterior mitral leaflet. One centimeter depth marks are inscribed on the right of the record. The designations of the parts of the echo complex are those proposed by Edler and Gustafson.[7] Shortly after the P wave of the electrocardiogram, atrial systole causes anterior movement of the leaflet into the ventricle to peak A. Peak A is followed by rapid movement posteriorly toward the atrium. This downstroke from A to C terminates at point C, which represents valve closure. This is the most posterior position reached by the valve. The A-C downstroke is initiated by atrial contraction and completed by ventricular systole. The velocity may change slightly at the time of ventricular systole (B). A gradual anterior movement (C-D) occurs during systole and re-

flects movement of the mitral annulus toward the apex of the left ventricle. A rapid anterior opening movement to peak E occurs at the beginning of diastole. Peak E is the most anterior position during the cardiac cycle. During rapid ventricular filling the leaflet executes a brisk movement toward a more closed position (F).

Mitral Stenosis. Many reports have confirmed Edler and Gustafson's studies showing the value of echocardiography in determining the severity of mitral stenosis.[7-12] A typical abnormal pattern obtained from a patient with mitral stenosis is shown in Figure 8-5. The distinctive feature of the pattern is a delay in posterior motion from peak E. This decrease in the E-F slope reflects delayed left ventricular filling and a persisting diastolic pressure gradient between the left atrium and left ventricle. In our laboratory the normal velocity of posterior movement from E is 85 to 180 mm. per second. Progressive decrease in velocity is found with increasingly severe narrowing of the mitral orifice. Posterior ve-

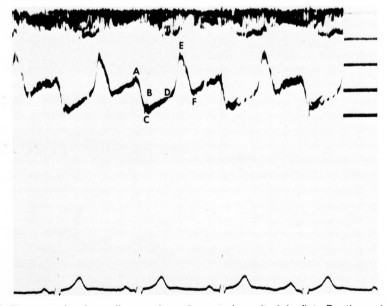

Figure 8-4. The normal echocardiogram from the anterior mitral leaflet; Depth marks of 1 cm. are recorded on the right. The designations of the various parts of the complex are those of Edler and Gustafson.[7] (Joyner, C. R.: Echocardiography of the atrioventricular valves and prosthetic valves. *In* Ultrasound in the Diagnosis of *Cardiovascular-Pulmonary Disease.* Copyright 1974 by Year Book Medical Publishers, Chicago. Used by permission.)

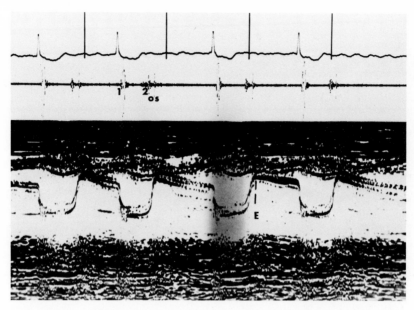

Figure 8-5. The mitral echocardiogram of a patient with mitral stenosis. There is a delay in descent from point *E. 1*, first heart sound; *2*, second heart sound; *OS*, opening snap.

locity from peak E in Figure 8-5 is 20 mm. per second. In one series of 80 patients from our laboratory, patients having mitral stenosis requiring surgery had a velocity less than 35 mm. per second.[10] Extremely severe stenosis was present when the E-F slope was less than 15 mm. per second.

Although the validity of the decrease in E-F velocity to assess the severity of mitral stenosis has been well accepted, reduction of this velocity may also be found in patients with decreased left ventricular compliance and a decrease in the rate of left ventricular filling. Examples are patients with hypertrophic subaortic stenosis or left ventricular hypertrophy due to aortic valve disease.[13] The difficulty of differentiating between valvular mitral stenosis and reduced diastolic velocity due to other conditions was greatly reduced when Duchak and associates reported the value of recording the echo from the posterior leaflet.[14] The anterior and posterior mitral leaflets move in opposite directions in normal subjects and in those patients in whom restricted anterior leaflet motion is due to poor ventricular compliance. In most pa-

tients with valvular mitral stenosis the leaflets move in the same direction. Figure 8-6 is the mitral valve echocardiogram and phonocardiogram from a patient with isolated aortic stenosis. The E-F slope is reduced to 55 mm. per second. Although this velocity is still faster than that found in patients with hemodynamically significant mitral stenosis, the anterior leaflet pattern alone would be considered to represent some mitral valve disease. However, the posterior mitral leaflet has a normal direction of movement opposite that of the anterior leaflet. In contrast, Figure 8-7 is the echocardiographic pattern from a patient with confirmed mitral stenosis. The transducer was angled to scan inferiorly from the anterior leaflet on the left to the anterior and posterior leaflets on the right. However, it should be noted that the posterior leaflet of some patients with mitral stenosis moves in a normal direction.[15] Figure 8-8 is a recording from a patient with moderately severe mitral stenosis and a posterior leaflet motion pattern that is a "normal" mirror image of the anterior leaflet echo. The leaflet echoes of many of

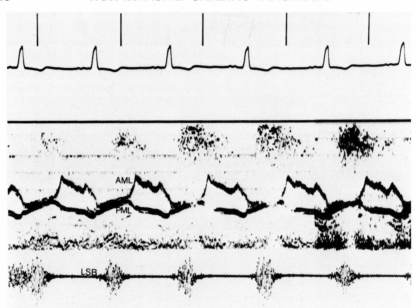

Figure 8-6. The electrocardiogram, echocardiogram of the anterior and posterior mitral leaflets and second left interspace phonocardiogram of a patient with aortic stenosis. The E slope is delayed, but the movement of the posterior mitral leaflet is opposite to that of the anterior mitral leaflet. *AML,* anterior mitral leaflet; *PML,* posterior mitral leaflet.

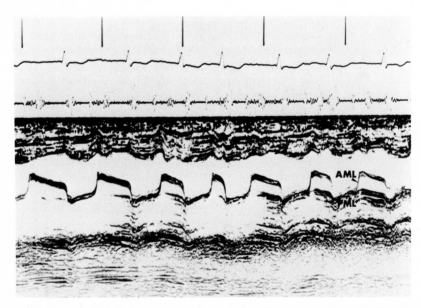

Figure 8-7. The echocardiogram of the anterior mitral leaflet on the left and both mitral leaflets on the right recorded from a patient with mitral stenosis. Both leaflets move in the same direction. AML, anterior mitral leaflet; PML, posterior mitral leaflet.

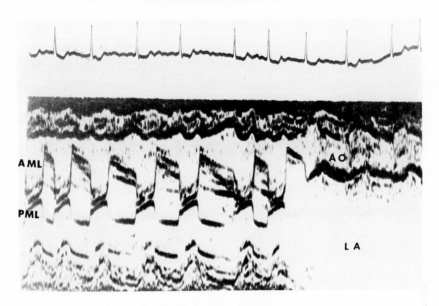

Figure 8-8. Echocardiographic scan through both mitral leaflets into the aorta and left atrium of a patient with mitral stenosis. The anterior and posterior leaflets move in opposite directions. The left atrium is enlarged. *AML,* anterior mitral leaflet; *PML,* posterior mitral leaflet; *AO,* aorta; *LA,* left atrium.

these patients show some thickening, and this aids in the diagnosis of true valvular stenosis regardless of the direction of leaflet motion.

In addition to assessing the severity of mitral stenosis, the echocardiogram may also give useful information for preoperative determination of mobility and thickness of the leaflet.[16,17] In our laboratory the normal anterior mitral leaflet presents an echo 1 to 3 mm. wide with a total anterior-posterior excursion of 2.5 to 3.5 cm. Stenotic valves with pliable leaflets show a 2- to 4-mm. echo with a near-normal range of anterior-posterior movement. A decrease in the anterior-posterior excursion and an increase in thickness of the echo from the leaflet indicates increased thickness or calcification of the valve.[16] The echocardiographic determination of the character of the leaflets has proved quite reliable in preoperative prediction of whether a commissurotomy or valve replacement will be required at the time of surgery. Figure 8-9 is the echocardiogram from a patient with an extremely thickened

valve, which required replacement with a prosthesis. This thick pattern is in marked contrast to the recording of the thin pliable stenotic valve shown in Figure 8-5.

Mitral Regurgitation. The echocardiogram has not proved reliable in assessing the severity of mitral regurgitation in patients with rheumatic heart disease. In those cases in which there is a fixed mitral orifice producing combined regurgitation and stenosis, the echocardiographic pattern from the anterior leaflet indicates the degree of stenosis.[18] In the presence of pure mitral regurgitation the echocardiogram may be entirely normal or may show an increase in anterior-posterior excursion and in the velocity of posterior movement from peak E. However, a similar pattern may be found in any condition producing rapid ventricular filling.

Some forms of mitral regurgitation produce specific echocardiographic patterns. Distinctive patterns have been described in patients with flail anterior or posterior leaflets due to ruptured chordae tendineae.[19,20] The echocardiogram in Figure

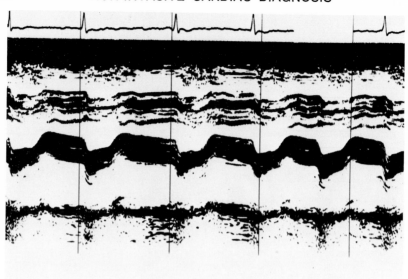

Figure 8-9. The mitral valve echocardiogram from a patient with an extremely thick, stenotic leaflet. The echo is extremely wide, and the anterior-posterior excursion is diminished.

8-10 was recorded from a patient with rupture of chordae to the posterior leaflet. The leaflet has an abnormal pattern and moves parallel rather than opposite to the anterior leaflet. In systole the posterior leaflet moves far posteriorly and remains widely separated from the anterior leaflet. In diastole there is an abnormal anterior motion into the ventricle and an irregular pattern of vibrations of the unsupported leaflet. The pattern of movement of a flail anterior leaflet is illustrated in Figure 8-11. There

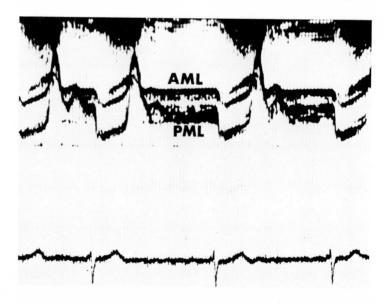

Figure 8-10. The anterior and posterior mitral echocardiogram from a patient with ruptured chordae of the posterior leaflet. The posterior leaflet motion is abnormal and unfurls anteriorly in diastole. (Joyner, C. R.: Echocardiography of the atrioventricular valves and prosthetic valves. *In* Ultrasound in the Diagnosis of Cardiovascular-Pulmonary Disease. Copyright 1974 by Year Book Medical Publishers, Chicago. Used by Permission.)

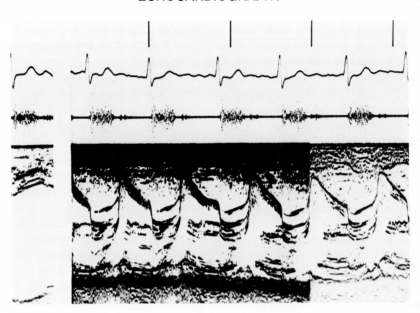

Figure 8-11. The pattern of motion of a flail anterior leaflet. The amplitude is increased, and there are multiple reduplicated echoes during systole. The control settings were changed on the right to show finer detail of the left side of the interventricular septum.

is increased amplitude of motion, and the anterior leaflet actually collides with the interventricular septum. The multiple reduplicated echoes during systole are also characteristic of this type of mitral regurgitation.

Echocardiography appears remarkably accurate for the diagnosis of the mitral valve prolapse syndrome.[21-24] Two echocardiographic patterns have been described in these patients. A typical example of one pattern is shown in Figure 8-12. An abrupt

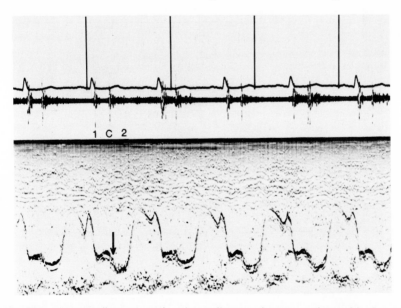

Figure 8-12. The phonocardiogram and echocardiogram from a patient with the mitral valve prolapse syndrome. There is abrupt posterior displacement of the mitral echo as the click and late systolic murmur develop. *1,* first heart sound; *C,* click; *2,* second heart sound.

posterior movement in midsystole is temporally related to the click and late systolic murmur. The second pattern that may be found in these patients is shown in Figure 8-13. There is a hammock configuration of pansystolic bowing producing maximum posterior displacement and apparent leaflet separation in midsystole.

Mitral Valvular Vegetations. Valvular vegetations due to bacterial endocarditis may also be detected by the echocardiogram.[25] Figure 8-13 shows vegetations on the mitral leaflet of a patient with the mitral leaflet prolapse syndrome. The vegetations are seen as shaggy, irregular echoes during diastole. The unevenly distributed vegetations are not in the beam path during systole when the valve appears thin. This feature distinguishes valve thickening due to vegetations from thickening due to rheumatic valvular disease.

The Mitral Echocardiogram in Aortic Regurgitation. The anterior mitral leaflet of some patients with aortic regurgitation demonstrates an unusual rapid oscillating vibration during diastole (Fig. 8-14).[26,27] This diastolic fluttering presumably is produced by the aortic regurgitant jet striking the leaflet or is a reflection of turbulence generated by the confluence of the aortic regurgitant and mitral inflow streams. These vibrations may contribute to generation of an Austin Flint murmur, although Fortuin and Craige suggest that the Austin Flint murmur is produced by an increase in antegrade flow velocity developing as the mitral valve is closed by the reflux of aortic blood.[28] Mitral diastolic fluttering may be recorded in some patients with modest aortic regurgitation and is not seen in some patients with massive regurgitation. The presence or absence of the vibrations probably is determined by the direction of the aortic regurgitant stream. Therefore, mitral diastolic flutter indicates some aortic regurgitation but cannot be relied upon for quantitative assessment of the volume of retrograde flow.

Premature mitral valve closure can be clinically useful in assessing the hemodynamic importance of aortic regurgitation.[29] Premature closure is most likely to be found in patients with aortic regurgitation of abrupt onset due to perforation or de-

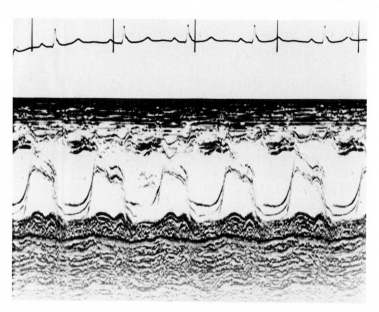

Fig. 8-13. Hammock-like configuration of pansystolic bowing in the mitral valve prolapse syndrome. Irregular thickened echoes representing valve vegetations are seen during diastole.

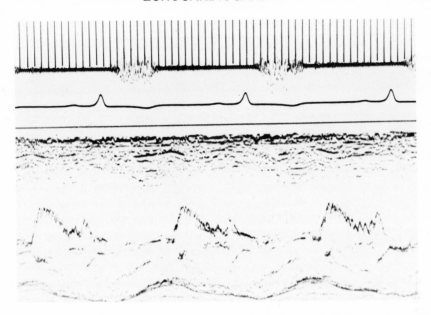

Figure 8-14. Rapid oscillating diastolic vibration of the anterior mitral leaflet of a patient with aortic insufficiency.

hiscence of a cusp. Early mitral closure occurs when the retrograde flow of a large volume of aortic blood rapidly increases left ventricular diastolic pressure to a level exceeding left atrial pressure. This condition is poorly tolerated, and most of our patients have required aortic valve replacement shortly after echographic detection of premature mitral closure.

Hypertrophic Subaortic Stenosis. The value of echocardiography in the diagnosis of idiopathic hypertrophic subaortic stenosis (IHSS) has been documented in many reports that have appeared over the past few years.[13,30-34] A characteristic systolic anterior motion of the mitral valve has been found in patients with significant subaortic obstruction. Figure 8-15 is the echocardiogram from a patient with IHSS and a resting left ventricular-aortic systolic gradient of 20 mm. Hg. Subsequent infusion of Isoproterenol increased the gradient to 110 mm. Hg. The echo pattern shows the classical pronounced anterior systolic motion of the mitral leaflets, a slow E-F velocity due to poor ventricular compliance and early diastolic collision of the

anterior leaflet with the left side of the septum. Recently it has been shown that systolic anterior motion may exist in the absence of a resting gradient.[33] Anterior systolic leaflet motion mimicking that found in IHSS may also be recorded from some patients with the mitral valve prolapse syndrome.[24] Care must be taken to avoid obtaining the mitral echogram from near the base of the leaflet in patients with mitral prolapse since this projection is particularly likely to give a pattern suggesting obstructive cardiomyopathy. Even if this error is made, proper interpretation is possible since the late systolic position of the valve is posterior to the C point in the mitral valve prolapse syndrome and anterior to this point in patients with IHSS.[24]

Asymmetric hypertrophy with an increase in septal thickness relative to that of the posterior wall has been suggested as the pathognomonic anatomic abnormality of hypertrophic cardiomyopathy with or without obstruction.[31,32] A septum–posterior wall ratio greater than 1.3:1 is considered abnormal. Figure 8-15 is not satisfactory for accurate measurement of

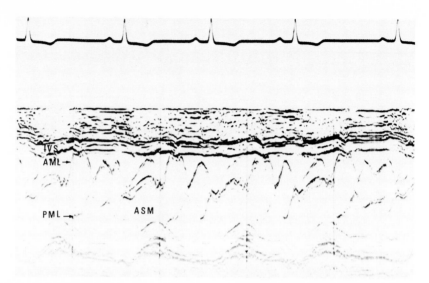

Figure 8-15. The echocardiogram in idiopathic hypertrophic subaortic stenosis. There is an anterior systolic movement of the mitral valve that moves forward to approach the ventricular septum. *IVS,* ventricular septum; *AML,* anterior mitral leaflet; *PML,* posterior mitral leaflet; *ASM,* anterior systolic motion.

the thickness of the interventricular septum since the ultrasound beam projection used for this recording failed to provide adequate definition of the right side of the septum. Figure 8-16, which is a recording from another patient with IHSS, shows asymmetric hypertrophy with a septal–posterior wall ratio of 2.7:1. However, disproportionate hypertrophy of the septum relative to the thickness of the posterior wall cannot be accepted as unequivocal proof of hypertrophic cardiomyopathy.

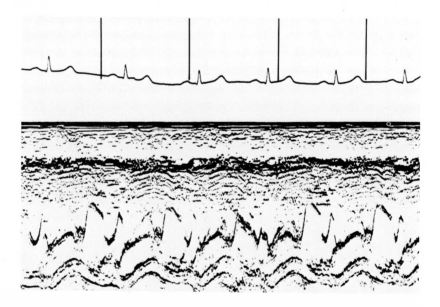

Figure 8-16. The echocardiogram of hypertrophic subaortic stenosis demonstrating the systolic anterior mitral motion and asymmetric hypertrophy with a septum–posterior wall ratio of 2.7:1.

Septum–posterior wall ratios greater than 1.3:1 have been found in some patients with primary pulmonary hypertension.[35]

Left Atrial Myxoma. Although not as common as mitral stenosis, a left atrial myxoma is a not infrequent cause for obstruction of the outflow from the left atrium. Many workers have reported the diagnostic accuracy of echocardiography in detecting these tumors.[36-39] The characteristic pattern of an atrial myxoma prolapsing into the mitral sleeve is shown in Figure 8-17. The multiple echoes from the tumor are contiguous with the anterior mitral leaflet in diastole but move away from the leaflet when ventricular systole pushes the tumor into the left atrium.

Close attention to technique is necessary to prevent false positive or false negative results of examination for an atrial myxoma. I have seen one patient in whom the diagnosis of mitral stenosis was made on the basis of an echocardiogram that was obtained with an improper, inordinately low gain setting. The gain was so low that there was insufficient ultrasound energy to penetrate the anterior mitral leaflet. The typical pattern of a left atrial myxoma was recorded when the echocardiogram was repeated with proper attention to control settings.[40] On the other hand, excess gain

setting can produce reduplication of echoes and change the pattern of valvular mitral stenosis to one that mimics a left atrial myxoma.[37] This error can be avoided by recording the motion of both leaflets of the mitral valve and also determining if the thick echoes remain contiguous with the mitral pattern in both systole and diastole. The posterior leaflet can be recorded in patients with mitral stenosis but usually is not seen in patients with an atrial myxoma. Confidence in the diagnosis of a left atrial tumor is increased by directing the beam into the left atrium where a large tumor can be seen to move into the beam during systole and recede during diastole. This is illustrated in Figure 8-18, which is the echogram from the left atrium of a patient whose mitral valve presentation of a myxoma is illustrated in Figure 8-17.

THE TRICUSPID VALVE ECHOCARDIOGRAM

The echocardiogram of the normal tricuspid valve has a configuration similar to that of the normal anterior mitral leaflet, and the abnormal pattern of tricuspid stenosis resembles the mitral pattern of mitral stenosis. The normal range for the tricuspid diastolic E-F slope velocity is 60 to

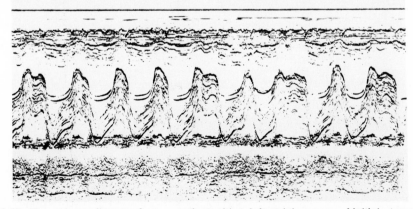

Figure 8-17. The echocardiogram from a patient with a left atrial myxoma. Multiple tumor echoes are seen posterior to and contiguous with the anterior mitral leaflet in diastole. The area immediately posterior to the valve becomes clear during systole as the myxoma moves into the atrium.

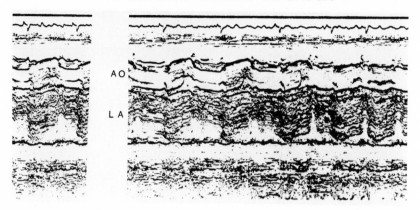

Figure 8-18. Echocardiogram from the left atrium of the patient whose mitral valve presentation of myxoma is shown in Figure 8-17 (see text).

125 mm. per second. Significant tricuspid stenosis is indicated by an E-F diastolic velocity of less than 30 mm. per second.[41] Visualization of tricuspid motion is important for the diagnosis of Ebstein's anomaly and other cardiac malformations. The tricuspid valve echocardiogram in these conditions will be discussed in the section on congenital heart disease.

THE AORTIC VALVE ECHOCARDIOGRAM

Normal. An echocardiogram from a normal aortic root and aortic valve is shown in Figure 8-19. Two parallel signals, representing the anterior and posterior aortic walls, move in an anterior direction during systole and in a posterior direction during diastole.[42,43] The mean normal adult aortic root diameter at the onset of systole is 3.4 cm.[44] The left atrial cavity is visualized immediately behind the aortic root. The aortic cusp echoes have a boxlike systolic configuration indicating brisk opening and closure of the valve. The cusps produce a central linear echo during diastole. In Figure 8-19 this is a single line pattern; however, two slightly separated diastolic components are recorded from many normal subjects.[42] The anterior valve echo is from the right coronary cusp, and the posterior echo is reflected from the noncoronary cusp.[42]

Aortic Stenosis. Aortic stenosis may be diagnosed by detecting thickened echoes and distortion of the normal boxlike pattern of valve motion. Figure 8-20 shows the second left interspace phonocardiogram, carotid pulse tracing and aortic valve echocardiogram from a patient with severe calcific aortic stenosis. There are thick valve echoes during systole and diastole, the systolic separation of the cusps is diminished, and the orifice is irregular.

Although echocardiographic quantitation of aortic stenosis does not approach the accuracy of ultrasonic measurement of mitral stenosis, Gramiak and Shah have reported some features that may be used for a general estimation of the severity of aortic obstruction.[44] Thickening of the valve complex to one third or more of the internal diameter of the aortic root usually indicates a left ventricular–aortic systolic gradient in the range of 75 mm. Hg. Thickened cusps that show no change in configuration during systole and diastole also suggest a high pressure gradient. If one cusp is seen to move well during systole the peak gradient is generally under 50 mm. Hg.

Yeh and associates have recently reported some correlation between the width of the systolic cusp separation and the transvalvular gradient.[45] The mean systolic separation in their normal subjects was 1.9

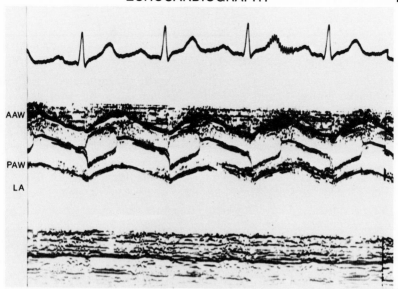

Figure 8-19. The echocardiogram of a normal aortic root and aortic valve. The anterior and posterior aortic walls have a parallel motion. Thin aortic cusps present a boxlike configuration in systole. The posterior aortic wall forms the anterior boundary of the left atrium. *AAW,* anterior aortic wall; *PAW,* posterior aortic wall; *LA,* left atrium.

cm. When the separation was measured as less than 0.6 cm., the transvalvular gradient was usually greater than 55 mm. Hg. A gradient of less than 35 mm. Hg was found in patients in whom cusp separation was greater than 1.3 cm. However, it should be noted that a decrease in valve excursion and cusp separation may be produced by a decrease in cardiac output without aortic stenosis. Also, a thick mass

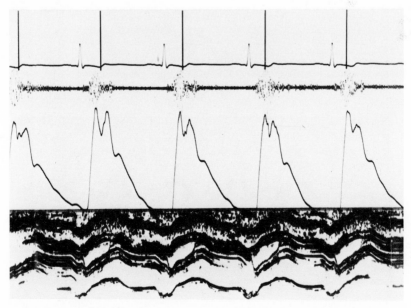

Figure 8-20. The second left interspace phonocardiogram, carotid pulse tracing and aortic valve echocardiogram of a patient with calcific aortic stenosis. In contrast to the normal, the aortic cusp echoes are thick, the systolic separation is diminished, and the orifice is irregular.

of echoes obscures the orifice and precludes measurement of the degree of systolic separation in many patients with
aortic stenosis.

Bicuspid Aortic Valve. Figure 8-21 is
representative of the abnormal pattern that
has been reported in patients with a bicuspid aortic valve.[46] There is eccentricity
of the cusp echoes in diastole (posterior
displacement in Fig. 8-21). The valves of
many patients also produce multiple-
layered diastolic echoes, which likely represent reflections from redundant valve
tissue.

Subaortic Stenosis. An abnormal pattern
of aortic systolic valve motion may be recorded from patients with idiopathic hypertrophic subaortic stenosis. The cusps
open normally, move to a closed position
in midsystole and reopen in late systole.[47]
The systolic closing apparently coincides
with the development of a high left ventricular–aortic pressure gradient and a
decrease in aortic flow. However, this
peculiar pattern cannot be considered unequivocally diagnostic of hypertrophic

cardiomyopathy. A similar pattern may
be found in some patients with discrete
subaortic stenosis.[48]

Aortic Regurgitation. The echocardiogram of the aortic root and aortic valve
is of limited value in the assessment of patients with aortic regurgitation. The aortic
root is usually slightly wider and the closing valve movement is somewhat more
rapid than in normal subjects. There may
be separation of the valve cusps during
diastole, but cusp separation may not be
visualized in some patients with severe re-
gurgitations.[43] Also, of course, some diastolic separation of the echoes is a frequent
finding in normal individuals. At the present time, aortic valve echocardiography
cannot be considered clinically useful for
quantitation of aortic regurgitation.

THE PULMONARY VALVE ECHOCARDIOGRAM

Normal. Ultrasound visualization of pulmonary valve motion is a relatively new
development that resulted from Gramiak,
Nanda and Shah's description of a satisfac-

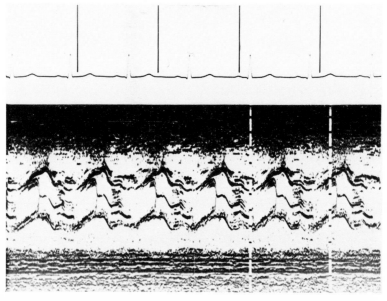

Figure 8-21. The echocardiogram in bicuspid aortic valve. There is eccentricity of the cusp echoes in diastole and a multiple layering of diastolic echoes. Depth marks of 1 cm. are recorded on the tracing.

tory recording technique.[6] The upward and oblique beam direction used for this examination most often visualizes only a single posterior cusp. With this projection, the valve is viewed from the right ventricular outflow tract. Therefore, opening movements into the pulmonary artery are recorded on the echocardiogram as posterior deflections, and valve closure is indicated by upward movement on the tracing (Fig. 8-22). There is a gradual posterior slope toward the pulmonary artery during diastolic filling of the right ventricle. A more pronounced posterior displacement (a dip) is temporally related to the P wave and represents transient valve movement produced by atrial ejection into the low-pressure right ventricle.

Pulmonary Hypertension. The movement of the pulmonary valve is abnormal in most patients with pulmonary hypertension.[49] The velocity of valve opening is increased since right ventricular pressure exceeds pulmonary artery pressure at a time when the right ventricular pressure is rapidly accelerating. Other changes in the pattern result from the increased diastolic pressure gradient across the pulmonary valve. The angle of the diastolic posterior slope is diminished, and the a dip is decreased or absent. However, an a dip may still be seen in patients with significant pulmonary hypertension and elevated right ventricular pressures. The preliminary reports are quite encouraging, but further studies are needed for final determination of the accuracy of the pulmonary valve echogram in the non-invasive quantitation of pulmonary hypertension.

PERICARDIAL EFFUSION

The detection of pericardial effusion has been one of the most widely employed and clinically useful applications of echocardiography. Edler first showed that pericardial fluid could be detected as a relatively echo-free area in front of the anterior heart wall.[50] The technique was quickly accepted for clinical diagnosis after the demonstration of the relative ease with which the

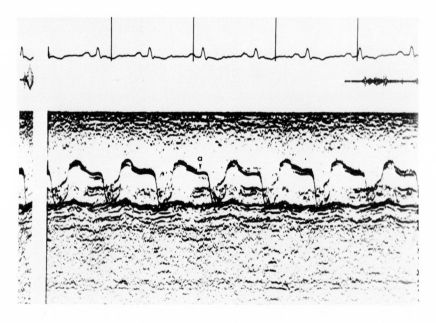

Figure 8-22. A normal pulmonary valve tracing. Opening movements are indicated as posterior deflections on the recording, and closure is inscribed as an upward deflection of the tracing. The a dip is a brief posterior displacement resulting from atrial ejection into the right ventricle.

presence of pericardial fluid between the posterior heart wall and the pericardium can be determined.[51-55] Nevertheless, meticulous attention to technique is required to avoid false positive or false negative findings. The reflected ultrasound examination is undertaken by directing the beam in a caudad and lateral direction from the mitral valve. This is the position that permits visualization of the interventricular septum and left ventricular posterior wall. The complete examination should include scanning the heart from near the cardiac apex to the left atrium. Since the demonstration of fluid is dependent upon recording a relatively sonolucent area between the epicardium and pericardium, it is necessary to vary the gain setting during the procedure. If the setting is too high, echoes may reflect from pericardial fluid and obscure the diagnosis. If the gain setting is too low, only the pericardial-lung interface may be recorded.

The gain setting was gradually increased from left to right during the recording of the echocardiogram shown in Figure 8-23. The structure labeled PW (posterior wall) is the epicardial echo on the left. The higher gain setting on the right demonstrates the myocardium, endocardium and chordal echoes anterior to the epicardium. The sonolucent posterior pericardial effusion is well seen on the left. On the right the increased gain produced echoes from the effusion similar in intensity to the reflection from the myocardium. Only gross quantitation of the amount of pericardial fluid is possible with this technique. In general, detection of anterior fluid indicates a rather large effusion since fluid tends to gravitate to the inferior-posterior parts of the pericardial sac.

CONGENITAL HEART DISEASE

Echocardiography has been used to record motion abnormalities resulting from distorted hemodynamics in congenital cardiac disease and has been employed to outline specific anatomic malformations. Although real-time two-dimensional echo-

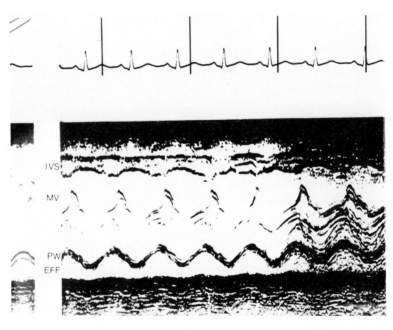

Figure 8-23. The echocardiogram from a patient with posterior pericardial effusion. *IVS,* interventricular septum; *MV,* mitral valve; *PW,* epicardium on the left and entire posterior wall structures on the right; *EFF,* pericardial effusion.

cardiographic systems that are now being developed will likely increase the accuracy of depicting anatomic structures, conventional M-mode echocardiography is now an essential diagnostic tool for the cardiologist who is entrusted with the diagnosis of congenital heart disease. In this section I will attempt to summarize the practical clinical use of M–mode reflected ultrasound in the assessment of some of the more common abnormalities.

Atrial Septal Defect and Right Ventricular Volume Overload. In 1971 Diamond and associates described an abnormal pattern of interventricular septal motion in patients with atrial septal defects and left-to-right shunts.[56] The normal septal motion is posterior during systole and anterior during diastole. Two types of abnormal motion are seen in patients with atrial septal defects. In type A (paradoxical) the septum moves anteriorly during systole and posteriorly during diastole. In the type B pattern the septal movement is diminished and flattened. Figure 8-24 shows type A paradoxical motion in a patient

with an atrial septal defect and a moderately large left-to-right shunt. The right ventricle, lying anterior to the septum, is dilated. The scan shows consistent paradoxical anterior interventricular septal movement paralleling the movement of the posterior left ventricular wall. In the initial report by Diamond it was emphasized that this pattern was not specific for an atrial defect but could be found in other situations in which there was volume overload of the right ventricle. This has been confirmed in several other studies, and a recent review summarizes the conditions of right ventricular diastolic overload that may produce abnormal septal motion. These include anomalous pulmonary venous drainage, tricuspid or pulmonic valve insufficiency, Ebstein's anomaly and partial atrioventricular canal.[57] However, it has also become apparent that not all patients with an atrial septal defect and a significant left-to-right shunt have an abnormal septal pattern. In one series, 5 of 21 patients who underwent surgery for an atrial septal defect had normal septal mo-

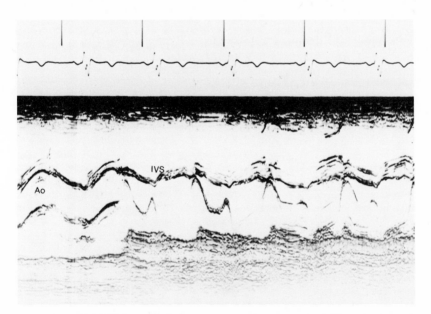

Figure 8-24. Type A paradoxical septal motion of a patient with an atrial septal defect and a left-to-right shunt. The septum moves anteriorly during systole and posteriorly during diastole. *Ao,* aorta; *IVS,* interventricular septum.

tion before closure of the defect.[58] Hagan and colleagues have reported an extensive analysis of septal motion in normal subjects and patients with right ventricular volume overload.[59] This report emphasizes the echocardiographic technique that should be employed for proper examination of septal motion. The upper one third of the septum normally moves anteriorly in systole. The inferior two thirds, below a pivot point, normally moves posteriorly during systole. The normal pivot point may be located below the plane of the mitral valve, and paradoxical motion should be diagnosed only if the abnormal movement is recorded when the beam is directed below the valve to the area of the chordae tendineae. In Hagan and coworkers' series, 8 of 21 patients with right ventricular volume overload had a pattern of the entire septum moving anteriorly (paradoxically) during systole. Normal septal motion was seen in 6 of the patients with volume overload of the right ventricle.

Paradoxical or flat septal movement may also be found in patients with left bundle branch block or disease of the left anterior descending coronary artery.[57,60] The configuration of the paradoxical movement resulting from left bundle branch block appears to be different from that seen in other conditions with systolic anterior movement.[60] This pattern is illustrated in Figure 8-25, which was recorded from a patient with mitral stenosis and ventricular ectopic contractions with a left bundle branch block configuration. An abrupt posterior motion of the septum shortly after the onset of the QRS is followed by paradoxical anterior movement during the remainder of ventricular systole. This is in contrast to the holosystolic paradoxical type A pattern (Fig. 8-24).

Therefore, not all patients with right ventricular volume overload have abnormal septal motion, and abnormal septal motion can be seen in conditions other than volume overload of the right ventricle. Nevertheless, if proper technique is employed and the echocardiogram is interpreted with the knowledge of all conditions that may influence septal motion, this pro-

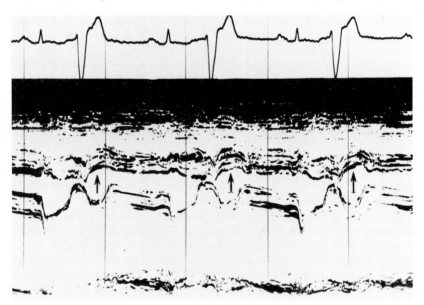

Figure 8-25. Abnormal septal motion produced by ventricular ectopic beats with a left bundle branch block configuration. A brisk posterior deflection immediately after the QRS is followed by abnormal anterior movement, indicated by arrows. The mitral valve echo shows the typical pattern of mitral stenosis.

cedure is still clinically useful for non-invasive screening of patients for right ventricular volume overload.

Ebstein's Anomaly. Abnormal motion of the interventricular septum and delayed closure of the large sail-like anterior tricuspid leaflet is the characteristic echocardiographic finding in Ebstein's anomaly.[61-63] Figure 8-26 shows a wide-amplitude excursion of the tricuspid valve, the paradoxical interventricular septal motion and the portion of the anterior mitral leaflet echo from one of our patients with this congenital abnormality. Delayed closure of the tricuspid valve is responsible for the abnormal late component of the first heart sound that is frequently heard in patients with Ebstein anomaly.[61]

Truncus Arteriosus and Tetralogy of Fallot. Chung and associates described the echocardiographic findings in truncus arteriosus and outlined the difficulties that may be encountered in distinguishing this condition from tetralogy of Fallot.[64] In a patient with a truncus arteriosus, there is a large aortic root overriding the ventricular septum and loss of the normal con-tinuity between the septum and the anterior aortic margin (Fig. 8-27). Similar overriding of the aorta may be seen in a patient with tetralogy of Fallot. If a pulmonic valve can be identified, it may be assumed that the diagnosis is tetralogy rather than truncus (Fig. 8-28). Inability to demonstrate the pulmonary valve cannot be accepted as unequivocally diagnostic of a truncus, but the demonstration of two semilunar valves will exclude the diagnosis.

Double-Outlet Right Ventricle. Mitral-semilunar valve discontinuity is present in patients with origin of both great vessels from the right ventricle.[65,66] The echocardiographic pattern shows the loss of mitral-semilunar valve continuity and the posterior border of the adjacent vessel located anterior to the mitral valve echo. The degree of the mitral-great vessel separation determined by echocardiography has agreed well with angiocardiographic measurements.[65]

The Hypoplastic Right and Left Heart Syndromes. A characteristic echocardiographic pattern has been found in patients

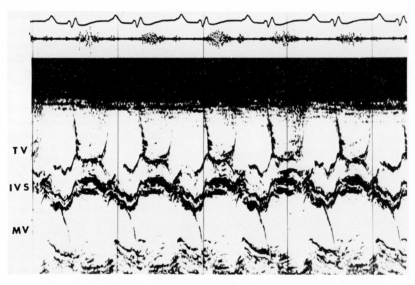

Figure 8-26. The echocardiogram of a patient with Ebstein's anomaly. There is wide amplitude of tricuspid valve excursion, late closure of the valve and paradoxical interventricular septal motion. *TV*, tricuspid valve; *IVS*, interventricular septum; *MV*, mitral valve.

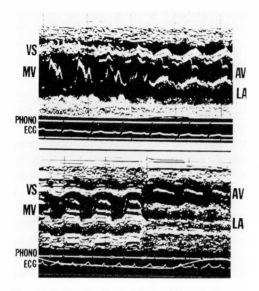

Figure 8-27. The top echocardiogram from a normal child shows continuity between the ventricular septum and the anterior aortic wall. The bottom echocardiographic scan from a patient with truncus arteriosus shows discontinuity between the ventricular septum and the anterior aortic wall, and a large aortic root. *VS,* ventricular septum; *MV,* mitral valve; *AV,* aortic valve; *LA,* left atrium. (Chung, K. J., Alexson, C. G., Manning, J. A., and Gramiak, R.: Echocardiography in truncus arteriosus—The value of pulmonic valve detection. Circulation 48:281, 1973. By permission of the American Heart Association).

with aortic atresia and a hypoplastic left ventricle.[67,68] The left ventricular dimension is quite small, while the right ventricular chamber is larger than normal. The mitral valve echo is markedly distorted or absent, and there is hypoplasia of the aortic root. In contrast, in patients with tricuspid atresia the right ventricular dimension is small, the left ventricular dimension is larger than normal, and there is no demonstrable tricuspid valve echo.

Single Ventricle. Meyer and Kaplan reported that single ventricle can be distinguished echocardiographically from the hypoplastic left or right heart syndrome.[66] They found that continuity of an atrioventricular valve and pulmonary root could not be demonstrated and that neither an aortic root nor a pulmonary root echo-

gram could be obtained. These two findings, and the failure to record a septal echo, were considered strongly indicative of a single ventricle. However, they have noted that it may be difficult to distinguish between a single ventricle and levotransposition of the great vessels when the ventricles lie side by side and the septal orientation is parallel to the ultrasonic beam.

Dextrotransposition of the Great Vessels. The altered spatial relationship of the great vessels that is characteristic of dextrotransposition may be demonstrated by conventional M-mode echocardiography.[69] The normal great vessel position and that present in transposition is shown in Figure 8-29. When the ultrasound transducer is directed from a left parasternal position, the normal aortic valve is located by directing the transducer in a medial and cephalad direction. The pulmonic valve is

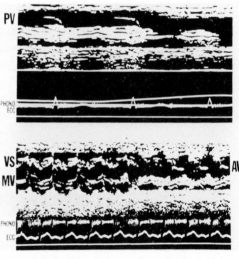

Figure 8-28. The echocardiogram in tetralogy of Fallot with a small pulmonary annulus. The top record of pulmonic valve motion differentiates tetralogy from truncus arteriosus. The bottom recording shows ventricular septal and anterior aortic wall discontinuity and a large aortic root, which is also seen in patients with truncus arteriosus. *PV,* pulmonic valve; *VS,* ventricular septum; *MV,* mitral valve. (Chung, K. J., Alexson, C. G., Manning, J. A., and Gramiak, R.: Echocardiography in truncus arteriosus—The value of pulmonic valve detection. Circulation 48:281, 1973. By permission of the American Heart Association.

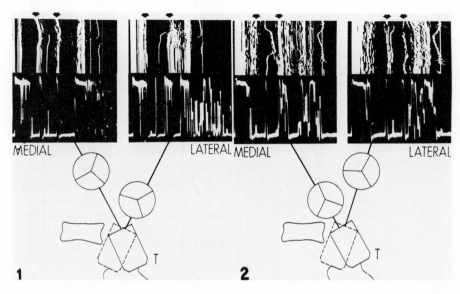

Figure 8-29. Schematic representation of the echocardiographic pattern showing normal great vessel relationship (*1*) and the altered relationship of dextrotransposition (*2*). With the transducer in a left parasternal position, the aortic valve is seen in a posterior-medial position, and the pulmonic valve is located in a lateral and anterior position. A- and M-mode recordings of valves are placed above the schematic representations. In transposition (*2*) medial beam direction demonstrates an anterior outflow vessel, and lateral direction demonstrates a posterior outflow vessel. (Gamiak, R., Chung, K. J., Nanda, N., and Manning, J.: Echocardiographic diagnosis of transposition of the great vessels. Radiology 106:187, 1973.)

located by directing the beam laterally, where the valve is recognized by its anterior position relative to the aorta. In contrast, in patients with dextrotransposition, medial angulation demonstrates an anteriorly situated outflow vessel. Lateral transducer angulation shows a deeply placed vessel. The diagnosis, therefore, is based upon the operator's knowledge of the angle of the transducer during the recording. The pattern obtained from the anterior vessel in transposition appears similar to the normal pulmonary echo, and the pattern of the posterior outflow vessel is similar to that obtained from an aorta in the normal location.

Two-dimensional cross-sectional echographic imaging instruments that produce a picture of anatomic relationships not possible with conventional M-mode one-dimensional scans will likely prove superior to M-mode examination for the definition of the relaton of the great vessels and

cardiac chambers in patients with congenital heart disease.[70]

THE ECHOCARDIOGRAPHIC EXAMINATION OF THE LEFT VENTRICLE

Interest in echocardiography escalated when it was demonstrated that this method of study could be used to evaluate left ventricular anatomy and some aspects of left ventricular function. Gross abnormalities such as left ventricular aneurysms can be diagnosed,[72] abnormal septal motion may be recorded in patients with disease of the left anterior descending coronary artery, and localized areas of myocardial asynergy may be detected.[57,71] Obviously, the visualization of a ventricular aneurysm or demonstration of asynergy by this non-invasive method gives useful clinical information. However, the possibility of using echocardiography to determine and monitor overall left ventricular performance has even greater interest for the clinician.

The many publications on the use of echocardiography to study left ventricular contractility and function have recently been reviewed.[73] Reports from several laboratories have shown a relationship between an interventricular septum–left posterior wall dimension and angiographically determined left ventricular volume.[74-76] An estimation of left ventricular volume has been derived by using the cube of the left ventricular internal dimension[74] or by using a regression formula.[75] This estimation of the systolic and diastolic volumes has been used to calculate the ejection fraction, stroke volume and mean rate of circumferential fiber shortening.[74,76-79]

It is not easy to master the technique of recording a satisfactory echogram from the left side of the interventricular septum and the endocardium of the left ventricular posterior wall. The examination begins with standard visualization of the mitral leaflet. For ventricular dimension studies, the transducer should be kept as close to the left sternal edge as possible in order to obtain optimal visualization of the left side of the septum. Slight caudad and lateral direction of the beam from the anterior leaflet projection visualizes the posterior leaflet. It has been suggested that reproducibility is best achieved by recording the septal-posterior wall dimension with a beam projection that traverses both the anterior and posterior leaflets.[4] However, in many patients, a satisfactory echo from the left side of the septum and endocardium can be obtained only if the beam is directed slightly inferior to the mitral valve. In fact, most publications on echocardiographic determination of left ventricular dimensions indicate a beam direction that passes through chordal echoes caudad to the mitral valve. If it is not possible to visualize the mitral leaflet during the dimension study, it is essential to record a chordal echo as close to the valve leaflet as possible. The far-gain of the ultrasonoscope must be adjusted to visualize a clean endocardial echo, and the near-gain is adjusted to depict the left side of the inter-

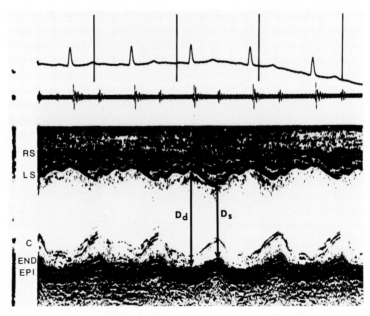

Figure 8-30. Left ventricular internal dimension (see text for details). *RS,* right side of the septum; *LS,* left side of the septum; *C,* chordae tendineae; *END,* endocardium; *EPI,* epicardium; *Dd,* end-diastolic dimension; *Ds,* end-systolic dimension.

ventricular septum. Measurements of the end-diastolic and end-systolic dimensions are made at the positions shown in Figure 8-30. The left ventricular internal end-diastolic dimension (Dd) is measured as the distance in centimeters between the left side of the septum and the left ventricular endocardium at the time of the R wave of the electrocardiogram. The left ventricular end-systolic dimension (Ds) is measured as the shortest vertical distance between the septum and endocardium.

The limitations inherent in attempting to derive volume from a single dimension of the complex left ventricular chamber was stated in one of the earliest reports[77] and has been confirmed in subsequent studies. The extrapolation of volume from the single linear measurement is based on the assumption that the ventricle is a symmetrically contracting structure with a configuration similar to a prolate ellipse. Incorrect values can be derived if there are regional areas of left ventricular asynergy or distortion of the assumed 2:1 ratio of the left ventricular long axis and transverse diameter.[80,81] Paradoxical motion of the interventricular septum precludes the echocardiographic determination of stroke volume and ejection fraction. The careful technique that is required for left ventricular dimension studies, the information that can be obtained and the errors that may occur are described in detail in a recent review.[82] If the examination is made with proper attention to technique and interpreted with background knowledge of the limitations, M-mode echocardiography can be used to obtain useful clinical information about left ventricular function.

SUMMARY

Twenty-one years after the introduction of echocardiography, this method of examination has become firmly established as an important technique for the diagnosis of cardiovascular disease. Today, a hospital or clinic that does not have facilities for echocardiographic examination cannot be considered an up-to-date diagnositc facility. In this chapter the techniques employed in the echocardiographic examination are reviewed. However, proficiency in performing studies and interpreting the echocardiographic patterns requires a long period of training and experience. When properly employed, the ultrasonic examination can detect abnormalities of cardiac function and structure that previously could be defined only by cardiac catheterization and angiocardiography. Even in situations in which the necessity for invasive studies is not obviated, the ultrasound examination will frequently provide information that supplements the data obtained in the catheterization laboratory.

There is no evidence that immediate or late harm results from the ultrasonic energy used in echocardiography. Therefore, repeated examinations can be performed to detect changes in anatomic structures and cardiac hemodynamics.

Reflected ultrasound has been used to study normal and abnormal motion of all four cardiac valves, define boundaries of the cardiac chambers and great vessels, detect pericardial effusion and evaluate certain aspects of ventricular function. We can anticipate that the development of new imaging systems will result in echocardiography becoming even more important in clinical cardiology. However, the value of M-mode echocardiography cannot be denied. Even if there were to be no further developments, Edler and Hertz made a remarkable contribution to cardiology in 1954.[1]

REFERENCES

1. Edler, I., and Hertz, C. H.: The use of ultrasonic reflectoscope for the continuous recording of movement of heart walls. Kungl. Fysiogr. Sallsk. i Lund Forhandl. 24:5, 1954.
2. Joyner, C. R., and Reid, J. M.: Applications of ultrasound in cardiology and cardiovascular physiology. Prog. Cardiovasc. Dis. 5:42, 1963.
3. Wells, P. N. T.: Physical Principles of Ultra-

sonic Diagnosis. New York, Academic Press, 1969.

4. Feigenbaum, H.: Clinical applications of echocardiography. Prog. Cardiovasc. Dis. 14:531, 1972.

5. Ludwig, G. D.: The velocity of sound through tissues and the acoustic impedance of tissues. J. Acoust. Soc. Am. 22:862, 1950.

6. Gramiak, R., Nanda, N. C., and Shah, P. M.: Echocardiographic detection of the pulmonary valve. Radiology 102:153, 1972.

7. Edler, I., and Gustafson, A.: Ultrasonic cardiogram in mitral stenosis. Acta Med. Scand. 159:85, 1957.

8. Edler, I., Gustafson, A., Karlefors, T., and Christensson, B.: Ultrasound Cardiography. Acta Med. Scand. (Suppl.) 370:1, 1961.

9. Joyner, C. R., Reid, J. M., and Bond, J. T.: Reflected ultrasound in the assessment of mitral valve disease. Circulation 27:506, 1963.

10. Joyner, C. R., and Reid, J. M.: Ultrasound cardiogram in the selection of patients for mitral valve surgery. Ann. N.Y. Acad. Sci. 118:512, 1965.

11. Segal, B. L., Likoff, W., and Kingsley, B.: Echocardiography—Clinical application in mitral stenosis. J.A.M.A. 195:161, 1966.

12. Zaky, A., Nasser, W., and Feigenbaum, H.: A study of mitral valve action recorded by reflected ultrasound and its application in the diagnosis of mitral stenosis. Circulation 37:789, 1968.

13. Shah, P. M., Gramiak, R., and Kramer, D. H.: Ultrasound Localization of Left Ventricular Outflow Obstruction in Hypertrophic Obstructive Cardiomyopathy. Circulation 40:3, 1969.

14. Duchak, J. M., Chang, S., and Feigenbaum, H.: The posterior mitral valve echo and the echocardiographic diagnosis of mitral stenosis. Am. J. Cardiol. 29:628, 1972.

15. Levison, J. A., Abbasi, A. S., and Pearce, M. L.: Posterior mitral leaflet motion in mitral stenosis. Circulation 51:511, 1975.

16. Joyner, C. R., Dyrda, I., Barrett, J. S., and Reid, J. M.: Preoperative determination of the functional anatomy of the mitral valve. Circulation 32:120, 1965.

17. Nanda, N. C., Gramiak, R., Shah, P. M., and DeWeese, J. A.: Mitral commissurotomy versus replacement—Preoperative evaluation by echocardiography. Circulation 51:263, 1975.

18. Edler, I.: Mitral valve functions studied by the ultrasound echo method. *In* Diagnostic Ultrasound, edited by C. Grossman, J. Holmes, C. Joyner, and E. Purnell. New York, Plenum Press, 1966.

19. Duchak, J. M., Chang, S., and Feigenbaum, H.: Echocardiographic features of torn chordae tendineae. Am. J. Cardiol. 29:260, 1972.

20. Sweatman, T., et al.: Echocardiographic diagnosis of mitral regurgitation due to ruptured chordae tendineae. Circulation 46:580, 1970.

21. Dillon, J., Haine, C., Chang, S., and Feigen-baum, H.: Use of echocardiography in patients with prolapsed mitral valve. Circulation 43:503, 1971.

22. Kerber, R. E., Isaeff, D. M., and Hancock, E. W.: Echocardiographic patterns in patients with the syndrome of systolic click and late systolic murmur. N. Engl. J. Med. 284:691, 1971.

23. DeMaria, A. N., et al.: The variable spectrum of echocardiographic manifestations of the mitral valve prolapse syndrome. Circulation 50:33, 1974.

24. Popp, R. L., Brown, O. R., Silverman, J. F., and Harrison, D. C.: Echocardiographic abnormalities in the mitral valve prolapse syndrome. Circulation 49:428, 1974.

25. Dillon, J. C., et al.: Echocardiographic manifestations of valvular vegetations. Am. Heart J. 86:698, 1973.

26. Joyner, C. R., Dyrda, I., and Reid, J. M.: The behavior of the anterior leaflet of the mitral valve in patients with the Austin Flint murmur. Clin. Res. 14:251, 1966.

27. Winsberg, F. et al.: Fluttering of the mitral valve in aortic insufficiency. Circulation 41:225, 1970.

28. Fortuin, N. J., and Craige, E.: On the mechanism of the Austin Flint murmur. Circulation 45:558, 1972.

29. Pridie, R. B., Benham, R., and Oakley, C. M.: Echocardiography of the mitral valve in aortic valve disease. Br. Heart J. 33:296, 1971.

30. Popp, R. L., and Harrison, D. C.: Ultrasound in the diagnosis and evaluation of therapy of idiopathic hypertrophic subaortic stenosis. Circulation 40:905, 1969.

31. Abbasi, A., MacAlpin, R. N., Eber, L. M., and Pearce, M. L.: Echocardiographic diagnosis of idiopathic hypertrophic cardiomyopathy without outflow obstruction. Circulation 46:897, 1972.

32. Henry, W. L., Clark, C. E., and Epstein, S. E.: Asymmetrical septal hypertrophy: Echocardiographic identification of the pathognomonic anatomic abnormality of idiopathic hypertrophic subaortic stenosis. Circulation 47:225, 1973.

33. Rossen, R., Goodman, D., Ingham, R., and Popp, R.: Echocardiographic criteria in the diagnosis of idiopathic hypertrophic suboartic stenosis. Circulation 50:747, 1974.

34. Rossen, R., Goodman, D., Ingham, R., and Popp, R.: Ventricular systolic septal thickening and excursion in idiopathic hypertrophic subaortic stenosis. N. Engl. J. Med. 291:1317, 1974.

35. Goodman, D., Harrison, D., and Popp, R.: Echocardiographic features of primary pulmonary hypertension. Am. J. Cardiol. 33:438, 1974.

36. Effert, S., and Domanig, E.: Diagnosis of Intra-atrial tumors by the ultrasonic echo method. Ger. Med. Mon. 4:1, 1959.

37. Wolfe, S. B., Popp, R. L., and Feigenbaum, H.: Diagnosis of atrial tumors by ultrasound. Circulation 29:615, 1969.

38. MacVaugh, H., and Joyner, C. R.: Mitral insufficiency due to calcified myxoma: Treated

by resection and mitral annuloplasty. J. Thorac. Cardiovasc. Surg. 61:287, 1971.

39. Schwarz, G. A., Schwartzman, R. J., and Joyner, C. R.: Atrial myxoma—Cause of embolic stroke. Neurology 22:1112, 1972.

40. Joyner, C. R.: Echocardiography (editorial). Circulation 46:835, 1972.

41. Joyner, C. R., et al.: Reflected ultrasound in the diagnosis of tricuspid stenosis. Am. J. Cardiol. 19:66, 1967.

42. Gramiak, R., and Shah, P. M.: Echocardiography of the normal and diseased aortic valve. Radiology 96:1, 1970.

43. Feizi, O., Symons, C., and Yacoub, M.: Echocardiography of the aortic valve—Studies of normal aortic valve, aortic stenosis, aortic regurgitation and mixed aortic valve disease. Br. Heart J. 36:341, 1974.

44. Gramiak, R. and Shah, P. M.: Echocardiography of the left ventricular outflow tract and aortic valve. *In* Ultrasound in the Diagnosis of Cardiovascular-Pulmonary Disease, edited by C. R. Joyner. Chicago, Year Book Medical Publishers, 1974.

45. Yeh, H. C., Winsberg, F., and Mercer, E.: Echographic aortic valve orifice dimension: Its use in evaluating aortic stenosis and cardiac output. J. Clin. Ultrasound 1:182, 1973.

46. Nanda, N., et al.: Echocardiographic recognition of the congenital bicuspid aortic valve. Circulation 49:870, 1974.

47. Gramiak, R., and Shah, P. M.: Cardiac ultrasonography: A review of current applications. Radiol. Clin. North Am. 9:3, 1971.

48. Davis, R., et al.: Echocardiographic manifestations of discrete subaortic stenosis. Am. J. Cardiol. 33:277, 1974.

49. Nanda, N. C., Gramiak, R., Robinson, T., and Shah, P. M.: Echocardiographic evaluation of pulmonary hypertension. Circulation 50:575, 1974.

50. Edler, I.: Diagnostic use of ultrasound in heart disease. Acta Med. Scand. (Suppl) 308:32, 1955.

51. Feigenbaum H., Waldhausen, J., and Hyde, L. P.: Ultrasound in diagnosis of pericardial effusion. J.A.M.A. 191:107, 1965.

52. Soulen, R. H., Lapayo, W., Kerm, S., and Gimenez, J. L.: Echocardiography in the diagnosis of pericardial effusion. Radiology 86:1047, 1966.

53. Klein, J. J., and Segal, B. L.: Pericardial effusion diagnosed by reflected ultrasound. Am. J. Cardiol. 22:57, 1968.

54. Feigenbaum, H.: Echocardiographic diagnosis of pericardial effusion. Am. J. Cardiol. 26:475, 1970.

55. Casarella, W. J., and Schneider, B. O.: Pitfalls in the ultrasonic diagnosis of pericardial effusion. Am. J. Roentgenol. Radium Ther. Nucl. Med. 110:760, 1970.

56. Diamond, M. A., et al.: Echocardiographic features of atrial septal defect. Circulation 43:129, 1971.

57. Assad-Morell, J., Tajik, A., and Giuliani, E.: Echocardiographic analysis of ventricular septum. Prog. Cardiovasc. Dis. 17:219, 1974.

58. Kerber, R. E., Dippel, W. F., and Abboud, F. M.: Abnormal motion of the interventricular septum in right ventricular volume overload. Circulation 48:86, 1973.

59. Hagan, A. D., et al.: Ultrasound evaluation of systolic anterior septal motion in patients with and without right ventricular volume overload. Circulation 50:248, 1974.

60. McDonal, G. I.: Echocardiographic demonstration of abnormal motion of the interventricular septum in left bundle branch block. Circulation 48:272, 1973.

61. Crews, T. L., Pridie, R. B., Denham, R., and Leatham, A.: Auscultatory and phonocardiographic findings in Ebstein's anomaly. Am. Heart J. 34:681, 1972.

62. Lundstrum, N.: Echocardiography in the diagnosis of Ebstein's anomaly of the tricuspid valve. Circulation 47:597, 1973.

63. Tajik, A. J., et al.: Echocardiogram in Ebstein's anomaly with Wolff-Parkinson-White pre-excitation syndrome. Type B. Circulation 47:813, 1973.

64. Chung, K. J., Alexson, C. C., Manning, J., and Gramiak, R.: Echocardiography in truncus arteriosus. The value of pulmonic valve detection. Circulation 48:281, 1973.

65. Chesler, E., Joffe, H., Beck, W., and Schrire, V.: Echocardiographic recognition of mitral-semilunar valve discontinuity. Circulation 43:725, 1971.

66. Meyer, R. A., and Kaplan, S.: Non-invasive technics in pediatric cardiovascular disease. Prog. Cardiovasc. Dis. 15:341, 1973.

67. Meyer, R. A., and Kaplan, S.: Echocardiography in the diagnosis of hypoplasia of the left or right ventricles in the neonate. Circulation 46:55, 1972.

68. Godman, M., Tham, P., and Langford-Kidd, B.: Echocardiography in the evaluation of the cyanotic newborn infant. Br. Heart J. 36:154, 1974.

69. Gramiak, R., Chung, K. J., Nanda, N., and Manning, J.: Echocardiographic diagnosis of transposition of the great vessels. Radiology 106:187, 1973.

70. King, D. L., Steeg, C. N., and Ellis, K.: Demonstration of transposition of the great arteries by cardiac ultrasonography. Radiology 107:181, 1973.

71. Jacobs, J. J., Feigenbaum, H., Corya, B., and Phillips, J.: Detection of left ventricular asynergy by echocardiography. Circulation 48:263, 1973.

72. Peterson, J. L., Johnston, W., Hessel, E. A., and Murray, J. A.: Echocardiographic recognition of left ventricular aneurysm. Am. Heart J. 83:244, 1972.

73. Feigenbaum, H.: Echocardiographic examination of the left ventricle. Circulation 51:1, 1975.

74. Pombo, J. F., Troy, B. L., and Russell,

R. O.: Left ventricular volumes and ejection fraction by echocardiography. Circulation 43:480, 1971.

75. Fortuin, N. J., Hood, W. P., Sherman, M. E., and Craige, E.: Determination of left ventricular volumes by ultrasound. Circulation 44:575, 1971.

76. Belenkie, I., et al.: Assessment of left ventricular dimensions and functions by echocardiography. Am. J. Cardiol. 31:755, 1973.

77. Popp, R. L., and Harrison, D. C.: Ultrasonic cardiac echography for determining stroke volume and valvular regurgitation. Circulation 41:493, 1970.

78. Fortuin, N. J., Hood, W. P., and Craige, E.: Evaluation of left ventricular function by echocardiography. Circulation 46:26, 1972.

79. Cooper, R. H., et al.: Comparison of ultrasound in cineangiographic measurements of the mean rate of circumferential fiber shortening in man. Circulation 46:914, 1972.

80. Teichholz, L. E., Kreulen, T. H., Herman, M. D., and Gorlin, R.: Problems in echocardiographic volume determinations: Echo-angiographic correlation. Circulation 46:1175, 1972.

81. Popp, R. L., Alderman, E. L., Brown, O. R., and Harrison, D. C.: Sources of error in calculation of left ventricular volumes by echography. Am. J. Cardiol. 31:152, 1973.

82. Popp, R. L., and Harrison, D. C.: Cardiac chamber size and volume: Echographic measurement of cardiac chamber dimensions, volume and ventricular function. *In* Ultrasound in the Diagnosis of Cardiovascular Pulmonary Disease, edited by C. R. Joyner. Chicago, Yearbook Medical Publishers, 1974.

Chapter 9

Phonocardiography[*]

MORTON E. TAVEL

Phonocardiography may be defined as the graphic representation of the sounds and pulses that originate in the heart and great vessels.[1] The sounds may be picked up from the surface of the body or, more directly, by placing a suitable apparatus within the heart or vascular structure where sound originates. In the ensuing discussion, I shall be concerned exclusively with the sounds as they are recorded from the body surface, corresponding to what the clinician hears through a stethoscope at the bedside. Although pulse recording comprises a part of phonocardiography, it will be dealt with herein only as an adjunct to sound recording.

There are three reasons why phonocardiography is performed: (1) To teach cardiac auscultation, (2) to provide diagnostic information that is difficult or impossible to obtain through auscultation, (3) to provide a permanent record with which subsequent comparison can be made. Recording heart sounds in a visual fashion allows one to correlate between auditory and visual representation. The student can then return to the bedside to reconstruct each perceptual phenomenon as it would appear if it were graphically recorded. Such a process enhances one's accuracy in predicting the graphic visual appearance and thereby sharpens diagnostic accuracy. Although most cardiac sounds and murmurs can be accurately recorded, these recordings are not a total substitute for the ear. The human ear is generally far more sensitive and discriminating than is a machine. Graphic recording is especially poor in the case of high-pitched murmurs such as those of aortic and mitral insufficiency, which if soft enough, tend to be lost in the baseline of most records and difficult to distinguish from ambient noise. Phonocardiography is more useful in recording low-frequency events such as gallop sounds and diastolic rumbles, the frequency range of which lies in an area difficult to perceive by ear. The phonocardiogram is especially accurate in the timing of sounds and other events, often with the aid of simultaneous pulse curves. Phonocardiography therefore provides an excellent adjunct to—but not a substitute for—bedside cardiovascular examination.

* Supported in part by the Herman C. Krannert Fund and by Grants HL-06308, HL-05363 and HL-05749 from the National Heart and Lung Institute of the National Institutes of Health, U.S. Public Health Service and the Indiana Heart Association.

171

Principles of Sound and Pulse Recording. Although human hearing ranges through a broad spectrum of 20 to 20,000 cycles per second, heart sounds and murmurs fall largely within the range of 20 to 300 cycles per second. After sonic vibrations are produced within the heart or great vessels, they are conducted outward through the tissues in a complex fashion, and most of the vibratory energy is propagated through the body tissue in the form of "transverse shear waves" that have a velocity of approximately 20 meters per second.[2] These waves are best conducted from the heart to the surface of the chest where the myocardial tissue lies in apposition to the chest wall, i.e., where the combination forms a relatively homogeneous mass through which conduction is best.

Standard phonocardiographic equipment registers waves and oscillations about a baseline. Upper deflections represent rela-

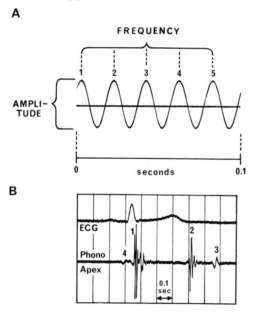

A, Oscillographic recording of a pure tone (sine wave), as might be produced by a tuning fork. **B,** Actual recording of heart sounds. Oscillations within the heart sounds are an uneven mixture of different frequencies and amplitudes.

Figure 9-1. A, Oscillographic recording of a pure tone (sine wave), as might be produced by a tuning fork. *B,* Actual recording of heart sounds. Oscillations within the heart sounds are an uneven mixture of different frequencies and amplitudes. (From Tavel, M. E.: Clinical phonocardiography. II. Its use in the evaluation of aortic stenosis. JAMA *202:*1093, 1967.)

tively high pressures, and downward deflections reflect low pressures, with respect to the medium in its resting state (Fig. 9-1A). Cardiovascular sound is basically a heterogeneous mixture of frequencies and generally "nonmusical" in nature, i.e., having no series of overtones with an arithmetic relationship to the fundamental tone. For this reason the oscillations and graphic recordings do not appear regular and smooth as one might see with a tuning fork or a musical instrument (Fig. 9-1B). Accurate breakdown of frequency components is not possible with commonly used equipment. For clinical purposes one is concerned primarily with the "outline" of sounds and murmurs, to wit, the point at which these phenomena begin and end, and whether a murmur is diamond shaped, plateau, etc.

In the cardiovascular system, low-frequency waves are produced and propagated to the skin surface in greater amplitude than are the higher frequencies. Consequently measurements made at the surface contain infrasonic components (0 to 20 CPS) of far greater magnitude than the audible sounds. Attempts to record the high-frequency sound vibrations are technically difficult since, in order to reduce the instrument's sensitivity to accommodate the large amplitude of the low-frequency waves, the relatively insignificant amplitudes of the superimposed audible sound are virtually lost from the record. Such a broad spectrum, or *linear*, recording will appear to be a slightly "tremulous" record of the low-frequency pulse waves, and the high-frequency data will be, for the most part, unreadable. One may, however, by the use of a filter, eliminate the infrasonic waves and then increase the instrument's sensitivity to allow measurement and interpretation of the audible data (Fig. 9-2).

All generally used phonocardiographic machines contain filters, which are electronic devices designed to eliminate vibrations of certain frequencies, primarily those

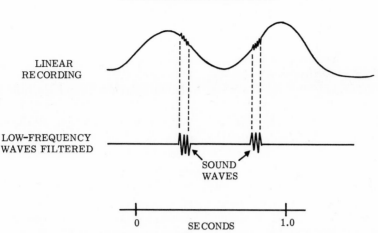

Figure 9-2. Schematic representation of the effect of a filter designed to rid the tracing of low-frequency vibrations. *Above,* "Linear" recording, i.e., a record that faithfully reproduces all waves in the same relative amplitudes as they might occur on the surface of the body. *Below,* After the large low-frequency waves have been eliminated with a filter, the higher-frequency sound waves can be amplified and studied in detail. (From CLINICAL PHONOCARDIOGRAPHY AND EXTERNAL PULSE RECORDING, 2nd ed. by Tavel, M. E. Copyright © 1972 by Year Book Medical Publishers, Inc., Chicago. Used by permission.)

in the lower range. The so-called high-pass filter allows only high-frequency waves to "pass" and to be registered (Fig. 9-3). A low-pass filter allows only registration of the low-frequency waves. Because of the natural dominance of low-frequency waves, it is generally not absolutely necessary to filter out the high-frequency waves, and therefore, low-pass filters are not necessary in clinical practice. A band-pass filter is that which allows only a certain frequency range to be registered, and it attenuates waves of frequencies above or below this range. Some machines employ multiple band-pass ranges in order to allow the clinician to obtain some idea where the major spectral energy of a sound or murmur lies. The rate at which waves are attenuated outside of the filter range is variable from filter to filter. With any specific filter, one

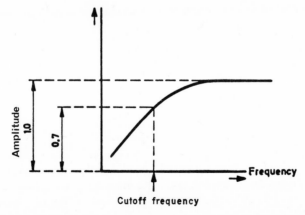

Figure 9-3. Typical characteristics of a high-pass filter. Above the cutoff frequency the waves are allowed to pass and be recorded with little loss of amplitude. The cutoff frequency is defined as the point at which the waves are reduced to an amplitude of 0.7 (minus 3 db.) of the original wave size. Below the cutoff frequency the lower frequencies are attenuated to a greater degree, the slope of which depends upon the characteristics of the specific filter.

can draw a curve that represents the intensity of waves of all frequencies that are allowed to pass. The so-called cutoff frequency is defined as the frequency in which the input is attenuated by 3 decibels. The further one moves into the filtered frequency spectrum the smaller becomes the recorded amplitude of the oscillations. The steepness of this filtration phenomenon, or rate of attenuation, is expressed in terms of decibels per octave, denoting the rate of intensity reduction for each octave above or below a given cutoff frequency. All filters tend to distort sounds to some extent; however, the steeper the filter's slope of attenuation, the greater will be this tendency to distort. As a rule, the best practical compromise is to use high-pass filters that have cutoff points in the low-frequency range and gradual slopes of attenuation.[3]

The human ear also functions as a filter. In general, it acts much as a high-pass filter, allowing higher frequency sounds to traverse the tympanic membrane and reach the brain with greater intensity than those in the lower frequencies. In order to obtain graphic recordings that approximate the sensory response, therefore, one must employ some filtration in the lower frequencies. This is especially important when phonocardiography is used for teaching purposes.

Recording Equipment. A phonocardiographic recorder is composed of four parts: (1) the microphone, (2) the amplifier, (3) the galvanometer and (4) the device used to print out the record.

The microphone converts the sound vibrations into electrical energy. The amplifier is an electronic apparatus that functions to amplify the electrical impulses coming from the microphone. The galvanometer is usually a moving coil that oscillates in response to the amplified electrical impulses. The oscillating part of the galvanometer is usually attached to some type of writing arm or mirror that inscribes the oscillations on a suitable moving-strip chart. The cathode-ray tube may also be used for this purpose. Galvanometers that are equipped with mirrors and register photographically or possess ink jets have relatively little inertia and therefore are capable of responding to all the sound frequencies of importance in cardiovascular work. On the other hand, some galvanometers are equipped for direct writing similar to an electrocardiographic machine, and possess considerable inertia. These machines are generally incapable of responding to the higher cardiovascular sound frequencies. For this reason they usually are supplied with internal correcting devices that allow the slower moving machine stylus to represent the amplitude of the higher frequency incoming waves. The machine actually records an outline or an "envelope" of the higher frequency sounds and murmurs, a display that is adequate for clinical use.

Technique of Recording. A quiet room should be used for recording. Two or more simultaneous channels must be available for recording. One channel should be capable of recording the electrocardiogram or the low-frequency pulse waves, while one or more channels record the sounds. It is helpful to have an oscilloscope available, allowing one to inspect visually the various registered phenomena prior to their graphic recording. It is also helpful to have a rapid writing process available, allowing for the immediate inspection of the registered signals. Recording speed generally ranges from 50 to 100 mm. per second, depending upon what type of information is desired.

Microphones are best applied to the chest wall by permitting them to lie free on the chest or afixing them to the chest surface with elastic straps or an Ace bandage.

Our recording technique encompasses the use of two or more simultaneously recorded sound channels from various locations on the surface of the chest, usually representing standard areas of auscultation (Fig. 9-4). Low-, medium- and high-frequency recordings are usually made. Although most recordings are made with held expiration, at least one tracing is taken from the pulmonary area during normal quiet breathing. In addition to sounds, various reference pulse tracings are recorded. These reference tracings include a carotid pulse, the jugular pulse and the apexcardiogram.

Accurate calibration of sound intensity is generally impractical. We have found it far more satisfactory to adjust the machine's gain by increasing the amplitude as much as possible, while still allowing a smooth baseline. This can be accomplished by gradually increasing the amplitude until the baseline (represented by quiet phases of the cardiac cycle) first becomes impure and then reducing the sensitivity to a level just below that point.

Ideally, the physician himself should record the phonocardiogram, but a well-trained technician can make reasonably good records. Under these circumstances, the physician should be available to instruct the technician, to perform provocative maneuvers if necessary and to check the quality of the record upon its completion.

Technique of Reading Phonocardiograms. Graphic recordings are best interpreted as part of the clinical evaluation. The interpreter should have prior knowledge of the results of the bedside examination and some grasp of the problems in need of solution. If possible, he should personally perform auscultation on the subject around the time of the recording. The greatest problem confronting the neophyte is in the separation of artifacts from cardiovascular sounds. To accomplish this, numerous cycles should be examined, and if the vibrations in question consistently parallel the cardiac cycle, they may be generally considered to be cardiovascular in origin. Artifacts such as bowel sounds or muscle movements do not bear this consistency.

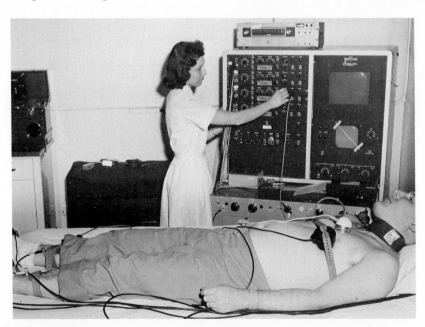

Figure 9-4. Recording a phonocardiogram. Microphones are allowed to lie free on flat portions of the chest (pulmonary area) or, where necessary, are affixed with an elastic strap (apex). Reference tracings include ECG (standard lead) and pulse tracing (carotid pulse being recorded via loosely applied neck cuff).

When one measures the timing of a sound (transient), he always uses the *onset* of the series of vibrations as the reference point.

HEART SOUNDS (TRANSIENTS)

First Heart Sound. This sound is normally composed of four major components (Fig. 9-5): (1) small low-frequency initial vibrations, which are probably caused by muscular contraction in the earliest phase of ventricular systole; (2) a group of larger, high-frequency vibrations caused by tension on the mitral valve and surrounding structures as it completes its closure; (3) a second group of high-frequency vibrations that follow the initial component by about 0.03 second (this sound probably relates to tricuspid closure,[4,5] although a contribution from early ejection into the great vessels may also play a major role); (4) small low-frequency vibrations that coincide with the acceleration of blood into the great vessels.

The entire first sound usually lasts from about 0.1 to 0.12 second, but at ausculta-

tion one usually hears only the two higher frequency components, i.e., the second and third components. Although numerous factors influence the intensity of the first sound, such as inotropic state, of major importance is the degree of opening of the atrioventricular valves at the time of ventricular systole. When the PR interval is less than 0.20 second, these valves are open at the onset of systole and the first sound is well heard (intensity and degree of opening vary inversely with the PR interval). When the P-R interval is 0.2 to 0.5 second, the first sound is virtually absent, owing to closure of the atrioventricular valves prior to ventricular systole. If the P-R interval becomes greater than 0.5 second, the atrioventricular valves are allowed to reopen at the time of ventricular systole.[5]

In mitral stenosis the high left atrial pressure maintains the mitral leaflets in a fully open position at the time of ventricular systole, resulting in a large rapid excursion of closure and a loud first sound.

The time elapsing from the onset of the

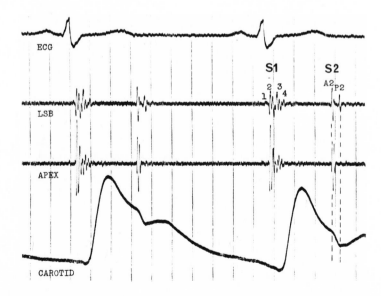

Figure 9-5. Normal first and second heart sounds recorded simultaneously from the lower left sternal border (*LSB*) and apex. The first sound (S_1) is divided into four components (*1* to *4*) and the second sound (S_2) into two (A_2 and P_2). ECG and carotid pulse included for reference (see text for explanation). (From CLINICAL PHONOCARDIOGRAPHY AND EXTERNAL PULSE RECORDING, 2nd ed. by Tavel, M. E. Copyright © by Year Book Medical Publishers, Inc., Chicago. Used by permission.)

Q wave to the beginning of the mitral first sound is designated the Q-1 interval. Mitral stenosis prolongs the interval in an amount roughly proportional to the diastolic pressure gradient across the mitral valve. The normal interval ranges from 0.03 to 0.07 second, and if the interval is prolonged greater than 0.07 second, significant mitral obstruction is usually present, and if 0.1 second or longer, the mitral valve area is likely to be 1.2 sq. cm. or less.[6]

Second Heart Sound. Sudden tension on the semilunar valve leaflets and surrounding structures following semilunar closure gives rise to the second heart sound. This sound is normally split sequentially into aortic followed by pulmonic component (Fig. 9-5). Quiet respiration increases the splitting interval up to 0.08 second, whereas during expiration the components are superimposed or split by 0.03 second or less. On held expiration, the splitting interval becomes slightly wider than during the expiratory phase of quiet respiration, but the splitting does not exceed 0.04 second.

Splitting of the second heart sound becomes less apparent or absent with advancing age, possibly owing to earlier and softer closure of the pulmonic valve.

Aortic closure is normally loud and radiates over the entire precordium. In a given patient, it precedes the dicrotic notch by a constant interval (range 0.02 to 0.05 second), depending upon the time required for the pulse wave to reach the neck. Pulmonic closure, on the other hand, is recorded normally only at the pulmonic area and below along the left sternal border and bears an inconstant relationship to the dicrotic notch.

Increases of relative intensity of either component may be brought about by hypertension within the systemic or pulmonary circuit, and decreases may be caused by hypotension within these vessels. Calcification of aortic or pulmonic valves may also cause softening of their closure.

Wide splitting of the components is usually brought about by late pulmonic closure, as seen in such conditions as volume overload of the right ventricle (i.e., atrial septal defect) or in complete right bundle branch block, wherein the electrical activation is delayed in the right heart. In the case of atrial septal defect the splitting is not only wide, but it is also "fixed," i.e., varying by less than 0.02 second with phases of respiration. Reversed splitting is usually caused by delay in aortic closure, as seen in left bundle branch block or aortic stenosis, and is recognized on graphic recordings by positive identification of sound components, i.e., their relationship to the arterial dicrotic notch, radiation to the apex and behavior with respiration.

Third Heart Sound. Third heart sounds are low-frequency events occurring 0.1 to 0.2 second after aortic closure and usually are seen best at the apex (Fig. 9-6; see also Fig. 9-17). They usually emanate from the left ventricle and coincide with the peak of the rapid filling wave on the apexcardiogram. When coming from the right ventricle, they are usually registered best at the lower left sternal border and coincide with a deep jugular Y trough. At present there is no practical way to distinguish patholo-

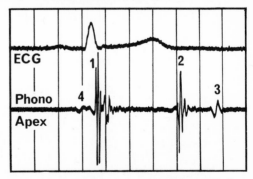

Figure 9-6. Third and fourth heart sounds in a normal individual. Time lines, 0.1 second (see text for explanation). (From CLINICAL PHONO-CARDIOGRAPHY AND EXTERNAL PULSE RE-CORDING, 2nd ed. by Tavel, M. E. Copyright © 1972 by Year Book Medical Publishers, Inc., Chicago. Used by permission.)

gic from physiologic third heart sounds phonocardiographically. Associated findings, such as abnormal systolic time intervals, marked accentuation of the apexcardiographic rapid filling wave or other signs of cardiac disease are most helpful in this regard.

Fourth Heart Sound. Fourth heart sounds are low-frequency vibrations coinciding with the a wave of the apexcardiogram (Fig. 9-6; see also Fig. 9-12). Originating in the left ventricle, they can usually be recorded at the apex (but probably not heard) in normal individuals if low-frequency filtration is employed. Therefore they cannot in themselves be considered pathologic. If the apical a wave is accentuated, however (greater than 15% of the total apex deflection), then the fourth heart sound is usually more easily recorded and more apt to be heard. These fourth heart sounds should be considered pathologic.

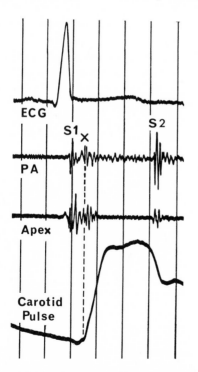

Figure 9-7. Ejection sound (X) in a patient with hypertension secondary to coarctation of aorta. Note that the sound's onset coincides with the onset of the carotid rise.

Right ventricular fourth heart sounds are occasionally seen and are best seen at the lower left sternal border, coinciding usually with a large jugular a wave.

Ejection Sounds (Clicks). Ejection sounds are high-frequency transients that follow the first heart sound, coinciding with the onset of ventricular ejection (Fig. 9-7). Their mechanism is twofold:[7] (1) sudden checking of the opening motion of stenotic aortic or pulmonic valves or (2) abrupt onset of pressure rise in the aorta or pulmonary artery, as might be found when the left or right ventricular pressures rise rapidly. The latter origin may simply represent intensification of the normally split first heart sound.

When these sounds have a valvular origin they often occur somewhat late, following the mitral first sound by 0.04 second or more. Valvular aortic sounds usually coincide with the onset of the carotid rise, whereas those originating in the aortic root may precede the rise by up to 0.03 second. Pulmonic ejection sounds may or may not coincide with the arterial upstroke. Since early ejection sounds closely resemble physiologic splitting of the first sound, their recognition in graphic records may be difficult or arbitrary. Their presence is suggested if they follow the mitral first sound by 0.04 second or more or radiate strongly to the base. In the case of pulmonic stenosis they often show marked inspiratory diminution or disappearance (see below).

Systolic "Nonejection" Sounds. Sounds occurring in mid or late systole are termed nonejection clicks.[8] These sounds are thought usually to result from mitral prolapse, and they may initiate or occur during late systolic murmurs (see Fig. 9-18). They often vary considerably in timing, occurring earlier with upright position or inspiration,[9] probably reflecting earlier prolapse as ventricular volume is decreased. Although nonejection clicks usually occur later in systole than do ejection sounds

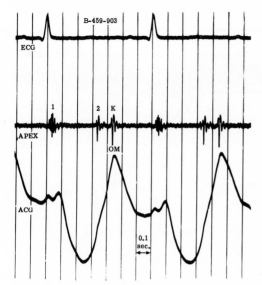

Figure 9-8. Pericardial knock in pericardial constriction. Following the second heart sound (2) by 0.1 second is a mid-frequency sound, the pericardial knock (*K*). Note also the apexcardiogram, which displays a systolic retraction and a sharp, early diastolic outward motion that stops abruptly at the time of the knock. (Tavel, M. E., and Stewart, J.: Usefulness and limitations of precordial phonocardiography and external pulse recordings. Cardiovasc. Clin. 6:41, 1974.)

(following well after the carotid rise), they occasionally appear early.[10] Usually they can be distinguished from ejection sounds by their tendency to vary with respiration.

Opening Snaps. The opening snap is usually caused by mitral stenosis and is a sharp, high-frequency transient following aortic closure by 0.04 to 0.13 second (see

Fig. 9-15). It is widely recorded but often best seen at the lower left sternal border. It corresponds with the 0 point of the apexcardiogram and is best distinguished from the split second heart sound by its greater radiation and lack of respiratory variation.

Miscellaneous Diastolic Sounds. Several varieties of diastolic sounds have been described.[11,12] The pericardial "knock" is a mid-frequency sound, following aortic closure by 0.09 to 0.12 second (Fig. 9-8). It is seen in constrictive pericarditis and corresponds to sudden arrest of ventricular expansion in early diastole.

The "tumor plop" is a low- to mid-frequency sound that also follows the second sound by about 0.08 to 0.13 second. It is seen in atrial myxoma and represents sudden checking of forward motion of the tumor on its stalk as it traverses the mitral or tricuspid annulus in early diastole.

MURMURS

Murmurs comprise prolonged series of vibrations that are probably caused by turbulence of blood as it passes through an abrupt narrowing or change of cross-sectional area. Murmurs are classified according to their location in the cardiac cycle and probable mechanism of production.

Systolic murmurs are best divided into two classes, i.e., mid systolic ejection murmurs and pansystolic regurgitant murmurs[13] (Fig. 9-9).

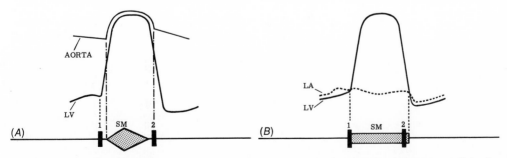

Figure 9-9. General categories of systolic murmurs. *A,* Ejection murmur. Murmur parallels flow velocity into the aorta (or pulmonary artery) with a crescendo-decrescendo pattern. *B,* Pansystolic regurgitant murmur. Prolonged plateau murmur that parallels regurgitation across mitral (or tricuspid) valve.

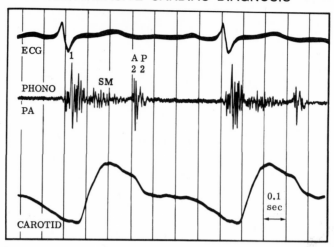

Figure 9-10. Innocent systolic ejection murmur seen at the pulmonary area (*PA*) of a normal 21-year-old man. Murmur is short and has a crescendo contour, peaking early in systole. (From CLINICAL PHONOCARDIOGRAPHY AND EXTERNAL PULSE RECORDING, 2nd ed. by Tavel, M. E. Copyright © 1972 by Year Book Medical Publishers, Inc., Chicago. Used by permission.)

Mid systolic ejection murmurs are caused by turbulence of blood as it flows through the outflow tract of the right or left ventricle. They are seen in most normal children and in many adults as well. When seen in normal individuals they are termed innocent murmurs and are short, crescendo-decrescendo murmurs that stop well before the second heart sound (Fig. 9-10).

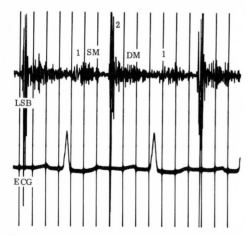

Figure 9-11. Aortic insufficiency—typical murmur. The diastolic murmur (*DM*) begins with the second heart sound (2), often intensifying slightly for a short time, but diminishing thereafter. Note the soft first heart sound and early systolic ejection murmur, both seen commonly in significant grades of aortic insufficiency.

When this type of murmur is caused by significant stenosis of the pulmonary or aortic orifice the murmur becomes longer, peaking later in systole (see below).

Pansystolic murmurs continue throughout systole and tend to encompass the second heart sound. Always abnormal, they reflect either mitral or tricuspid insufficiency or ventricular septal defect. A special subcategory of the pansystolic murmur is the so-called late systolic murmur. This murmur begins midway throughout the systolic period and continues through the second sound (see below).

Diastolic murmurs may be caused by insufficiency of the semilunar valves, in which case they begin with the second heart sound and tend to diminish throughout most of diastole (Fig. 9-11). Another category of the diastolic murmur is that related to forward flow of blood through atrioventricular valves. These murmurs begin after a brief pause following the second heart sound. When they are caused by rapid flow states, i.e., mitral insufficiency or shunt lesions with large atrioventricular flow, they usually are initiated by a third heart sound and diminish rapidly thereafter—with no subsequent presystolic accentuation. Murmurs caused by stenotic leaflets, i.e., mitral stenosis, usually begin shortly after the opening snap and generally continue throughout the remainder of diastole, intensifying prior to the next first heart sound if normal sinus rhythm is present (see Fig. 9-15).

Continuous murmurs are defined as those murmurs that continue from systole to beyond the second heart sound. They originate from vessels outside of the heart, usually from shunting of blood from a high-pressure to a low-pressure vessel, i.e., patent ductus arteriosus or peripheral arteriovenous shunt. Occasionally, high-grade obstructive lesions in the peripheral arteries can cause murmurs of this type (see below).

PHONOCARDIOGRAPHIC EVALUATION OF SPECIFIC CARDIOVASCULAR LESIONS

In the following section are presented several of the more common cardiovascular conditions in which phonocardiography may offer clinical assistance.

Valvular Aortic Stenosis. Phonocardiography provides an excellent means to obtain semiquantitative data about the presence or degree of valvular aortic obstruction. The clinician is often confronted by the patient possessing a systolic ejection murmur, often quite loud, that radiates to the carotid vessels. The phonocardiogram may help to localize the murmur to the aortic valve by demonstrating that the murmur is ejection in type (crescendo-decrescendo), that it stops before aortic closure and that it is associated with a carotid pulse that is distorted, i.e., has anacrotic notching or superimposed vibrations (shudder) or a slow rise with a prolonged ejection time (Fig. 9-12A). The presence of an aortic ejection sound helps to indicate that the obstruction is valvular in nature, although in older individuals with valvular calcification the ejection sound

may be lost, and the aortic second sound often becomes quite soft.

After one is satisfied that a given ejection murmur is emanating from the aortic outflow tract, one must then decide whether the murmur indicates significant outflow obstruction. Ejection murmurs may be totally innocent or may represent a wide spectrum of severity of aortic obstruction. Unfortunately, physical examination is often inaccurate in evaluating this problem. Phonocardiography is especially useful in identifying those patients with innocent murmurs or hemodynamically unimportant mild aortic stenosis and in separating these from the group with severe obstruction. In this connection the three most useful indices are: (1) the timing of the peak intensity of the systolic murmur, (2) the left ventricular ejection time (carotid pulse) and (3) the maximum rate of rise of the carotid pulse.[14]

The timing of the systolic murmur (Q wave of the electrocardiogram to the peak murmur intensity) is the most valuable single measure in assessing the severity. If this interval exceeds 0.24 second, the aortic stenosis is almost always severe, whereas patients with innocent murmurs do not possess intervals as long as 0.24 second.[14] Occasional patients with severe aortic stenosis, however, have values lower than 0.24 second.

Prolongation of the left ventricular ejection time also bears a significant relationship to the presence and severity of aortic stenosis when the values are corrected for rate.[14,15] If one obtains a corrected value of greater than 0.43 second, the presence of severe aortic stenosis is quite likely.[14] Occasional patients with severe aortic stenosis have values in a lower range of 0.39 to 0.43 second. Maximal rate of rise of the carotid pulse (determined indirectly) is also helpful in assessing the severity of aortic stenosis.[14] Almost all normal persons possess rates of rise greater than 500 mm. Hg per second. If the rate is 400 mm. Hg

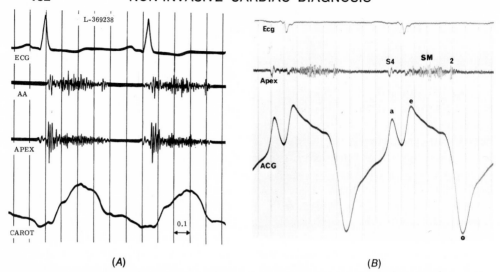

(A) *(B)*

Figure 9-12. A, Aortic stenosis, valvular, severe, in a 62-year-old man. A pressure gradient across the aortic valve measured 85 mm. Hg; the valve was calcified and barely mobile. A prolonged crescendo-decrescendo systolic murmur (*SM*) is seen, together with a slowly rising carotid pulse which has an anacrotic shoulder and superimposed coarse vibrations (shudder) near its crest. AA, aortic area; CAROT, carotid pulse. Time lines = 0.1 second.
B, Aortic stenosis, severe, with fourth heart sound (S_4) and accentuated apical a wave in the apexcardiogram (*ACG*). This patient was a 70-year-old man with a transvalvar aortic pressure gradient of 100 mm. Hg. (Tavel, M. E., and Stewart, J.: Usefulness and limitations of precordial phonocardiography and external pulse recordings. Cardiovasc. Clin. 6:41, 1974).

or less, then severe aortic stenosis is probable. Occasional patients with severe stenosis have normal rates (up to 1000 mm. Hg per second), probably indicating stiff distal arteries in an aged arteriosclerotic population. Combining the three most highly correlated indices yields the most clinically useful information, particularly in assessing severity of aortic stenosis. Values outside all three selected limits (ejection time greater than 0.42 second, maximum rate of rise less than 500 mm. Hg per second and Q peak of murmur exceeding 0.19 second) are highly suggestive of severe aortic stenosis.

The presence of a fourth heart sound and large apical a wave usually indicates a transvalvular aortic gradient of 75 mm. Hg or more (Fig. 9-12B).[16] Some workers have stated that a fourth heart sound is often present in an elderly population with arteriosclerotic heart disease, thus invalidating such a finding in those patients over

the age of 40 with suspected aortic stenosis.[17] However, our experience does not agree entirely with this conclusion.[18] We believe that, although soft fourth heart sounds may be recorded often in the normal population of all ages, when the fourth sound is fairly intense and accompanied by a large a wave (15% or more of the total height of the complex of the apexcardiogram), aortic stenosis is almost always in the severe range (greater than 75 mm. Hg gradient). Unfortunately, however, about 55% of individuals with severe aortic stenosis have small fourth sounds and normal-sized a waves.[18]

The phonocardiogram is especially helpful in suggesting the presence of aortic stenosis in patients with congestive heart failure.[19] When congestive heart failure results from tight aortic stenosis, the murmur may become quite soft, and the usual physical findings are obscured if not absent. If congestive heart failure results from myocardial disease, such as that seen in hypertensive cardiovascular disease, ischemic heart disease or primary cardiomyopathy, the pre-ejection period (PEP) is long, the left ventricular ejection time (LVET) is short, and the PEP:LVET ratio is high.[20] (PEP is the interval from beginning of QRS to carotid rise, corrected for delay in pulse transmission by subtracting A_2-dicrotic notch interval.) On the other hand, when aortic stenosis causes congestive heart failure, the pre-ejection period remains within normal range or somewhat shorter, the left ventricular ejection time tends to be prolonged, and the mean PEP:LVET ratio averages 0.24 (range 0.19 to 0.28), which is below the lower limit of normal in most cases (normal = 0.35 ± 0.08 second). In our experience, all patients fall below the accepted lower limits for congestive heart failure due to myocardial disease (0.41 second).[21] These findings are not valid in the presence of left bundle branch block, for this conduction delay causes, in itself, prolongation of the PEP.[22]

Subvalvular Aortic Stenosis, Muscular (Idiopathic Hypertrophic Subaortic Stenosis). This type of subvalvular obstruction has received increased attention in recent years, representing a relatively common form of heart disease. The obstruction to left ventricular outflow is caused by disproportionate hypertrophy of the interventricular septum in the region of the outflow tract, which, together with an anteriorly deviated anterior mitral valve leaflet, causes a dynamic, and often variable, form of obstruction to left ventricular outflow. The obstruction becomes manifest only during the middle and late phases of ventricular contraction, when the offending structures move closely together in the left ventricular outflow tract. As one might expect, the abnormal spatial orientation of the mitral valve often results in mitral insufficiency during the latter part of systole.

The murmur resulting from the aortic outflow obstruction is a prolonged, dia-mond-shaped murmur, having its maximal intensity at the lower left sternal border and apex.[23] It may be increased by certain maneuvers such as upright position, Valsalva maneuver and amyl nitrite inhalation. If a resting outflow pressure gradient is present the carotid pulse has a peculiar double peak (spike and dome) appearance, usually possessing a prolonged ejection time (Fig. 9-13). In milder cases this change can be brought to light through the use of the Valsalva maneuver or amyl nitrite. A fourth heart sound (atrial gallop) is present in about 90% of patients, reflecting the fact that the left ventricle is usually generally hypertrophied and stiff and resists diastolic filling. The apexcardiogram usually shows an accentuated a wave and in some instances a late systolic outward movement. We regard the presence of the typical murmur—together with the typical

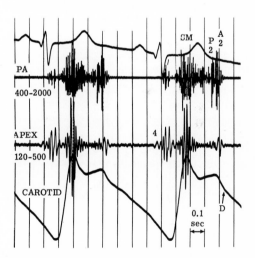

Figure 9-13. Idiopathic hypertrophic subaortic stenosis. An intense mid-systolic crescendo-decrescendo murmur (*SM*) appears at the pulmonary area (*PA*), a fourth heart sound (*4*) at the apex, and a carotid pulse, after an initial rapid rise, displays a double-peaked contour and prolonged ejection time. *D,* dicrotic notch. Because of the prolonged ejection time, reversed splitting of the second heart sound is manifest. (From CLINICAL PHONOCARDIOGRAPHY AND EXTERNAL PULSE RECORDING, 2nd ed. by Tavel, M. E. Copyright © 1972 by Year Book Medical Publishers, Inc., Chicago. Used by permission.)

bifid arterial pulse (spike and dome) and accentuated apical a waves—as being virtually diagnostic of hypertrophic subaortic stenosis. On the other hand, it is usually not possible to diagnose the coexistence of mitral insufficiency through phonocardiography, inasmuch as the murmur of subvalvular stenosis dominates the picture and probably obscures the mitral murmur.

Pulmonic Stenosis. Valvular pulmonic stenosis is a frequently encountered congenital lesion, often being discovered in young adulthood or later. The resulting murmur is ejection in type, i.e., diamond shaped and often prolonged beyond aortic closure (Fig. 9-14). The hallmark of this lesion is a delay of pulmonic closure (often marked). This component is also usually softer than normal. A pulmonic ejection sound is usually present but may appear so early that it becomes indistinguishable from the latter part of the normal first heart sound. This ejection sound may soften or disappear with inspiration, owing to premature diastolic opening of the pulmonic valve with phasic inspiratory rises

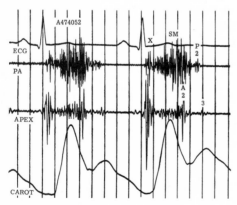

Figure 9-14. Severe valvular pulmonic stenosis in a 16-year-old boy (right ventricular systolic pressure 147 mm. Hg). A prolonged systolic ejection murmur (*SM*) follows an early systolic ejection sound (*X*) and continues beyond A_2, seen only at the apex. P_2 is soft and widely separated from A_2. Time lines = 0.1 second. (From CLINICAL PHONOCARDIOGRAPHY AND EXTERNAL PULSE RECORDING, 2nd ed. by Tavel, M. E. Copyright © 1972 by Year Book Medical Publishers, Inc., Chicago. Used by permission.)

of right ventricular diastolic pressure. The murmur contour, together with the splitting interval of the second heart sound and degree of prematurity of the ejection sound, forms a basis to evaluate the severity of pulmonic obstruction.[24,25] The phonocardiogram is especially useful in grading the severity of the outflow obstruction, inasmuch as these morphologic features and time intervals may be carefully assessed in such tracings. A fourth heart sound (right atrial gallop) indicates severe obstruction.

The murmur of pulmonic stenosis is often so prolonged that it extends well past the aortic second sound at the base, stopping before a late and soft P_2. Such a duration often evokes confusion in distinguishing this murmur from pansystolic murmurs, particularly those due to ventricular septal defects. One can usually make the distinction by noting the absence of an ejection sound and a well-preserved or loud P_2 in ventricular septal defect.

Tetralogy of Fallot also causes a pulmonary ejection systolic murmur that may, in milder cases, be prolonged.[25] This murmur, however, almost never goes beyond A_2, and P_2 is almost always totally absent from the recording, thus allowing distinction of tetralogy from both pulmonary stenosis with intact septum and ventricular septal defect without pulmonic stenosis.

Innocent Systolic Ejection Murmur. One of the most common problems in phonocardiography is in distinguishing ejection murmurs caused by organic disease from the innocent systolic murmur found in a large number of individuals of all ages.[26] The innocent murmur is a short, early systolic ejection murmur (see Fig. 9-10) that is unassociated with other markers of organic disease, such as abnormal splitting of the second sound, the ejection sound or distortion of the arterial or other pulses. These murmurs are usually recorded best over the pulmonary area or along the lower left sternal border but often are noted well at the aortic area and conducted into the arteries of the neck as well. The entire clinical examination is otherwise normal in the individual who has an innocent systolic ejection murmur.

Aortic Insufficiency. The high-frequency diastolic blowing murmur of aortic insufficiency is often difficult to record graphically; it tends to be soft and obscured by high-pitched extraneous ambient noises. Hence, mild degrees of aortic insufficiency are more easily recognized at the bedside than with phonocardiography. Grading the severity of aortic insufficiency is possible graphically in a rough fashion inasmuch as the murmur tends to diminish more rapidly with more severe gradients of insufficiency.[27] Severe degrees of insufficiency cause enlargement of the apical a wave, which tends to be abnormally broad and usually is not associated with a fourth heart sound.[28] On the other hand, as the degree of aortic insufficiency becomes even more extreme, the apical a wave may be reduced or totally lost. This latter effect results from the high left ventricular diastolic pressure, which renders atrial contraction no longer able to open the mitral valve or cause ventricular filling.

The presence of an Austin Flint murmur or a bisferious arterial pulse suggests severe insufficiency. In significant grades of insufficiency the first heart sound may be soft or absent, presumably because of premature mitral closure, which results from elevation of left ventricular diastolic pressure. Also in significant aortic insufficiency, an early systolic ejection murmur is usually found, reflecting the large stroke output of the volume-loaded left ventricle (Fig. 9-11).

Mitral Stenosis. The timing of the first heart sound and the mitral opening snap in mitral stenosis are time-honored measurements and can yield valuable information concerning the diastolic pressure gradient across the mitral valve (Fig. 9-15). As the gradient becomes higher the first sound is delayed, and the opening snap comes earlier. Various formulas have been applied in the effort to render these measurements more accurate in assessment, probably the best of which is subtraction of the 2-OS from the Q-1 intervals.[29] Several other factors must be taken into account in arriving at an accurate estimate of pressure gradient, such as the systolic

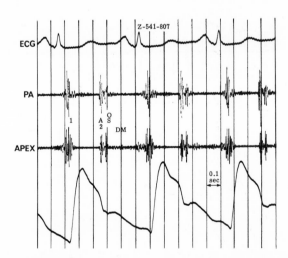

Figure 9-15. Severe mitral stenosis in a 37-year-old woman. Tracing demonstrates an intense opening snap (*OS*), which follows A_2 by about 0.05 second. A diastolic murmur (*DM*) follows the opening snap and intensifies before the first sound. (Tavel, M. E., and Stewart, J.: Usefulness and limitations of precordial phonocardiography and external pulse recording. Cardiovasc. Clin. 6:41, 1974).

systemic blood pressure, cardiac rate and presence of other lesions (e.g., aortic insufficiency or mitral insufficiency). One must realize also that, while these indices allow a prediction of gradient, they do not necessarily indicate mitral valve area. As a rule of thumb, if Q-1 — 2-OS is + 0.02 second or greater, tight mitral stenosis is almost always present. Values more negative than —0.01 second generally represent mild stenosis (valve areas greater than 1.5 sq. cm.).

Duration of the mitral rumble is of some help in predicting severity of pressure gradient, being longer with more severe stenosis. The apexcardiogram tends to show a reduced rapid filling wave in mitral stenosis[30] but is somewhat variable and, in our experience, has been limited in the prediction of severity of mitral stenosis.

Tricuspid Stenosis. The murmur of tricuspid stenosis simulates the diastolic murmur of mitral stenosis, although it is more easily recorded at the lower left sternal border (Fig. 9-16).[31] In addition, the presystolic accentuation is often earlier than that of mitral stenosis, with which it is commonly associated. The finding of two opening snaps may also suggest the concomitant presence of tricuspid stenosis. This latter finding is often difficult to recognize on graphic tracings. The jugular pulse is especially useful in the diagnosis of tricuspid stenosis, displaying large a waves and often some reduction in Y descent, with little or no subsequent diastolic rise from the Y trough.

Mitral Insufficiency. The murmur of mitral insufficiency is characteristically pansystolic, i.e., extending evenly from the first to the second heart sound (Fig. 9-17).[32] Although its contour is often even or flat, it may follow a decrescendo or crescendo pattern. Very soft murmurs are often seen in mild mitral insufficiency and tend to have a high-frequency or "blowing" quality. These murmurs may be difficult or impossible to record graphically. More severe grades of mitral insufficiency may give rise to third heart sounds that are often followed by short diastolic rumbles (without presystolic accentuation). The carotid pulse may display a single peak with a rapid fall in late systole, reflecting

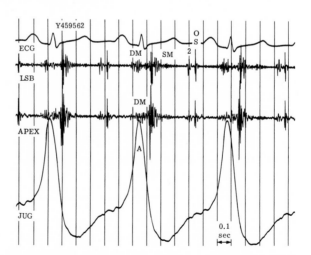

Figure 9-16. Tricuspid stenosis in a 42-year-old woman. Mitral stenosis was also present. The tricuspid diastolic murmur increases earlier, before the first sound at the left sternal border (*LSB*), in comparison to the mitral murmur seen at the apex. Note the giant jugular A waves. A single opening snap is recorded, probably originating from the mitral valve. (From CLINICAL PHONO-CARDIOGRAPHY AND EXTERNAL PULSE RECORDING, 2nd ed. by Tavel, M. E. Copyright © 1972 by Year Book Medical Publishers, Inc., Chicago. Used by permission.)

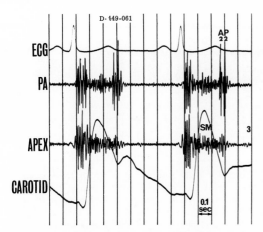

Figure 9-17. Severe mitral insufficiency in a 40-year-old man. An intense pansystolic murmur is seen. In addition, there is a third heart sound and a prominently split second heart sound (seen at pulmonic area) with an intense P_2. (Tavel, M. E., and Stewart, J.: Usefulness and limitations of precordial phonocardiography and external pulse recordings. Cardiovasc. Clin. 6:41, 1974.)

difficulty on the part of the left ventricle in sustaining forward ejection of flow throughout the latter part of systole.

When mitral insufficiency arises as a result of ballooning of one or both leaflets (usually posterior) of the mitral valve, or in association with papillary muscle dysfunction, the murmur so produced is often confined to late systole and may be associated with one or more mid systolic (nonejection) clicks (Fig. 9-18).[8] One of these clicks often introduces the late systolic murmur.

Although the fourth heart sound is not a part of the picture of chronic mitral insufficiency, when the mitral leak is recently acquired the ventricle often possesses insufficient ability to dilate. This results in a functionally "stiff," relatively small ventricle that produces a fourth heart sound in response to a vigorous left atrial contraction.[33]

Significant grades of mitral insufficiency frequently give rise to wide splitting of the second heart sound, a finding that is readily demonstrated on graphic recordings. De-

creased left ventricular stroke volume with early closure of the aortic valve accounts for the wide splitting interval in this condition.

Atrial Septal Defect. The combination of an early systolic ejection murmur plus wide, fixed splitting of the second heart sound (less than 0.02-second respiratory variation) helps the clinician confirm his suspicion of an atrial septal defect (ASD; Fig. 9-19). Unfortunately, however, the murmur itself is not distinguishable from the innocent systolic ejection murmur, and occasionally individuals with atrial septal defect have normal splitting of S_2.[34] Owing to large tricuspid flow, a mid diastolic rumble may be recorded at the lower left sternal border and laterally in patients with large left-to-right shunts. This murmur has a crescendo-decrescendo contour following pulmonic closure and seldom does one record a discrete third heart sound.[35] A peculiar jugular pulse abnormality is seen in about 40 to 50% of all patients with atrial septal defect and is characterized by high, peaked V waves (Fig. 9-16).[36] When

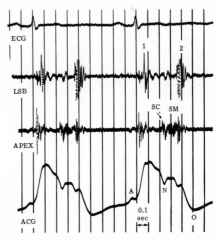

Figure 9-18. Mid systolic click (*SC*) with late systolic murmur (*SM*) in a 46-year-old asymptomatic man believed to have a prolapsing mitral valve with mitral regurgitation. The apexcardiogram (*ACG*) displays a retraction (*N*) at the time of the click. (Tavel, M. E., and Stewart, J.: Usefulness and limitations of precordial phonocardiography and external pulse recordings. Cardiovasc. Clin. 6:41, 1974).

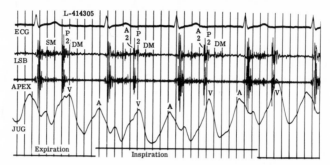

Figure 9-19. Atrial septal defect in a 24-year-old male. An early systolic ejection murmur is seen together with a widely split second sound. The splitting of the second sound shows no signifi-cant respiratory variation. A diastolic murmur (*DM*) follows P_2 and signifies a large tricuspid flow that increases with inspiration. The jugular pulse displays large V waves, typical of this condition. Times lines = 0.1 second. (Tavel, M. E., and Stewart, J.: Usefulness and limitations of precordial phonocardiography and external pulse recordings. Cardiovasc. Clin. 6:41, 1974).

present they are virtually diagnostic of atrial septal defect (or partial anomalous pulmonary venous drainage).

Because of the problems detailed above, the phonocardiogram is helpful in diagnos-ing atrial septal defect but does have some shortcomings as a screening method. In this conjunction, echocardiography is ex-

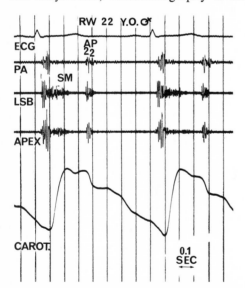

Figure 9-20. Muscular ventricular septal defect in a 22-year-old asymptomatic woman with early systolic decrescendo murmur, recorded best at the lower left sternal border. (From Tavel, M. E.: CLINICAL PHONOCARDIOGRAPHY AND EX-TERNAL PULSE RECORDING, 2nd ed. by Tavel, M. E. Copyright © 1972 by Year Book Medical Publishers, Inc., Chicago. Used by permission.)

tremely useful as a screening tool, demon-strating a large, volume-overloaded right ventricle with reversed or flat septal motion in almost all atrial septal defects with left-to-right shunting.[37]

Ventricular Septal Defect. The murmur of ventricular septal defect is typically a pansystolic murmur, recorded best along the left sternal border, maximum intensity being over the level of the defect. The mur-mur may display other contours, particu-larly if the defect is located within the mus-cular septum, in which case the murmur may display a descrescendo pattern and may stop before the second sound (Fig. 9-20).[38] If the defect is moderate to large in size the second sound may be widely split, owing to large right ventricular stroke volume with delay of pulmonic closure. The splitting usually varies with respira-tion, but the degree of variation may be abnormally small.[39] With large left-to-right shunting and large mitral flow, one fre-quently encounters a prominent left ven-tricular third heart sound, which may intro-duce a diastolic rumbling murmur. The entire picture of ventricular septal defect, with its pansystolic murmur, third heart sound and widely split second heart sound, may closely simulate the picture of mitral insufficiency. Differentiation between the two on graphic tracings may be impossible.

In this regard, other clinical findings, plus location of maximum intensity of the murmur, may be decisive in determining a correct diagnosis.

Extracardiac Murmurs (Including Patent Ductus Arteriosus). Murmurs that arise beyond the heart often are delayed in onset and may continue beyond the second heart sound or even throughout the entire cardiac cycle (Fig. 9-21). The duration of such a murmur depends upon how long a pressure gradient is maintained at the murmur's origin. Thus, in the case of patent ductus arteriosus or arteriovenous shunt the pressure difference between the systemic arterial side and the pulmonary artery or peripheral veins is great and continuous, rendering the murmur both continuous and long. Severe arterial obstruction may yield a similar murmur. A mild arterial obstructive lesion, on the other hand, gives rise to a short crescendo-decrescendo murmur, analogous to the innocent intracardiac systolic ejection murmur. Phonocardiography, therefore, offers potential aid in the clinical distinction between inconsequential and severe obstructive arterial lesions.[40,41] A murmur that occupies the entire systolic period or longer suggests severe arterial narrowing (90% or more), whereas a short murmur occupying approximately half of the systolic period denotes a minimal or nonobstructing condition of the vessels.

Myocardial Disease. In general, graphic recordings of sounds and pulses in myocardial disease are limited in value. Soft third or fourth heart sounds may be recorded even when they are not heard.

Use of systolic time intervals has been of some additional value in assessing malfunction of the left ventricle in most myocardial diseases[20] and will be discussed elsewhere in this book.

Use of Pharmacologic Agents in Diagnosis.[1] Amyl nitrite, which induces a fall in systemic pressure, tachycardia, and increased cardiac output, has proved to be

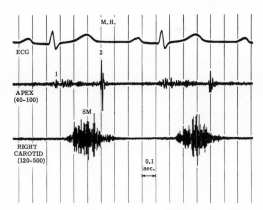

Figure 9-21. Peripheral arterial murmur caused by severe obstruction of right common carotid artery in a 48-year-old woman. The peripheral murmur begins late in relationship to the first heart sound and has a duration equal to the entirety of systole. (From CLINICAL PHONOCARDIOGRAPHY AND EXTERNAL PULSE RECORDING, 2nd ed. by Tavel, M. E. Copyright © 1972 by Year Book Medical Publishers, Inc., Chicago. Used by permission.)

a helpful adjunct in cardiac diagnosis. It intensifies most systolic ejection murmurs and diastolic mitral or tricuspid flow murmurs. It decreases regurgitant systolic murmurs of mitral insufficiency and ventricular septal defect and diastolic murmurs of aortic insufficiency. Because of these effects, amyl nitrite is especially useful in differentiation of aortic stenosis (increase) from mitral insufficiency (decrease), pulmonic stenosis (increase) from small ventricular septal defect (decrease) and organic mitral stenosis (increase) from the Austin Flint murmur of aortic insufficiency (decrease). Table 9-1 summarizes the effect of amyl nitrite on the various murmurs.

Methoxamine and phenylephrine are vasopressors that, when given intravenously, elevate systemic vascular resistance without affecting appreciably the pulmonary circuit. They intensify systolic murmurs of mitral insufficiency or ventricular septal defect while those due to aortic stenosis are unchanged or reduced. Diastolic murmurs of aortic insufficiency or the Austin Flint murmur are increased whereas

TABLE 9-1

Effect of Amyl Nitrite and Vasopressors on Various Murmurs[1]

Diagnosis	Amyl Nitrite	Methoxamine or Phenyle-phrine
Systolic Murmurs		
Mitral insufficiency	Decrease	Increase
Ventricular septal defect	Decrease	Increase
Patent ductus arteriosus	Decrease	Increase
Fallot's tetralogy	Decrease	Increase
Atrial septal defect	Increase	Increase or no change
Idiopathic hypertrophic subaortic stenosis	Increase	Decrease
Aortic stenosis (valvular)	Increase	No change
Pulmonic stenosis (valvular and muscular)	Increase	No change
Tricuspid insufficiency	Increase	No change
Systolic ejection murmur (innocent)	Increase	Decrease
Diastolic Murmurs		
Aortic insufficiency	Decrease	Increase
Austin Flint murmur	Decrease	Increase
Mitral stenosis	Increase	Decrease
Pulmonic insufficiency	Increase	No change
Pulmonic insufficiency secondary to Eisenmenger's syndrome	Decrease	Increase
Tricuspid stenosis	Increase	No change

those of organic mitral stenosis are reduced. The effect of vasopressors is summarized in Table 9-1.

SUMMARY

Phonocardiography provides one of a growing list of valuable intermediary studies between physical examination and cardiac catheterization. It not only provides a medium for instruction in physical examination but also allows one to make certain diagnoses and assess severity of numerous cardiovascular lesions. It is especially valuable in the evaluation of all valvular stenoses, especially aortic stenosis. One can also use phonocardiography for screening and diagnosis of idiopathic hypertrophic subaortic stenosis. It is also a helpful adjunct in the study of several con-genital abnormalities and in diagnosis of pericardial constriction.

REFERENCES

1. Tavel, M. E.: Clinical Phonocardiography and External Pulse Recordings, ed. 2. Chicago, Year Book Medical Publishers, 1972.
2. Von Gierke, H. E.: Transmission of vibratory energy through human body tissue. Proc. First Nat. Biophysics Con., 1957, p. 647.
3. Van Vollenhoven, E., Beneken, J. E. W., Reuver, H., and Dorenbos, T.: Filters for phonocardiography. Med. Biol. Eng. 5:127, 1967.
4. Lakier, J. B., Bloom, K. R., Pocock, W. A., and Barlow, J. B.: Tricuspid component of first heart sound. Br. Heart J. 35:1275, 1973.
5. Burggraf, G. W., and Craige, E.: The first heart sound in complete heart block: Phono-echocardiographic correlations. Circulation 50: 17, 1974.
6. Surawicz, B.: Effect of respiration and upright position on the interval between the two components of the second heart sound and that between the second heart sound and mitral opening snap. Circulation 16:422, 1957.
7. Whittaker, A. V., Shaver, J. A., Gray, S., and Leonard, J.: Sound-pressure correlates of the aortic ejection sound. Circulation 39:475, 1969.
8. Barlow, J. B., Bosman, C. K., Pocock, W. A., and Marchand, P.: Late systolic murmurs and non-ejection ("mid-late") systolic clicks. Br. Heart J. 30:203, 1968.
9. Fontana, M. E., Pence, H. L., Leighton, R. F., and Wooley, C. F.: The varying clinical spectrum of the systolic click–late systolic murmur syndrome. Circulation 41:807, 1970.
10. Hutter, A. M., Dunsmore, R. E., Wilkerson, J. T., and DeSanctis, R. W.: Early systolic clicks due to mitral valve prolapse. Circulation 44:516, 1971.
11. Martinez-Lopez, J. I.: Sounds of the heart in diastole. Am. J. Cardiol. 34:594, 1974.
12. Rothbaum, D. A., DeJoseph, R. L., and Tavel, M. E.: Diastolic heart sound produced by mid-diastolic closure of the mitral valve. Am. J. Cardiol. 34:367, 1974.
13. Leatham, A.: A classification of systolic murmurs. Br. Heart J. 17:574, 1955.
14. Bonner, A. J., Jr., Sacks, H. N., and Tavel, M. E.: Assessing the severity of aortic stenosis by phonocardiography and external carotid pulse recordings. Circulation 48:247, 1973.
15. Weissler, A. M., Peeler, R. G., and Roehill, W. H.: Relationship between left ventricular ejection time, stroke volume and heart rate in normal individuals and in patients with cardio-vascular disease. Am. Heart J. 62:267, 1961.
16. Goldblatt, A., Aygen, M., and Brunwald, E.: Hemodynamic phonocardiographic correlations of the fourth heart sound in aortic stenosis. Circulation 26:92, 1962.
17. Caulfield, H., Perloff, J. K., and DeLeon,

A. C.: The hemodynamic significance of atrial sounds in aortic stenosis. Am. J. Cardiol. 28:179, 1971.

18. Kavalier, M. A., Stewart, J., and Tavel, M. E.: The apical A wave versus the fourth heart sound in assessing the severity of aortic stenosis. Circulation 51:324, 1975.

19. Bonner, A. J., and Tavel, M. E.: Systolic time intervals: Use in congestive heart failure due to aortic stenosis. Arch. Intern. Med. 132:816, 1973.

20. Weissler, A. M., Lewis, R. P., and Leighton, R. F.: The systolic time intervals as a measure of left ventricular performance in man. *In* Progress in Cardiology. Philadelphia, Lea & Febiger, 1972, p. 155.

21. Weissler, A. M., Harris, W. S., and Schoenfeld, C. D.: Systolic time interval in heart failure in man. Circulation 37:149, 1968.

22. Baragan, J., et al.: Chronic left complete bundle-branch-block. Br. Heart J. 30:196, 1968.

23. Braunwald, E., et al.: Idiopathic hypertrophic subaortic stenosis. Circulation 30:3, 1964.

24. Leatham, A., and Weitzman, D.: Auscultatory and phonocardiographic signs of pulmonary stenosis. Br. Heart J. 19:303, 1957.

25. Vogelpoel, L., and Schrire, V.: Auscultatory and phonocardiographic assessment of Fallot's tetralogy. Circulation 22:73, 1960.

26. Caceres, C. A., and Perry, L. W.: The innocent murmur. Boston, Little, Brown & Co. 1967.

27. Watanabe, H., and Sakamoto, T.: Clinical and phonocardiographic study of aortic regurgitation. Jap. Heart J. 2:7, 1961.

28. Parker, E., Craige, E., and Hood, W. P., Jr.: The Austin Flint murmur and the A wave of the apexcardiogram in aortic regurgitation. Circulation 43:349, 1971.

29. Davies, J. P. H.: A simple phonocardiographic formula for predicting left atrial pressure in mitral stenosis. Br. Heart J. 29:843, 1967.

30. Benchimol, A., Dimond, E. G., Waxman, D., and Shen, Y.: Diastolic movements of the precordium in mitral stenosis and regurgitation. Am. Heart J. 60:417, 1960.

31. Lisa, C. P., and Tavel, M. E.: Tricuspid stenosis: Graphic features which help in its diagnosis. Chest 61:291, 1972.

32. Perloff, J. K., and Harvey, W. P.: Auscultatory and phonocardiographic manifestations of pure mitral regurgitation. Prog. Cardiovasc. Dis. 5:172, 1962.

33. Cohen, L. S., Mason, D. T., and Braunwald, E.: Significance of an atrial gallop sound in mitral regurgitation. Circulation 35:112, 1967.

34. Cohn, L. H., Morrow, A. G., and Braunwald, E.: Operative treatment of atrial septal defect: Clinical and haemodynamic assessments in 175 patients. Br. Heart J. 29:725, 1967.

35. Nadas, A. S., and Ellison, R. C.: Phonocardiographic analysis of diastolic flow murmurs in secundum atrial septal defect and ventricular septal defect. Br. Heart J. 29:684, 1967.

36. Tavel, M. E., et al.: The jugular venous pulse in atrial septal defect. Arch. Intern. Med. 121:524, 1968.

37. Diamond, M. A., et al.: Echocardiographic features of atrial septal defect. Circulation 43:129, 1971.

38. Evans, J. R., Rowde, R. D., and Keith J. D.: Spontaneous closure of ventricular septal defects. Circulation 22:1044, 1960.

39. Harris, C., Wise, J., Jr., and Oakley, C. M.: "Fixed" splitting of the second heart sound in ventricular septal defect. Br. Heart J. 33:428, 1971.

40. Kesteloot, H., Sluzta, R., and Van Houte, O.: A phonocardiographic study of the physiological and pathological vascular murmurs. Acta Belg. Militari 13:16, 1967.

41. Ueda, H., et al.: Quantitative assessment of obstruction of the aorta and its branches in "aortitis syndrome." Jap. Heart J. 7:3, 1966.

Chapter 10

Pulse Tracings and Apexcardiography

GORDON A. EWY

Graphic recordings of venous, arterial and precordial impulses enable the physician to document, identify, time and semiquantitate these cardiovascular physical findings. By confirming or denying subjective impressions and providing educational feedback, these techniques have helped to move the bedside cardiovascular examination from an art to a science. Occasionally the recordings are diagnostic of specific disease entities. They usually provide information that has diagnostic importance.

The major limitation of graphic recordings is the qualitative nature of the derived information. Attempts at quantitation were initially limited by inadequate response characteristics of the recording instruments. In recent years these problems have been partially overcome. It is now clear that groups of patients with hemodynamic abnormalities can be differentiated from normal patients by non-invasive techniques.

Environment. Non-invasive recording can be made in the patient's room if his condition demands. Routine tracings should be obtained in a quiet room with proper temperature and lighting controls and enough privacy so that the gowned patient is completely relaxed. A hospital bed is ad-

vantageous as the head of the bed can be raised and lowered with ease.

Recorders. A multichannel recorder is necessary so that venous, arterial and precordial pulsations can be recorded individually or simultaneously with the electrocardiogram, phonocardiogram, echocardiogram or all three. An oscilloscope interfaced with a direct writing recorder assures a quality recording with minimal usage of paper. With recorders using photographic processing, an oscilloscope is an essential component of the machine. The recorder should be capable of multiple speeds, i.e., 10, 25, 50 and 100 mm. per second.

The pickup device, transducer and amplifier used will vary with the type of recording being made. The frequency response characteristics of the instrumentation are of utmost importance. Unfortunately instrumentation incorporating ideal frequency response characteristics is expensive. When low-frequency recordings such as venous, arterial or precordial pulsations are made, the time constant should be at least several seconds in duration. The time constant is defined as the time it takes for a signal to decay to 37% of its initial amplitude. To test the time constant of the recording system, a constant pressure is applied to the pickup device. If the recording system has a good time constant, the resultant tracing will remain elevated or will decay only slightly until the pressure is released, at which time it will return to the baseline without negative overshoot. Recording systems with less than ideal response characteristics will result in distorted tracings. A time constant less than 3 or 4 seconds is probably not acceptable if low-frequency events are not to be recorded. The time constant is only one of the important response characteristics—phase shift and overshoot are two others. Although related to the time constant, phase shift and overshoot should be tested as well. Special instrumentation is needed to test these characteristics. Therefore, before purchasing a multichannel recorder one should be sure that there is no phase shift or overshoot in the frequency range of 0 to 100 cycles per second. Examples will be shown later of the marked variation in recording that result when units with inadequate response characteristics are used.

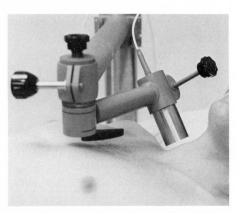

Figure 10-1. Technique of recording displacement of the jugular venous pulsations utilizing the Wayne Kerr system. The pickup probe is placed within ¼ inch of the skin. Changes in the distance between the probe and the skin result in changes in capacitance, thereby changing the voltage output. Electronic circuitry is used to make the output linear over the recording distance.[1]

Personnel. Most recordings should be made by the physician, since the majority of venous, arterial and precordial tracings are made to confirm or deny clinical impressions. The design of the study has to be based on the clinical evaluation and planned accordingly. The type of recording, patient position, location of the transducer and the instrumentation used must be chosen according to the information needed. A technician can be trained to make adequate routine tracings, such as systolic time intervals (see next chapter).

Indications. One reason for recording pulsations is to teach their recognition at the bedside. A well-trained clinical cardiologist usually does not need tracings to discern the configuration of venous, arterial or precordial pulsations. Recordings are made for documentation, illustrations or precise timing of the events. Occasionally the recordings are diagnostic of a specific disease state. This is usually not the case, and hence they must be interpreted in the context of the history, other physical findings and other laboratory findings.

JUGULAR VENOUS PULSATIONS

Recording Methods. Jugular venous pulsations (JVPs) reflect right atrial hemodynamics but may be modified by superimposed carotid pulsations. Ideally the recording system used for JVPs should depend upon the purpose of the recording. If the records are to be used to teach ourselves and students to recognize venous wave forms at the bedside, a system should be chosen that accurately records these low-frequency, low-pressure pulsations without touching and, therefore, without distorting them (Fig. 10-1). These devices are not in common use. They include instruments that employ reflected light or those that utilize the capacitance principle.[1,2] In this chapter, illustrations recorded by this latter method (Fig. 10-1) are referred to as displacement recordings.

The second reason for making phlebo-

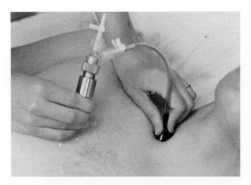

Figure 10-2. Technique of recording the indirect jugular pulse (see text).

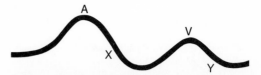

Figure 10-4. Graphic illustration of the A and V waves and X and Y descents of phlebograms.

grams is to obtain wave forms similar to right atrial pressure tracings and thereby obtain information regarding right atrial and right ventricular hemodynamics. A popular method is to record internal jugular pulsations from the base of the neck, utilizing a funnel or conical shaped pickup (Fig. 10-2). The recording is usually made with the patient supine. The patient's head should be supported by a small pillow so that the neck muscles will be relaxed. The hand-held funnel pickup is placed at the base of the neck above the medial end of the right clavicle. The open end of the funnel is directed downward and medially toward the heart. This method tends to minimize interference from carotid pulsations.[3]

External jugular pulsations can be recorded with a double-rimmed cup (Fig.

10-3). Suction is applied to the outer chamber that holds the cup onto the skin over the external jugular vein.[4] The patient and the cup are positioned so that the cup overlies the top of the venous column. Pressure volume changes in the inner compartment of the pickup are slight and, therefore, a sensitive transducer, such as a piezoelectric crystal microphone, is necessary to obtain tracings of suitable amplitude.

Normal Jugular Venous Pulsations. The jugular venous pulsations are classically taught to consist of two crests, the A and V waves, and two troughs that mark the end of the X and Y descents (Fig. 10-4). The A wave is caused by atrial contraction. The X descent results from atrial relaxation and movement of the floor of the atrium toward the right ventricle during ventricular systole. The trough of the X descent is normally the lowest point of the jugular venous tracing. The V wave is formed by passive filling of the right atrium during ventricular systole while the tricuspid valve is closed and peaks soon after the second heart sound. The Y descent is formed by the fall in atrial pressure that occurs when the tricuspid valve opens. The C wave (Fig. 10-5) may interrupt the X descent. It is usually unimpressive but may be the dominant wave.

Illustrations of the normal venous pulse with high-amplitude A and V waves tend

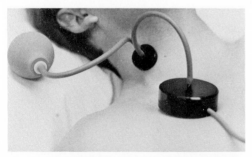

Figure 10-3. Suction-held cup for recording external jugular venous pulsations. Suction is applied via the bulb to the outer compartment. Volume undulations in the inner compartment result in small pressure changes that are transformed into electronic signals by the piezoelectric microphone.

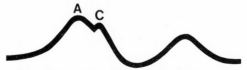

Figure 10-5. Graphic illustration of the C wave of the venous pulse.

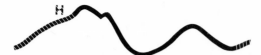

Figure 10-6. Graphic illustration of the H wave of the venous pulse.

to confuse the student or careful observer who fails to see these events in the normal venous pulse. At the bedside, distinct A and V waves may be difficult to appreciate in normal individuals. Instead, the dominant venous motion is systolic collapse or retraction of the pulse with gentle venous motion preceding and following. This dominant retraction is the X descent. The other waves are less obvious partly because of the H wave (Fig. 10-6). The H wave represents passive filling of the atrium and ventricles in diastole and results in a gradual increase in the venous pressure before the A wave. The appearance of the jugular venous pulsations is best represented by low-amplitude recording made with instruments that do not touch or distort the venous pulse (Figs. 10-1 and 10-7).

A Wave. An increase in the height of the A wave occurs when there is an increase in the force of atrial contraction or increased resistance to atrial contraction or

both. Examples of the latter are tricuspid stenosis and decreased compliance of the right ventricle. Thus, common causes of increased A waves are pulmonary hypertension, pulmonary valve stenosis or right ventricular hypertrophy secondary to chronic left ventricular failure. As the A wave increases in height it becomes more conspicuous and is then termed a giant A wave. A prominent A wave is not invariably present in patients with severe right ventricular hypertrophy. Patients with cyanotic Fallot's tetralogy seldom have a giant A wave even though the right ventricular pressure is equal to left ventricular pressure.

Small A waves occur because of either a decreased force of atrial contraction or a decreased resistance to atrial contraction. Damage of the atrial muscle from chronic stretch will result in a decrease in the force of atrial contraction. Decreased resistance to atrial contraction may occur with first-degree heart block. When atrial contraction occurs soon after the tricuspid valve opens at a time when the right ventricle is relatively empty, the A wave is very small. In atrial flutter, small rapid waves that have been designated F waves can be recorded.

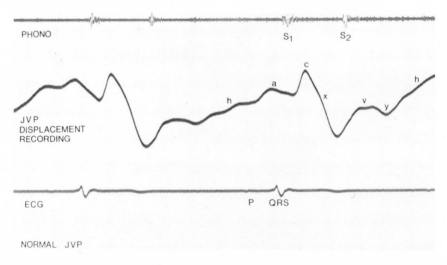

Figure 10-7. Displacement recording of the jugular venous pulse (*JVP*) in a normal young male. Simultaneous phonocardiogram (*PHONO*) and electrocardiogram (*ECG*) serve as reference tracings. Note that the dominant motion is the X descent.

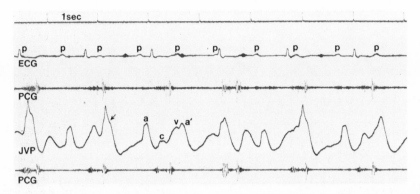

Figure 10-8. Cannon A waves were present in this patient with complete heart block. Jugular venous pulsation recorded with the funnel pickup air coupled to a Statham pressure transducer as pictured in Figure 10-2. One of the cannon A waves is marked with an *arrow*. An A not occurring during systole is marked *a'*. Simultaneous 1-second time lines, electrocardiogram *(ECG)* and phonocardiogram *(PCG)* are recorded as reference tracings.

The A waves completely disappear with atrial fibrillation or atrial standstill.

Cannon A Waves. When the right atrium contracts against a closed tricuspid valve the full force of atrial contraction is transmitted into the venous system. The resultant impulse is a cannon A wave or cannon wave (Fig. 10-8). These waves differ from giant A waves in two respects. First, the cannon A wave is systolic in timing, whereas the giant A wave is presystolic. Second, cannon A waves tend to have a more rapid rate of rise and appear as flickering of the venous pulse.

Intermittent cannon A waves commonly occur with premature ventricular contractions (Fig. 10-9), complete heart block, atrial-ventricular dissociation, including that occurring with ventricular pacemakers, and rarely with premature atrial contractions.

X Descent. The origin of the X descent has been the subject of some controversy. Since it is often decreased in patients with

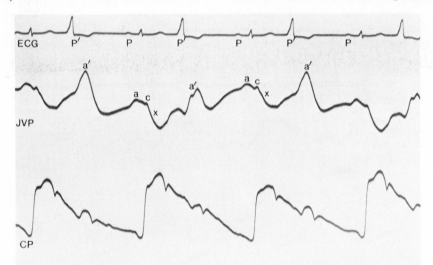

Figure 10-9. Cannon A waves in a patient with frequent premature ventricular contractions. Simultaneous electrocardiogram *(ECG)* with *P'* indicating P waves masked by the QRS of the premature beat, jugular venous pulsation *(JVP)* with cannon A waves marked *a'* and carotid arterial pulse *(CP)*.

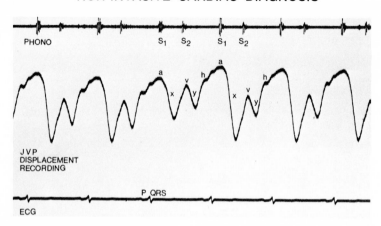

Figure 10-10. Prominent X and Y descents in a 39-year-old man with constrictive pericarditis. Simultaneous recording of phonocardiogram (*PHONO*), jugular venous pulse (*JVP*) displacement recording and electrocardiogram (*ECG*).

atrial fibrillation, it has been thought to be related to atrial relaxation. However, it is not invariably absent in atrial fibrillation and may be quite pronounced in patients with atrial fibrillation and constrictive pericarditis. For this reason, systolic descent of the tricuspid valve, or "descent of the floor of the right atrium," has been postulated as another etiology of the X descent. The JVP recording from a patient with constrictive pericarditis is shown in Figure 10-10.

Some authors divide the X descent into two components, designating the descending limb of the A wave prior to its interruption by the C wave as the X descent and the continued descent following the C wave as the X′ descent (Fig. 10–11).

C Wave. The C wave of the venous pulsation was originally ascribed to the transmitted carotid pulse by MacKenzie. Wood agreed with this opinion as he could not find a wave of similar magnitude in right atrial pressure tracings. A recent study by

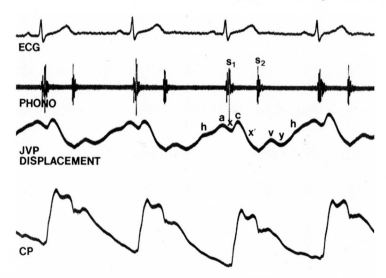

Figure 10-11. Simultaneous recordings of electrocardiogram (*ECG*), phonocardiogram (*PHONO*), jugular venous pulsation (JVP) and carotid arterial pulsations (CP) in a normal young man. Note the X′ descent is the continuation of the X descent following the C wave.

Rich and Tavel revealed that the C wave of the JVP occurred a similar distance from the QRS complex in both controls and patients with left bundle branch block, whereas the onset of the carotid pulse was significantly delayed in the latter group.[5] They concluded that the C wave was not transmitted from the carotid. Their method of recording the jugular venous pulse was by the technique illustrated in Figure 10-2, in which the funnel-shaped pickup is held with some pressure over the internal jugular bulb and directed posteriorly and caudally. As noted earlier, this type of tracing produces records that tend to resemble the right atrial pressure tracings. Devices that work on the capacitance principle (Fig. 10-1) record the JVP higher in the neck and produce tracings that more closely resemble the JVP as it appears at the bedside. In patients with aortic insufficiency the JVP recorded with this method has C waves of much greater amplitude than that found in right atrial pressure tracings (Fig. 10-12). Therefore, as emphasized by Colman, there are in all probability two mechanisms that produce the C wave in the jugular venous pulse.[6]

V Wave. Normally the A wave is the dominant venous wave. In patients with an atrial septal defect (ASD) the V wave is increased in height so that the A and V waves are of equal amplitude.[7] The most common cause of an increased V wave is incompetence of the tricuspid valve. These waves are more than an augmented V wave. Since they usually begin with or soon after the C wave, they are often referred to as CV waves, or regurgitant CV waves. The appearance of the CV wave will depend not only upon the amount of blood regurgitated into the atrium during right ventricular contraction but also upon the compliance or stiffness of the right atrium. With mild degrees of tricuspid regurgitation the only abnormality might be the obliteration of the X descent. With increasing degrees of tricuspid regurgitation, the height of the CV wave will increase, provided the right atrium does not become extremely large and compliant. Patients with severe degrees of tricuspid regurgitation can have such prominent CV waves that they result in motion of the ear lobe.

Patients with aortic insufficiency have forceful carotid and peripheral pulses and

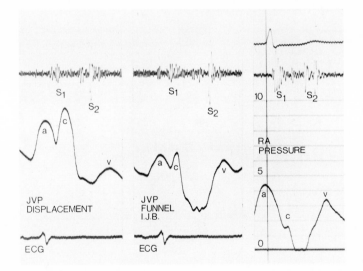

Figure 10-12. Recordings of the JVP in a 50-year-old man with aortic regurgitation by displacement recording (Fig. 10-1) and funnel pickup (Fig. 10-2). These are compared to pressure recording from his right atrium.

prominent systolic venous pulses. It may be difficult to tell if the waves are transmitted C waves or CV waves due to coexistent tricuspid insufficiency. This problem may be resolved by recording the hepatic pulse—another way of indirectly recording the right atrial hemodynamic events.[8]

Y Descent. The most obvious abnormality in the venous wave form of patients with constrictive pericarditis or restrictive myocardial disease is usually the striking diastolic collapse. There is also a rapid Y ascent that follows the rapid Y descent (Fig. 10-10). The Y descent is also prominent in patients with large regurgitant CV waves of tricuspid insufficiency, provided there is no associated tricuspid stenosis.

CAROTID ARTERIAL PULSE TRACINGS

The carotid pulse tracings reflect changes in carotid pressure and volume once the artery has been slightly compressed by the recording pickup device. The resultant tracing bears a striking resemblance to intra-aortic (ascending aorta) pressure pulses (Fig. 10-13). These tracings are used as timing references for phonocardiographic events, for timing hemodynamic events (such as measurements of systolic time intervals) and for contour analysis.

The non-invasive devices generally used for recording the carotid arterial pulse are either the hand-held funnel (Fig. 10-14) or a pediatric blood pressure cuff Fig. 10-15). The tracings that result from the two methods are comparable (Fig. 10-16) if the transducer, amplifier and recording systems are similar.

There are two minor disadvantages of the cuff method. First, venous artifacts are recorded if the venous pressure is elevated and, second, minor discomfort and anxiety result in some patients when the cuff is placed around the neck and inflated. The first problem can usually be overcome by raising the patient's thorax and head so that the neck is elevated above the venous pressure. The second can be minimized by inflating the cuff to only 5 or 10 mm. Hg, and never more than 20 mm. Hg pressure.

A third device used for recording carotid

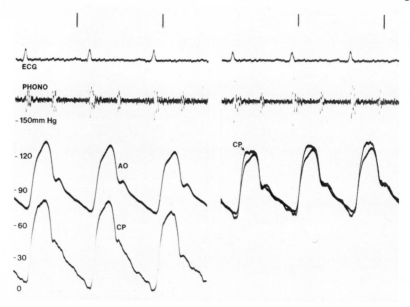

Figure 10-13. Simultaneous electrocardiogram (*ECG*), phonocardiogram (*PHONO*), intra-aortic (*AO*) pressure pulse with a fluid-filled catheter system and external carotid pulse tracing (*CP*). *Left,* pulse tracings separated; *right:* superimposed AO and CP tracings.

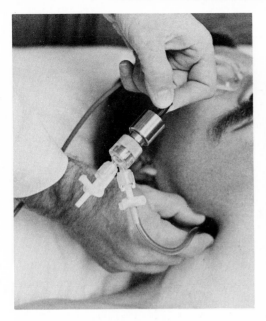

Figure 10-14. Technique of recording carotid arterial pulsation with hand-held funnel pickup device air coupled to a Statham pressure transducer.

arterial pulsations is a piezoelectric or other pressure sensitive transducer with a button type of pickup. The device is hand held and placed on the skin over the palpable carotid pulse.

Reference Tracings. The carotid pulse is commonly used as a reference tracing for timing of the aortic component of the second heart sound. In patients with severe aortic stenosis the aortic component of the second heart sound may be very difficult to hear or record by phonocardiography. Yet, in the absence of left bundle branch block, paradoxical or reversed splitting of

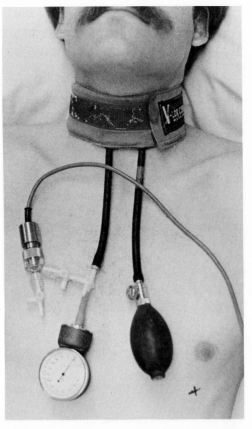

Figure 10-15. Technique of recording carotid arterial pulsations with cuff method. The cuff is inflated to less than 20 mm. Hg and is air coupled to an appropriate transducer. Illustrated is a Statham pressure transducer.

the second heart sound is one of the better clinical indicators of the severity of the stenosis. If the recorded second heart sound is more than 0.05 second before the dicrotic notch, the sound probably represents the pulmonic and not the aortic com-

EXTERNAL RECORDINGS: CARTOID PULSE

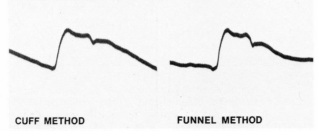

CUFF METHOD   FUNNEL METHOD

Figure 10-16. External recordings of the carotid arterial pulse with the two recording methods illustrated in Figures 10-14 and 10-15.

ponent of the second heart sound. In this situation, paradoxical or reversed splitting of the second heart sound is present, suggesting severe aortic stenosis.

Another suggested use of the indirect carotid pulse tracing is for left-sided ejection sounds and nonejection systolic clicks.

Because of the transmission delay the aortic component of the second heart sound occurs 0.01 to 0.05 second before the dicrotic notch (Fig. 10-17). Left-sided ejection sounds can be present in patients with valvular aortic stenosis or in patients with dilated aortic roots. The elegant studies reported from the University of Pittsburgh have shown that ejection sounds without aortic valve stenosis coincide with the upstroke of intra-aortic pressure pulse recorded with transducer-tipped catheter, whereas those associated with valvular aortic stenosis occur 0.024 to 0.040 second later and coincide with the anacrotic notch.[9]

In Figure 10-17 the transmission delay between the aortic component of the second heart sound and the dicrotic notch is about 0.05 second. If the carotid pulse tracing were redrawn so that the dicrotic notch corresponds to the second heart sound, the ejection sound (E) in this patient with

clinically mild aortic insufficiency would coincide with the anacrotic notch of the carotid pulse tracing, suggesting that it might be valvular in origin. Because of the many sounds that may occur near the upstroke of the carotid pulse, i.e., the high-frequency second component of the normal first heart sound, right-sided ejection sounds and early clicks of mitral valve prolapse, employing the upstroke of the carotid pulse as a timing reference is not extremely useful.

CONTOUR ANALYSIS

It has classically been taught that the carotid arterial pulse contour is composed of the percussion wave, tidal wave and dicrotic wave (Fig. 10-18A). I prefer the designation of Freis and associates who proposed the designations flow wave, pressure wave and dicrotic wave (Fig. 10-18B).[10] Simultaneous recordings of the carotid pulse and intra-aortic blood flow and pressure reveal that the early systolic peak in the carotid artery corresponds to peak aortic flow and the late systolic peak to peak aortic pressure. In clinical conditions in which flow is slower, such as aortic stenosis, the early wave or flow is de-

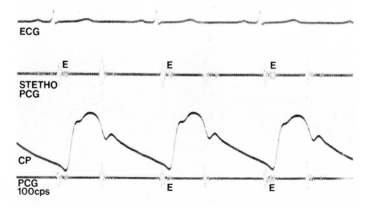

Figure 10-17. Carotid pulse tracings as timing reference for an ejection sound (*E*) and the aortic component of the second heart sound. Simultaneous electrocardiogram (*ECG*), phonocardiogram (*PCG*) at stetho frequency filtration, carotid arterial pulse (*CP*) and phonocardiogram (*PCG*) filtered at 100 cycles per second (*cps*). Patient has mild aortic insufficiency and a prominent left-sided ejection sound (*E*). In this patient the aortic component of the second heart sound precedes the dicrotic notch by about 0.05 second.

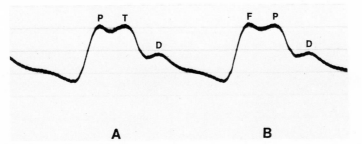

Figure 10-18. Arterial pulsations showing typical peaks or waves. *A,* percussion wave (*P*), tidal wave (*T*) and dicrotic wave (*D*). *B,* flow wave (*F*), pressure wave (*P*), and dicrotic wave (*D*).

creased in height and referred to as an anacrotic notch. In patients given an isoproterenol infusion, or in patients with idiopathic hypertrophic subaortic stenosis, conditions in which flow is rapid in early systole, this early wave is accentuated (Fig. 10-19). The pressure wave is increased with hypertension, age and disease processes that make the vascular system less compliant. With infusion of a pressure agent, such as phenylephrine, the pressure peak will increase relative to the flow peak (Fig. 10-20), whereas inhalation of amyl nitrite will decrease the height of the pressure wave relative to the flow wave. In some patients the flow and pressure peaks are not distinctive (Fig. 10-21).

Carotid Upstroke. Because the upstroke of the carotid pulse is usually slow in patients with aortic stenosis, several authors have attempted to predict the severity of aortic stenosis by analysis of the pulse contour. Since the height of the recorded pulse varies with the gain setting, analyses have been made by measuring the arterial half-rise time (T time), the upstroke time (U time), or the maximal rate of rise of the carotid upstroke.[11–13]

The T time (Fig. 10-22A) is the time required for the pulse to reach one half of its total height. The U time is the time from onset to the peak of the carotid pulse (Fig. 10-22B). The T time varies slightly and the U time varies greatly when the flow and pressure waves vary slightly in relative height. The maximal rate of rise of the carotid pulse (Fig. 10-22C) is obtained by

fitting a line to the steepest portion of the carotid upstroke. This line is extrapolated from the onset to the peak of the carotid tracing. The time to reach maximum pulse pressure along this line is then divided into the pulse pressure. The pulse pressure is obtained by careful sphygmomanometer measurement of brachial arterial blood pressure immediately before and after the carotid pulse recording.[13]

Correlations can be made between a decreased carotid upstroke, measured by T time,[11] U time,[12] maximal rate of rise or all three,[13] and the severity of aortic stenosis in groups of subjects. The carotid up-

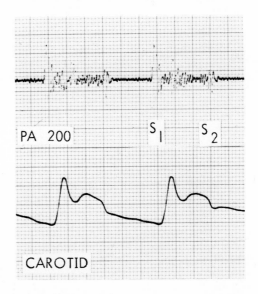

Figure 10-19. Simultaneous phonocardiogram and pulse tracing in a patient with idiopathic hypertrophic subaortic stenosis. Note the accentuated flow wave.

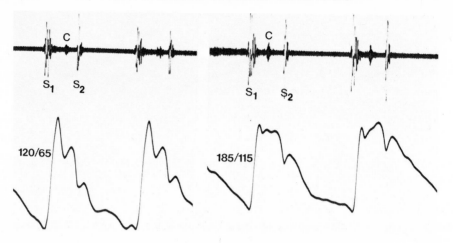

Figure 10-20. Simultaneous phonocardiogram and carotid pulse tracing from a patient with a mid systolic click. The patient was given an infusion of phenylephrine, raising his blood pressure from normal of 120/65 to 185/115 mm. Hg. Note the change in contour of the carotid pulse, with the second systolic wave or pressure wave increasing in height relative to the first systolic wave or flow wave.

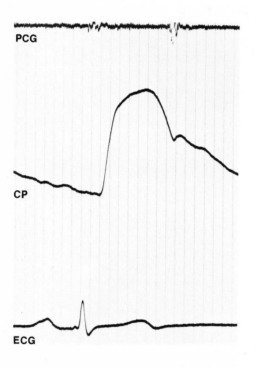

Figure 10-21. Simultaneous phonocardiogram (*PCG*), carotid pulse recording (*CP*) and electrocardiogram (*ECG*). Note that the carotid pulse does not have distinctive flow and pressure waves.

stroke is not diagnostic in the individual patient because the rate of rise of the ca-

rotid pulse is dependent not only upon the degree of stenosis but also on other factors, such as myocardial contractility and vessel stiffness. The rate of rise of the carotid pulse is decreased by impaired myocardial contractility and increased in a noncompliant vascular system as occurs in the aged, in patients with diffuse arteriosclerosis and in patients with coexistent systemic hypertension.

Bonner and coworkers found that a decrease in the maximum rate of rise of the arterial pulse in conjuction with prolonged ejection time and a late-peaking aortic stenotic murmur was indicative of severe aortic stenosis.[14] In their patients with varying degrees of aortic stenosis, when all three of these parameters were outside the delineated limits (ejection time index greater than 0.42 second, maximum rate of rise of carotid pulse less than 500 mm. Hg per second and the onset of QRS of the electrocardiogram to the peak of the murmur greater than 0.19 second) 27 of 28 patients had severe aortic stenosis. These authors also confirmed the finding that a normal rate of rise of the carotid pulse can be present in older patients (age 58 to 69 years) with severe aortic stenosis.

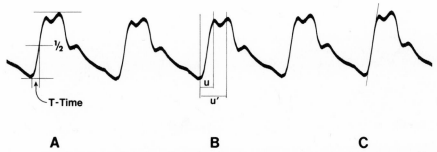

A   **B**   **C**

Figure 10-22. Arterial pulse indicating methods of measuring the T time or arterial half-rise time, the U time or upstroke time, and the maximal rate of rise. The T time is the time between the onset of the carotid upstroke and the point where the pulse reaches one half of its height. Note that the T time would vary slightly if the F or the P wave were dominant. The U time is the time between the onset of the carotid upstroke and the peak of the pulse. Note that the U time varies considerably, depending upon the relative height of the F or P waves. These differences are illustrated by the difference in the duration of U and U'. The maximal rate of rise of the carotid pulse is measured by drawing a line to the steepest portion of the carotid upstroke. This line is extrapolated from the onset to the peak of the carotid tracing. The time from the onset to peak of this line is divided into the pulse pressure obtained by routine arm blood pressure obtained by cuff.

BISFERIOUS AND DICROTIC ARTERIAL PULSES

Bisferious carotid pulsations are present in patients with aortic regurgitation (Fig. 10-23), idiopathic hypertrophic subaortic stenosis (Fig. 10-19) and in some young anxious, hyperkinetic individuals.

Another twin-peaked pulse is the di-

crotic pulse. In contrast to the bisferious arterial pulse, the dicrotic pulse has one impulse in systole and the other in diastole (Fig. 10-24 and 10-25, left). The systolic pulse is of short duration with a slow rate of rise. These features result in an abnormally long pre-ejection period (PEP), a shortened left ventricular ejection time (LVET) and thus an abnormal PEP/

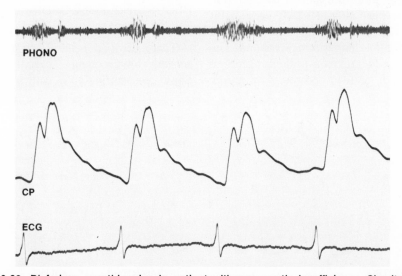

Figure 10-23. Bisferious carotid pulse in patient with pure aortic insufficiency. Simultaneous recording of phonocardiogram (*PHONO*), carotid pulse (*CP*) and electrocardiogram (*ECG*). The systolic flow murmur was impressive, but there was no systolic gradient across the aortic valve at cardiac catheterization.

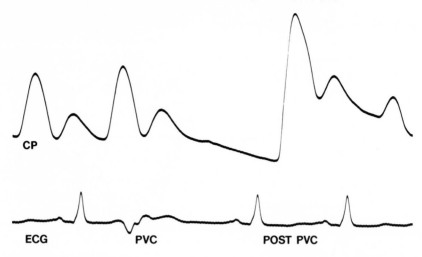

Figure 10-24. Dicrotic carotid pulse. Note that the dicrotic notch is low, near the foot of the pulse, and that the dicrotic wave is accentuated. The more forceful post premature beat has a more normal pulse contour.

LVET. Other features of the dicrotic arterial pulse are that the dicrotic notch is low and the dicrotic wave is markedly increased.[15] The dicrotic pulse is found in patients who have a small stroke volume relative to the capacitance of the arterial system. Patients with dicrotic arterial pulses have a low cardiac output, small stroke volume and elevated peripheral vascular resistance.[15] The contour of dicrotic arterial pulsations normalizes with the post premature beat (Fig. 10-24), presumably because the more forceful post premature beat results in a larger stroke volume. This contrasts with the twin-peaked bisferious pulse, which tends to become more promi-

nent with the post premature beat. Decreasing the peripheral resistance of the artery by administration of a peripheral dilating agent will also normalize the contour of the dicrotic pulse (Fig. 10-25).

Inspection of the pulse contour may provide qualitative information about the patient's hemodynamic status. Quantitative analysis of carotid pulse by systolic time intervals is considered in Chapter 11.

RECORDING PRECORDIAL PULSATIONS

There are two general methods of recording low-frequency precordial pulsations: *apexcardiography,* and displacement

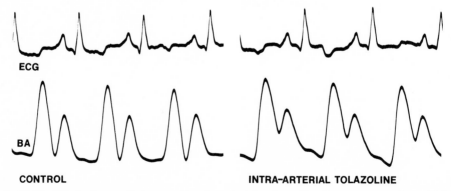

Figure 10-25. Effect of vasodilator on dicrotic arterial pulse. Simultaneous recording of electrocardiogram and brachial arterial pulse. *Left,* control; *right,* following intra-arterial injection of tolazoline.

recordings, or *kinetocardiography*. The apexcardiogram is a recording of the motion of a circumscribed area of the precordium *relative* to the motion of surrounding chest wall. A displacement recording, or kinetocardiogram, records precordial motion relative to a fixed point off the chest wall. Kinetocardiograms more accurately record diffuse precordial motion, whereas a localized impulse can usually be recorded with either the apexcardiogram or kinetocardiogram. In apexcardiography the method of applying the pickup device to the apex impulse can alter the shape and magnitude of the tracing. If the pickup device is rigidly hand held the motion recorded tends to be more relative to a fixed point off the chest wall. If the pickup device is held lightly or strapped and rides on the chest wall the recorded motion tends to be relative to the chest wall or the rim of the recording device.

Apexcardiography. The apexcardiogram is widely used to record low-frequency vibrations of the precordium. Its major virtue is its simplicity and ease of application. Satisfactory tracings can be obtained in the majority of patients with a modicum of practice. Exceptions are those patients who are obese or who have pulmonary emphysema.

The apexcardiogram is usually recorded with the patient in the left lateral position. The patient is positioned until the most forceful apical impulse is located by careful

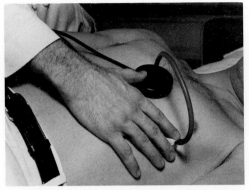

Figure 10-27. Apexcardiography using a hand-held 2.5-cm. open-ended funnel air coupled to a pulse wave crystal microphone.

palpation. The pickup device is then strapped or hand held over this area (Figs. 10-26 to 10-29). At times there is marked variation in the intensity of impulse related to inspiration. As the diaphragm moves up and down, the cardiac impulse moves behind a rib and then into the interspace. The apexcardiogram is best recorded with the impulse in the interspace. The patient is asked to suspend breathing for short periods in the appropriate phase of respiration so that good recordings can be obtained.

Various types of pickup devices are used

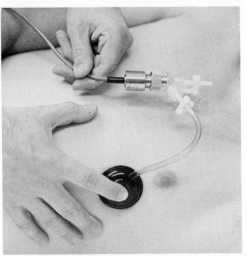

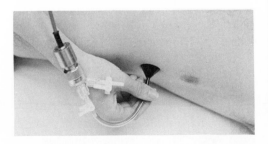

Figure 10-26. Technique of apexcardiography using a hand-held 2.5-cm. open-ended funnel air coupled to a Statham physiologic pressure transducer.

Figure 10-28. Apexcardiography using a 5.0-cm. cup air coupled to a Statham physiologic pressure transducer.

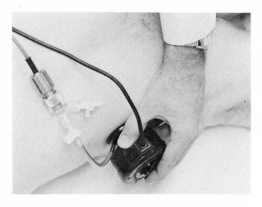

Figure 10-29. Apexcardiography and apex phonocardiography. The 5.0-cm. cup is attached to a crystal microphone and air coupled via a side arm to the transducer.

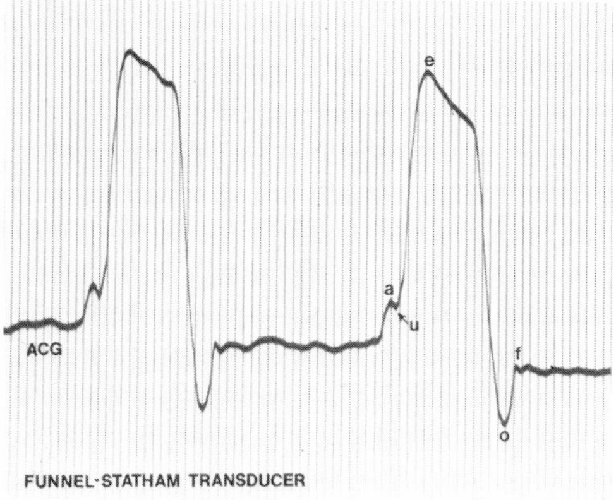

Figure 10-30. Apexcardiogram with wave forms labeled (see text).

to make contact with the chest wall. A commonly used pickup is the conical or funnel-shaped device with a small-diameter (2.5 cm.) open end (Figs. 10-26, 10-27). The larger 5.0-cm. diameter pickup is referred to as the cup. It can be hand held (Fig. 10-28) or connected to the phonocardiographic microphone for simultaneous recordings of the apexcardiogram and apex phonocardiogram (Fig. 10-29). Other pickup devices have button–shaped chest wall contact pieces connected to piezoelectric crystals, and still others are plunger-type pickups that work on an inductance principle.

With the patient in sinus rhythm, the apexcardiogram consists of an A wave, E point, O point and F point (Fig. 10-30). The wave between the O point and the F wave is the *rapid filling wave* and the wave between the F point and the next A wave is the *slow filling wave*. The A wave relates to atrial systole and reflects distention of the ventricle by atrial contraction. It is absent in atrial fibrillation and may be absent in patients with mitral stenosis in spite of forceful left atrial contraction, since the stenotic valve prevents the atrial systolic pressure from being transmitted to the ventricle. The onset of outward motion following the A wave is sometimes referred to as the U or upstroke point. The U point

is said to coincide with the onset of left ventricular isovolumetric contraction. The E point is usually the dominant systolic wave and is said to correspond with the onset of ventricular ejection. The E point is not always clearly demarcated and often varies significantly from the onset of left ventricular ejection. The O point occurs near the opening of the mitral valve. It follows the left ventricular-left atrial pressure crossover during early diastole by an interval up to 50 msec. The F point occurs at the end of rapid passive ventricular filling. In spite of these minor variations the apexcardiogram has found its greatest utility as a timing reference for phonocardiograms.[16] The A wave coincides with the atrial diastolic gallop sound, or fourth heart sound (S₄), the E point with left-sided ejection sounds, the O point with the opening snap of mitral stenosis and the F point with the ventricular diastolic gallop, or third heart sound (S₃). Soon after the onset of the outward systolic wave there may be a notch that corresponds to the first heart sound (Fig. 10-31).

Over the past two decades the apexcardiogram has received enthusiastic support from some centers while being on the fringes of medical respectability in others. Observations made in one laboratory could not consistently be confirmed by another.

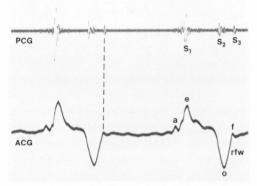

Figure 10-31. Simultaneous phonocardiogram (*PCG*) and apexcardiogram (*ACG*), illustrating the relationship of the F point and the third heart sound (S₃). Note the notch on the upstroke of the systolic wave that corresponds to the high-frequency components of the first heart sound.

The failure of apexcardiography to gain widespread acceptance was related in part to problems of instrumentation. Distortions in the apexcardiogram result from the use of instrumentation with poor response characteristic and, in some cases, air leaks.[17-20] References 17 to 20 are a reading "must" for any physician interested in apexcardiography. Figure 10-32 illustrates some of the variations in configurations of the apexcardiogram that can be obtained from the same individual simply by using different transducers and different pickup devices. The variations are due to both different diameter pickup devices and different transducers. The most marked difference in contour relates to transducers with differences in time constants. The ACGs in Figures 10-30, 10-31 and 10-32 were recorded from the same individual. The sharpened peaks and valleys of apexcardiograms recorded with instruments with short time constants (Fig. 10-31) are distortions of the true complex (Fig. 10-30). The time constant of the entire recording system determines the resultant contour. This is best illustrated when a Statham physiologic pressure transducer is attached to a crystal microphone for simultaneous recording of the apexcardiogram and apex phonocardiogram (Fig. 10-29).

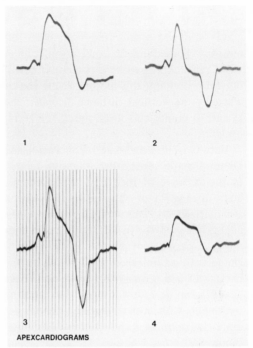

APEXCARDIOGRAMS

Figure 10-32. Apical precordial motion recorded with different instrumentation. *1,* Funnel-type 2.5-cm. pickup air coupled to a Statham physiologic pressure transducer, as in Figure 10-26. *2,* Funnel pickup air coupled to crystal microphone, as illustrated in Figure 10-27. *3,* Cup-type 5.0-cm. pickup air coupled to a Statham physiologic pressure transducer, as in Figure 10-28. *4,* Displacement recording with Wayne Kerr device, as in Figure 10-1.

Even though the time constant of the Statham transducer is long, when connected to the crystal microphone the overall time constant is shortened.

A Wave Ratio. In spite of problems with instrumentation, some qualitative but clinically useful information has evolved from recordings of the apex impulse. The A wave of the apexcardiogram was shown to correspond to the left ventricular presystolic filling wave caused by atrial contraction. Large or accentuated A waves of the apexcardiogram correlated with directly recorded left ventricular presystolic waves of the LV pressure pulse and thus were thought to relate to diminished left ventricular compliance.[21-23] Since the absolute height of the A wave of the apexcardiogram varies with recording gain, the A wave ratio was most often used when attempting hemodynamic correlation. The A wave ratio expressed as a percent is calculated by dividing the amplitude of the A wave by the vertical distance between the E and O points and multiplying the result by 100.

Between 1961 and 1966 Benchimol and Dimond made several observations related to the A wave of the ACG and ischemic heart disease. Their observations have been summarized by Dimond as follows: "In angina an increase in left ventricular end-diastolic pressure occurs . . . and is associated with an enlarged atrial wave on the chest wall and a fourth heart sound. These changes can be returned toward normal by treatment with nitroglycerine, venous 4-limb tourniquets, and tight abdominal binders."[24]

The magnitude of the A wave ratio of the apexcardiogram appears to be influenced by left ventricular end-diastolic pressure, volume and compliance or stiffness.[25,26] Voight and Friesinger found that the A wave ratio of the apexcardiogram predicted the *magnitude* of the left ventricular presystolic wave more than the absolute left ventricular end-diastolic pressure.[25] They found that an A wave ratio equal to or greater than 15% indicated elevated left ventricular end-diastolic pressure (Fig. 10-33) but that a normal A wave ratio did not rule out elevated left ventricular end-diastolic pressure.

An abnormal A wave ratio was found to have diagnostic significance in patients being evaluated for chest pain syndrome, especially when combined with a third or fourth heart sound; 90% of patients with these findings had significant coronary artery disease.[27] The sensitivity of the A wave in predicting abnormalities may be improved by postexercise recordings.[21,24,28,29]

Another use for analysis of the A wave ratio is in patients with aortic insufficiency and associated low-frequency apical murmurs. Most patients with aortic insufficiency and an Austin Flint murmur had A wave ratios of 11 to 25%, whereas patients with aortic insufficiency and associated mitral stenosis did not.[20,30] In the few patients with Austin Flint murmur and normal A wave ratios the A wave ratio was increased after inhalation of amyl nitrite.[31] Thus the apexcardiogram may be helpful in patients with aortic insufficiency to differentiate an Austin Flint murmur from that of associated mitral stenosis.

Quantitative Apexcardiography. In recent years attempts have been made to obtain more quantitative information from the apexcardiogram. Sutton and Craige used a standard impulse produced by a simple calibrator applied to the tambour of their transducer.[32] Using this technique, they have been able to show differences in the amplitude of systolic impulses, and have divided the systolic apical impulses into normal, hyperdynamic and sustained (see below).

Others have reported on further at-

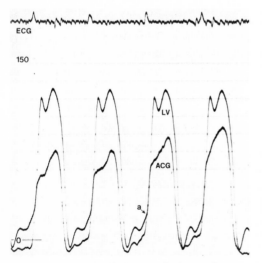

Figure 10-33. Simultaneous electrocardiogram (*ECG*), left ventricular pressure pulse (*LV*) and apexcardiogram (*ACG*) recorded with 2.5-cm. funnel pickup air coupled to a Statham physiologic pressure transducer. The patient was in the left lateral position. The A wave of the ACG is increased in height with an A wave ratio of about 15%. The LV and diastolic pressure was elevated to 26 mm. Hg.

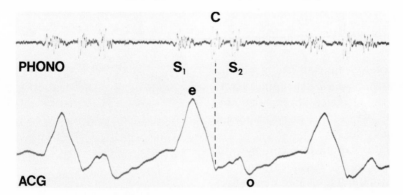

Figure 10-34. Simultaneous phonocardiogram (*PHONO*) and apexcardiogram (*ACG*) from a patient with a floppy or prolapsed mitral valve syndrome. Note the correlation between the midsystolic click (*C*) and systolic retraction of the ACG.

tempts at quantitation of the ACG by quantitating the force with which the pickup device is held against the apical impulse and noting the difference between applied and peak pressures. More recently, simultaneously recorded ACG and the first derivative of the ACG have been made in attempts to standardize or normalize the ACG.[33-37]

Systolic Impulses. Analysis of the systolic waves of the apexcardiogram has been avoided until recently, as the short time constants of the recording equipment turned sustained impulses into tracings with nonsustained waves. Another problem is that the force with which the pickup is held against the apical impulse will also alter the systolic waves of the ACG.

The basic types of apical impulses are normal, hyperdynamic, sustained[33] and bifid. In the *normal,* a declining plateau is noted during systole (Fig. 10-30). The *hyperdynamic* apical impulse differs from the normal only in amplitude and is found in patients with volume overload of the left ventricle such as aortic and mitral regurgitation. The *sustained* impulse is characterized by a plateau that is horizontal, or rising (Fig. 10-33), during ventricular ejection.[33] This type of impulse is found in patients with aortic stenosis, systemic hypertension, primary myocardial disease and ventricular aneurysms.[38] The *bifid* sys-

tolic impulse is found in idiopathic hypertrophic subaortic stenosis (IHSS) and in the floppy, or prolapsed, mitral valve syndrome (Fig. 10-34).[39,40,41]

Displacement Recordings. Displacement recordings are particularly useful in studying systolic impulses[42-44] (Fig. 10-35). With the patient in the *supine* position, the left ventricular apex impulse is normally nonsustained. When sustained, left ventricular hypertrophy or left ventricular akinesis or dyskinesis is present. In a study in which the recorded displacement of the left ventricular apical impulse was compared with the left ventricular mass determined by

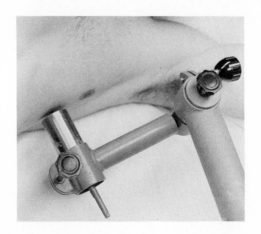

Figure 10-35. Technique of recording displacement of the point of maximal cardiac impulse. This type of recording results in tracings very similar to the kinetocardiogram.

cineangiography, Conn and Cole found that when the left ventricular apical impulse was nonsustained, i.e., early systolic only, 78% of the patients had a normal left ventricular mass. If the impulse was holosystolic or sustained throughout systole (Fig. 10-36), 88% had an increased left ventricular mass.[44]

Precordial displacement recordings, or kinetocardiograms, can document the presence of abnormal impulses that may reflect physiologic or anatomic ventricular aneurysm.[45,46]

Left Parasternal Recordings. When displacement of the left parasternal area is being recorded the patient is instructed to exhale maximally and stop breathing (Fig. 10-37). The dominant left parasternal motion in the normal patient is a gentle retraction. A slight outward motion in early systole, during the isovolumetric or pre-ejection period, is usually recorded. Increased retraction of the left parasternal impulse is found in patients with aortic regurgitation.

There are two general abnormalities of left parasternal displacement associated with right ventricular abnormalities, the *accentuated* parasternal impulse and the *sustained* parasternal impulse. An impulse

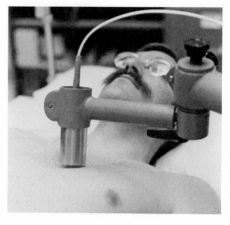

Figure 10-37. Technique of recording precordial displacement. Tracings obtained are similar to kinetocardiograms.

in the left parasternal area that is forceful and sustained is associated with right ventricular hypertrophy or right ventricular dysfunction. Recordings show these impulses to begin in early systole and remain sustained throughout systole. Patients who have volume overload of the right ventricle, such as atrial septal defect, have an accentuated impulse that occurs early in systole. These accentuated impulses are nonsustained. Similar left parasternal impulses may be present in patients with the straight back syndrome.

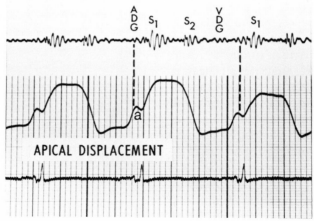

Figure 10-36. Sustained apical impulse. Simultaneous recording of phonocardiogram (*top*), displacement tracing recording from the point of maximal impulse over the left ventricle (*APICAL DISPLACEMENT*) and electrocardiogram (*bottom*). The atrial diastolic gallop (*ADG*) or S₁ coincides with the wave of the displacement tracing.

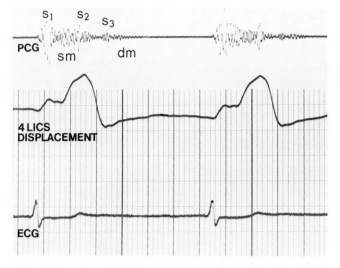

Figure 10-38. Simultaneous phonocardiogram (*PCG*), displacement recording from the fourth left intercostal space (*4LICS*) and electrocardiogram (*ECG*) in a man with severe mitral regurgitation. Note the dominant late systolic outward motion. This is seen in patients with severe mitral regurgitation.

Patients with mitral regurgitation frequently have a prominent parasternal impulse. Because of this, concomitant right ventricular hypertrophy is frequently over-diagnosed. Displacement recordings reveal that the left parasternal impulse of mitral regurgitation peaks in late systole (Fig. 10-38). Timing of the late systolic parasternal impulse of mitral regurgitation indicates that it coincides with the late systolic regurgitant V wave in the left atrial pressure pulse.[47] It has been postulated that the regurgitant flow of blood from the left ventricle into the left atrium and pulmonary veins is initially accepted by the left atrium with little increase in pressure. As systole and the regurgitation progress and the left atrium and pulmonary veins expand to their limit, there is a sharp rise in pressure near the end of systole. The expanding left atrium and the pulmonary veins force the heart anteriorly in late systole. Recently recordings have also been made from the parasternal area with devices used to record apexcardiograms and the findings reported to correlate with the regurgitant volume.[48]

SUMMARY

Non-invasive graphic techniques, although predominantly qualitative in nature, have contributed to the assessment of cardiovascular disease. The clinical applications of many of these recordings will probably decrease as advancements in echocardiography are made. In some conditions it appears that simultaneous recordings of pulse tracings will enhance the diagnostic value of the echocardiogram.

Every cardiovascular patient requires clinical evaluation. It is probable that the principal use of these tracings in the future, as it has been over the past decades, will be to teach the bedside diagnosis of cardiovascular disease.

REFERENCES

1. Podolak, E., Kinn, J. B., and Westura, E. E.: Biomedical applications of a commercial capacitance transducer. IEEE Trans. Biomed. Eng. 16:40, 1969.
2. Cole, J. S., and Conn, R. D.: Assessment of cardiac apex impulse using fiber optics. Br. Heart J. 33:463, 1971.
3. Hartman, H.: The jugular venous tracing. Am. Heart J. 59:698, 1960.

4. Feder, W., and Cherry, R. A.: External jugular phlebogram as reflecting venous and right atrial hemodynamics. Am. J. Cardiol. 12:383, 1963.

5. Rich, L. L., and Tavel, M. E.: The origin of the jugular C wave. N. Engl. J. Med. 234:1309, 1971.

6. Coleman, A. L.: Jugular C wave. N. Engl. J. Med. 235:462, 1971.

7. Tavel, M. E., et al.: The jugular venous pulse in atrial septal defect. Arch. Intern. Med. 121:524, 1968.

8. Calleja, H. B., Rosenow, O. F., and Clark, T. E.: Pulsations of the liver in heart disease. Am. J. Med. 30:202, 1961.

9. Whittaker, A. V., et al.: Sound pressure correlates of the aortic ejection sound. Circulation 39:475, 1969.

10. Freis, E. D., et al.: Changes in the carotid pulse that occur with age and hypertension. Am. Heart J. 71:757, 1966.

11. Epstein, E. J., and Coulshed, N.: Assessment of aortic stenosis from external carotid pulse wave. Br. Heart J. 26:84, 1964.

12. Duchosal, P. W., et al.: Advance in the clinical evaluation of aortic stenosis by arterial pulse recordings of the neck. Am. Heart J. 51:861, 1956.

13. Lyle, D. P., et al.: Slopes of the carotid pulse wave in normal subjects, aortic valvular disease and hypertrophic subaortic stenosis. Circulation 43:374, 1971.

14. Bonner, A. J., Sacks, H. N., and Tavel, M. E.: Assessing the severity of aortic stenosis by phonocardiographic and external carotid pulse recordings. Circulation 48:247, 1973.

15. Ewy, G. A., Rios, J. C., and Marcus, F. I.: The dicrotic arterial pulse. Circulation 39:655, 1969.

16. Benchimol, A., Dimond, E. G., and Carson, J. D.: The value of apexcardiogram as a reference tracing in phonocardiography. Am. Heart J. 61:485, 1961.

17. Mashimo, K., et al.: An instrumental aspect of apexcardiography decay characteristics of transducers and its clinical implication. Jap. Heart J. 7:536, 1966.

18. Kesteloot, H., Willens, J., and Van Vollenhoven, E.: On the physical principles and methodology of mechanocardiography. Acta Cardiol. 24:147, 1969.

19. Johnson, J. M., Siegel, W., and Blomquist, G.: Characteristics of transducers used for recording the apexcardiogram. J. Appl. Physiol. 31:796, 1971.

20. Kastor, J. A., et al.: Air leaks as a source of distortion in apexcardiography. Chest 57:163, 1970.

21. Benchimol, A., and Dimond, E. G.: The apexcardiogram in normal older subjects and in patients with arteriosclerotic heart disease. Effect of exercise on the "A" wave. Am. Heart J. 65:789, 1963.

22. Benchimol, A., and Dimond, E. G.: The apexcardiogram in ischemic heart disease. Br. Heart J. 61:251, 1968.

23. Martin, C. E., Shaver, J. A., and Leonard, J. J.: Physical signs, apexcardiography, phonocardiography systolic time intervals in angina pectoris. Circulation 46:1098, 1972.

24. Dimond, E. G.: The exercise apexcardiogram: A clinical test in angina pectoris. Am. J. Cardiol. 27:120, 1971.

25. Voigt, G. C., and Friesinger, G. C.: The use of apexcardiography in the assessment of left ventricular diastolic pressure. Circulation 41:1015, 1970.

26. Gibson, T. C., et al.: The A wave of the apexcardiogram and left ventricular diastolic stiffness. Circulation 49:441, 1974.

27. Cohn, P. F., et al.: Diastolic heart sounds and filling waves in coronary artery disease. Circulation 44:196, 1971.

28. Ginn, W. M., et al.: Apexcardiography: Use in coronary heart disease and reproducibility. Am. Heart J. 73:168, 1967.

29. Aronow, W. S., Cassidy, J., and Uyeyawa, R. R.: Resting and post exercise apexcardiogram correlated with maximal treadmill stress test in normal subjects. Circulation 44:397, 1971.

30. Parker, E., Craige, E., and Hood, W. P., Jr.: The Austin Flint murmur and the A wave of the apexcardiogram in aortic regurgitation. Circulation 43:349, 1971.

31. Fortuin, N. J., and Craige, E.: On the mechanism of the Austin Flint murmur. Circulation 45:558, 1972.

32. Sutton, G. C., and Craige, E.: Quantitation of precordial movement: I. Normal subjects. Circulation 35:476, 1967.

33. Sutton, G. C., Prewitt, T. A., and Craige, E.: Relationship between quantitated precordial movement and left ventricular function. Am. J. Cardiol 29:667, 1972.

34. Vetter, W. R., Sullivan, R. W., and Hyatt, K. H.: Assessment of quantitative apexcardiography: A noninvasive index of LV function. Am. J. Cardiol. 29:667, 1972.

35. Willens, J., De Geest, H., and Kesteloot, H.: A new approach to the recording of low frequency precordial vibrations. Acta Cardiol. 26:263, 1971.

36. Denef, B., et al.: On the clinical value of calibrated displacement apexcardiography. Circulation 51:541, 1975.

37. Motomura, M., et al.: An apexcardiographic index "(Peak DA/DT)/A" for the assessment of left ventricular function. Jap. Circ. J. 37:1355, 1973.

38. McGinn, F. X., Gould, L., and Lyon, A. F.: The phonocardiogram and apexcardiogram in patients with ventricular aneurysm. Am. J. Cardiol. 21:467, 1968.

39. Benchimol, A., Legler, J. F., and Dimond, E. G.: The carotid tracing and apexcardiogram in subaortic stenosis and idiopathic myocardial hypertrophy. Am. J. Cardiol. 11:427, 1963.

40. Spencer, W. H., Behar, V. S., and Orgain, E. S.: Apexcardiogram in patients with prolapsing mitral valve. Am. J. Cardiol. 32:276, 1973.

41. Ahuja, S. P., and Gutterrez, M. R.: Apexcardiography in the elucidation of a double or multiple impulse apex beat. Am. J. Cardiol. 19:468, 1967.

42. Bancroft, W. H., Jr., and Eddleman, E. E., Jr.: Methods and physical characteristics of the kinetocardiographic and apexcardiographic systems for recording low frequency precordial motion. Am. Heart J. 73:756, 1967.

43. Beilin, L., and Mounsey, P.: The left ventricular impulse in hypertensive heart disease. Br. Heart J. 24:409, 1962.

44. Conn, R. D., and Cole, J. S.: The cardiac apex impulse: Clinical and angiographic correlations. Ann. Intern. Med. 75:185, 1971.

45. Harrison, T. R., and Huges, L.: Precordial systolic bulges during anginal attacks. Trans. Assoc. Am. Physicians 71:174, 1958.

46. Eddleman, E. E., Jr., and Langley, J. O.: Paradoxical pulsations of the precordium in myocardial infarction and angina pectoris. Am. Heart J. 63:579, 1962.

47. Tucker, W. T., Knowles, J. L., and Eddleman, E., Jr.: Mitral insufficiency: Cardiac mechanics as studied with the kinetocardiogram and ballistocardiogram. Circulation 12:278, 1955.

48. Basta, L. L., et al.: The value of left parasternal impulse recordings in the assessment of mitral regurgitation. Circulation 43:1055, 1973.

Chapter 11

Systolic Time Intervals

ERNESTO E. SALCEDO AND WAYNE SIEGEL

Ventricular systole is defined as that period of the cardiac cycle beginning with electrical depolarization of the interventricular septum and ending with closure of the semilunar valves. The initial electrical event during which depolarization of the ventricles occurs in sequential order is the period of electromechanical delay. Isovolumic systole begins with ventricular myocardial contraction, and the subsequent rise in ventricular pressure above the pressures in the pulmonary artery and aorta opens the semilunar valves. This ends the period of isovolumic contraction. As soon as the pulmonic and aortic valves open the ejection period starts and continues until ventricular pressures fall below the great vessel pressures. The termination of systole occurs with closure of the semilunar valves.

The timing of ventricular systole can be precisely determined without cardiac catheterization, and these data provide information related to left ventricular performance, preload and afterload. Right-sided systole is usually evaluated by cardiac catheterization. Recently Hirschfeld and associates, employing echocardiographic studies of the pulmonic valve, were able to obtain right ventricular systolic time intervals in a group of children.[1] The value of this technique for the adult population will prove cumbersome and requires confirmation.

Even though analysis of the radial pulse as an indicator of health or disease has been attempted for centuries, it was not until 1860 that Marey analyzed the arterial pulse for the diagnosis of specific cardiovascular disorders.[2] Garrod described the inverse relationship between ejection time and heart rate.[3] In 1923 Katz and Feil introduced the use of simultaneous photographic recordings of the electrocardiogram, heart sounds and central arterial pulse to measure the systolic phases of the cardiac cycle.[4] The influence of sex and posture on duration of ejection was first described in 1926 by Lombard and Cope.[5] This technique received little attention as a clinical tool until Weissler and coworkers made an enormous contribution in the understanding and clinical use of the systolic time intervals (STIs).[6-12] Benchimol and Dimond renewed interest in apexcardiography and in 1962 introduced this technique for the evaluation of systolic events.[13]

At present there are three approaches

for the measurement of STIs by non-invasive methods.

1. Use of the electrocardiogram, carotid pulse and phonocardiogram with which total electromechanical systole (QS_2), left ventricular ejection time (LVET) and pre-ejection phase (PEP) are derived, as described by Weissler and coworkers.[9] Most of the information on STIs in normal subjects and in patients with cardiac abnormalities has been obtained by this method.

2. Other investigators have indicated that the apexcardiogram is essential for the exact determination of STIs since the precise onset of left ventricular contraction can only be determined externally by defining the U point of the apexcardiogram.[14-16] With this information, the electromechanical delay (QU) and the isovolumic contraction time (IVCT) can be measured.

3. Measurement from a high-speed strip chart recording of the aortic valve echocardiogram. By this method the QS_2 is calculated from the beginning of ventricular depolarization to the aortic valve closure in the echocardiogram. The LVET is measured as the interval from the opening of the aortic valve to its closure. The PEP is obtained indirectly by subtracting LVET from QS_2.[17] The few studies that have compared this echocardiographic method with the conventionally measured STIs have demonstrated an excellent correlation of values.[1,17,18] This technique offers an alternative method of recording STIs in patients in whom the carotid pulse or high-frequency components of the second heart sound cannot be adequately recorded. Because of the technical difficulties in obtaining high-quality aortic valve studies in

all patients, there are definite limitations to this approach.

RECORDING EQUIPMENT

We use a six-channel photographic recorder for the following determinations:

1. A bipolar chest lead is used for determining the onset of ventricular depolarization.

2. Carotid pulse tracing is obtained with an inductance displacement transducer (Hewlett-Packard APT-16) recorded with a 5-second time constant amplifier (Elema Schonander, Solna, Sweden) for evaluating LVET.

3. One microphone is placed in the second left intercostal space to record the initial high-frequency components of the second heart sound and another at the cardiac apex for recording the initial low-frequency components of the first heart sound.

4. The apexcardiogram is recorded at the apex impulse with an inductance displacement transducer (Hewlett-Packard APT-16) and a 5-second time constant amplifier (Elema Schonander Solna, Sweden) (Fig. 11-1).

MEASUREMENT TECHNIQUES

1. Total electromechanical systole. The QS_2 is measured from the onset of ventricular depolarization to the initial high-frequency vibrations of the aortic component of the second heart sound.

2. Left ventricular ejection time. The LVET is measured from the beginning of the upstroke to the dicrotic notch of the carotid pulse.

3. Pre-ejection period. The PEP is obtained indirectly by subtracting LVET from QS_2 interval.

4. Electromechanical delay. The QU interval begins with the onset of ven-

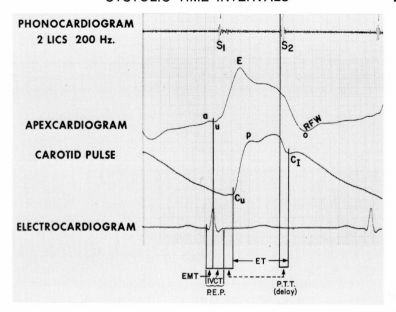

Figure 11-1. Systolic time intervals commonly measured with important points to identify on the electrocardiogram, phonocardiogram, carotid, and apex pulses. *EMT,* electromechanical delay; *IVCT,* isovolumic contraction time; *PEP,* pre-ejection phase; *ET,* ejection time; *PTT,* pulse transmission time from the aortic valve to the carotid artery; *2 LICS,* second left intercostal space

tricular depolarization and ends at the beginning of contraction; it is measured from the beginning of ventricular depolarization to the U point of the apexcardiogram.

5. Isovolumic contraction time. The IVCT begins with ventricular contraction and ends with the beginning of ejection. This is measured from the U point of the apexcardiogram to the beginning of the upstroke of the carotid pulse corrected for the pulse transmission time (Table 11-1).

PHYSIOLOGIC BASIS FOR THE SYSTOLIC TIME INTERVALS

The understanding and interpretation of systolic time intervals is difficult, since multiple factors and variables affect total duration and different phases of ventricular systole (Table 11-2). The first factor recognized was the effect of heart rate. This problem has been partially resolved by the description of curves that correct for different heart rates. Regression equations for

PEP, OS_2 and LVET have been developed for a wide range of heart rates.[6]

Other variables are more difficult to evaluate, and these may present more serious problems in the interpretation of the systolic time intervals. These include the effects of preload and afterload of the ventricles and the inotropic state of the heart.

TABLE 11-1

Measurement of Systolic Time Intervals

Total electro-mechanical systole (QS_2)	From the onset of ventricular depolarization to the initial high-frequency vibrations of A_2
Left ventricular ejection time (LVET)	From the beginning of upstroke to the dicrotic notch of the carotid pulse
Pre-ejection period (PEP)	Measured by subtracting LVET from QS_2
Electromechanical delay (QU)	From the beginning of ventricular depolarization to the U point of the apexcardiogram
Isovolumic contraction time (IVCT)	From the U point of the apexcardiogram to the beginning of the upstroke of the carotid pulse corrected for pulse transmission time

TABLE 11-2

Factors That Alter Systolic Time Intervals

	Chronotropism		Inotropism		Afterload		Preload	
	Increased	Decreased	Increased	Decreased	Increased	Decreased	Increased	Decreased
PEP	↓	↑	↓	↑	±	↓	↓	↑
LVET	↓	↑	↑	↓	↑	±	↑	↓
QS₂	↓	↑	±	±	↑	±	±	±

↑ = lengthen; ↓ = shorten; ± = variable or no change.

Since these variables affect the systolic time intervals, it is essential to understand their role in normal and abnormal cardiac function. In the following discussion we present the STI changes by grouping the physiologic and pathophysiologic processes that affect primarily the preload, afterload or the inotropic state of the heart (Table 11-3). Clinically, overlap occurs with multiple variables in effect producing a "composite" measured set of systolic intervals.

At present there is enough information to validate externally recorded STIs as an accurate measure of left ventricular systolic events.[12,19,20] Van De Werf and colleagues, on studying 26 patients, found that LVET and PEP measured internally and externally were strongly correlated, but they found that at rest external LVET was 4 to 4.5 msec. shorter, external PEP 5.5 to 6 msec. longer than corresponding intervals measured internally.[20] At heart rates above 100 the relationship was reversed.

TABLE 11-3

Factors That Alter Cardiac Dynamics

A. Chronotropism
   Adrenergic stimuli
   Vagal blockade
   Atrial pacing
   Exercise
   Arrhythmias
B. Inotropism
   Primary myocardial disease
   Arteriosclerotic cardiovascular disease
   Thyroid state
   Drugs: digitalis, isoproterenol, epinephrine, nor-
      epinephrine, propranolol
C. Afterload
   Aortic stenosis
   Idiopathic hypertrophic subaortic stenosis
   Hypertension
   Drugs
D. Preload
   Aortic insufficiency
   Mitral insufficiency
   Mitral stenosis
   Left atrial myxoma
E. Miscellaneous
   Age
   Sex
   Position
   Diurnal change
   Conduction abnormalities: LBBB, RBBB, and
      LAHB
   Pericardial disease
   Chronic lung disease
   Pregnancy

EFFECTS OF VENTRICULAR PRELOAD

Preload is the diastolic stretch of the ventricle just before the beginning of systole, with greater stretch producing more powerful and faster contraction. In hemodynamic terms, this would mean that larger end-diastolic volumes would be associated with larger stroke volumes. Expressed in terms of STIs, increased preload produces shortening of the IVCT. For example, in atrial fibrillation the longer the preceding cycle with greater diastolic preload, the shorter the IVCT. This means that the larger the preload or presystolic stretch, the faster the contraction velocity and greater the shortening of the IVCT. Simultaneously, lengthening of the LVET occurs because of a larger ejected volume. The overall duration of systole is essentially unaltered. The classical alteration producing an increased left ventricular preload occurs in patients with aortic insufficiency when bidirectional diastolic blood flow into the left ventricle produces a large end-diastolic volume. Because of this increased preload and because of low central aortic diastolic pressure (decreased afterload) the PEP is characteristically reduced.[9] There is a long LVET as a consequence of an increased stroke volume. Heart failure in patients with aortic insufficiency tends to normalize the PEP and LVET.

In mitral stenosis the preload is reduced because the diastolic flow to the left ventricle is obstructed. This results in a reduced stroke volume and shortening of the LVET.[21-23] Mitral closure is delayed because of the additional time required for the left ventricle to generate enough pressure to exceed the raised left atrial pressure. This results in prolongation of the Q-S_1 interval. The amount of Q-S_1 prolongation correlates roughly with the amount of diastolic pressure gradient across the mitral valve; therefore, the Q-S_1 interval has been suggested as an index of the severity of mitral stenosis.[24-26] The Q-S_1 interval measurement is of limited value in quantitating mitral obstruction because it is affected by multiple factors such as the variations of electromechanical interval from individual to individual, the length of the preceding cycle and the individual variations of the rate of pressure rise (inotropic state) within the left ventricle.[27] In studying 36 patients with mitral stenosis, Oreshkov found the initial phase of ventricular contraction (C-MI interval, from the U point of the apexcardiogram to the mitral component of the first sound) to be lengthened, and the pressure elevation time (MI-E interval, from the onset of mitral component of the first sound to the onset of ejection) to be shortened.[28] The isovolumic contraction was normal.

Garrard and associates demonstrated that the relation between PEP/LVET and ejection fraction is retained in patients with mitral stenosis, but this correlation is not as good as the one obtained in patients with myocardial disease.[21]

In left atrial myxoma, the tumor obstructs the diastolic blood flow to the left ventricle. The left atrial pressure is increased and the Q-S_1 interval is prolonged by a similar mechanism as in mitral stenosis.[27]

The STIs in mitral regurgitation are not as well understood as other valve lesions. It is of interest that despite the large total stroke volume ejected by the left ventricle, a prolonged LVET is distinctly uncommon.[21-23] Indeed, the STIs are often normal. Prolonged PEP and shortened LVET are strongly suggestive of abnormal left ventricular function in the patient with mitral regurgitation.[9]

EFFECTS OF VENTRICULAR AFTERLOAD

Afterload is determined by aortic impedance and peripheral resistance. In practical terms this can be considered as the diastolic pressure in the aorta prior to aortic valve opening. It is apparent that the higher the diastolic aortic pressure, the longer will be the interval between the onset of the ventricular pressure rise and the opening of the semilunar valves. Conversely, when the diastolic pressure is low, isovolumic contraction is abbreviated. Severe aortic stenosis is often accompanied by prolongation of the LVET despite a normal or decreased stroke volume.[22,23,29] This is primarily related to reduced ejection velocity. In addition, this may reflect the relatively low ventricular pressure necessary to begin and end ejection as a consequence of lowered aortic pressure. In patients with aortic stenosis the PEP is frequently shorter than normal and LVET is often prolonged. The PEP/LVET ratio is strikingly reduced in these patients.[9] With left ventricular decompensation, one may expect prolongation of the PEP and shortening of the LVET. However, since the

PEP is initially shortened and the LVET prolonged, these deviations due to left ventricular dysfunction may simply normalize the systolic time intervals.

The duration of LVET may also be useful in predicting the presence or absence of significant dynamic outflow obstruction in hypertrophic subaortic stenosis.[30] Outflow obstruction prolongs LVET as in valvular aortic stenosis, and maneuvers that increase the outflow gradient such as catecholamine administration may lengthen the LVET in these subjects.

In chronic hypertensive disease with compensated left ventricular performance, PEP and LVET are usually normal.[11] In patients with severe hypertension the QS_2 has been found to be prolonged.[31] As left ventricular failure supervenes, there is prolongation of the PEP and abbreviation of the LVET.

EFFECTS OF CONTRACTILE PERFORMANCE

Cardiac performance is also affected by changes in the inotropic state of the myocardium. In contrast to the quantitative change in myocardial function resulting from alteration of the preload and afterload, enhanced contractility causes a qualitative change in the contraction of myocardial fibers. Myocardial contractility is generally assessed directly by cardiac catheterization. The determinations are based primarily upon the rate of rise of left ventricular pressure (DP/DT)[32] or velocity of circumferential fiber shortening. With heart rate and peripheral resistance kept constant, increased cardiac contractility shortens the isovolumic phase and prolongs LVET but has little or no effect on the duration of total systole. Conversely, diminished cardiac contractility prolongs the isovolumic phase and shortens LVET.[32] In the presence of diminished cardiac contractility and low stroke volume with elevated peripheral resistance, as is the case in congestive heart failure, there

is prolongation of the PEP and IVCT, abbreviation of LVET and virtually an unaltered duration of total electromechanical systole.[6] Both periods of the pre-ejection phase are prolonged in heart failure. The principal cause for this prolongation is the diminished rate of rise in isovolumic left ventricular pressure. The possibility of contribution by an increased electromechanical delay has not been excluded but appears to be theoretically unimportant.

There is a close relationship between the changes in left ventricular function and changes in duration of the different phases of systole, especially isovolumic contraction time. This may imply that prolongation of IVCT and left ventricular dysfunction may be caused by the same underlying defect in the mechanical performance of the heart. The intrinsic contractile state of the myocardium from failing hearts as reflected in the decreased maximum isotonic velocity, isometric tension and in the active length tension curves is present in heart failure.[33] Abnormalities in myocardial contractility as well as possible defects in the number, organization and synchrony of the myofibers may be primary causes of the altered systolic time intervals in patients with heart failure. The time required for the intraventricular pressure to reach aortic diastolic pressure is prolonged because of a deficient velocity of myocardial force. This, regardless of the end-diastolic volume, results in prolongation of the PEP period.[6,33]

Decreased inotropism results in increased PEP and shortening of LVET. In this respect, the most practical use of STI has been the one derived from the excellent correlation found between the ratio of PEP/LVET and ejection fraction in evaluating left ventricular performance.[21] This ratio is not influenced by heart rate within the range of 50 to 110 beats per minute.[9] Diminished left ventricular performance results in increased PEP/LVET ratio.[7] This results in a positive correlation for prolonged PEP and an abbreviated LVET. The degree of correlation of this ratio with the ejection fraction is excellent;[21] thus, the PEP/LVET ratio reflects the combined influence of the directionally opposite relationship of each of the systolic intervals to the ejection fraction.

There is less significant correlation of this ratio with angiographically determined end-diastolic volume and poor correlation with left ventricular end-diastolic pressure and stroke volume.[21] However, it should be stressed that left ventricular disease does not imply that STI will be abnormal. Patients with clinically recognizable primary myocardial disease usually have abnormal STI, but patients with coronary artery disease may not.[9] It is not uncommon to find patients with angina pectoris with normal STI.

Acute myocardial infarction produces changes in the STI that may be clinically helpful. Diamant and Killip, in studying 100 patients with acute myocardial infarction, found that the QS_2 interval was shortened, especially on the day of admission.[34] The PEP was found to be prolonged during the first 5 days, and this was more evident in patients with transmural infarcts. This resulted from prolongation of both the QS_1 and IVCT. Other investigators have found the QS_1 and IVCT to be shortened in the first few days after myocardial infarction, probably due to catecholamine release.[35-37] Gradual lengthening accompanies recovery as one would expect from the diminution of the release of catecholamines.[35] Hamosh and coworkers correlated STIs with direct hemodynamic measurements in patients with acute myocardial infarction and found that patients with significantly elevated left ventricular end-diastolic pressure and clinical signs of congestive heart failure usually had prolonged PEP as compared with normal subjects or patients with myocardial failure.[38]

The measurement of systolic time intervals has contributed to the understanding of the inotropic effect of certain drugs on cardiovascular dynamics. For example, Weissler and associates studied 30 normal men and found that after the administration of 1.6 mg. deslanoside (Cedilanid D) intravenously there was significant abbreviation in the duration of all phases of left ventricular systole when compared to control levels.[10] The degree of shortening of each phase of ventricular systole remained relatively constant during the first 8 hours following the administration of deslanoside, and during the following 5 days there was a progressive increase of the systolic phases. The changes in the phases of ventricular systole during the first 4 hours following drug administration were accompanied by relative bradycardia. This was not the case in 8 hours or the subsequent 5 days of observation. In overt heart failure, the same group demonstrated that the administration of deslanoside was followed by prompt shortening of the STI.[11] The duration of isovolumic contraction is dependent upon the left ventricular end-diastolic pressure, the arterial diastolic pressure and the rate of left ventricular pressure rise during the isovolumic period. Digitalis appears to decrease the left ventricular end-diastolic pressure and has no effect on aortic diastolic pressure. Thus the diminution and duration of the isovolumic period probably reflect an increase in the rate of rise of left ventricular pressure during the isovolumic interval. It appears that the vagal effect of deslanoside is transient and may be of shorter duration compared to contractile effects of the drug.[11]

The PEP has also been found to be shortened by isoproterenol, norepinephrine and epinephrine,[39] all of which activate beta-adrenergic receptors. The shortening of the PEP reflects an increased velocity of ventricular contraction induced by these inotropic agents, since PEP is not altered by changes in heart rate induced by atropine or atrial pacing. In addition to the positive inotropic actions of isoproterenol and epinephrine, peripheral vessel dilatation and resultant lowering of aortic diastolic pressure may also contribute to the shortening of the PEP induced by these agents. The shortening of PEP is greatest with isoproterenol, a drug with virtually pure beta-adrenergic receptor–activating properties. Lesser abbreviation of PEP is observed with epinephrine, a drug with predominant beta-adrenergic but also considerable alpha-adrenergic properties. A minimal shortening of PEP is measured after administration of norepinephrine, a drug with minor cardiac beta-adrenergic receptor–activating properties and potent vasoconstrictive action. The degree of shortening of PEP by these three agents appears to be related directly to the cardiac and vascular beta-adrenergic effects and inversely related to the alpha-adrenergic or vasoconstrictive effects.

Harris and associates studied normal resting subjects after intravenous administration of 10 mg. propranolol and found that this lengthened the PEP an average of 10 msec.[39] After beta blocking, isoproterenol had little effect on the PEP, whereas epinephrine and norepinephrine actually prolonged it. This effect of epinephrine and norepinephrine that emerges during beta blocking is presumably due to residual alpha-adrenergic receptor–stimulating properties of these two agents. This concept was supported by the observation that angiotensin, a nonadrenergic vasoconstricting agent, lengthened the PEP both before and after administration of propranolol. Thus, vasoconstriction with resultant increases in cardiac afterload prolongs the PEP. In contrast, beta-adrenergic activity is characterized by shortening of the PEP, an effect that propranolol blocks.

Although the chronotropic effect of thyroid hormone on the myocardium was clearly demonstrated by Yater[41] and by Markovitz and Yater,[40] the possible inotropic effects of thyroid hormone have remained controversial. Buccino and asso-

ciates have shown that the thyroid state exerts positive inotropic effect on the isolated papillary muscle of hyperthyroid and hypothyroid cats.[42] The accelerated rate of muscular shortening and abbreviation of time to peak tension in hyperthyroid muscles and the opposite situation in hypothyroid muscles were demonstrated. Morteza and colleagues recently studied a group of patients with different thyroid states and found LVET to be shortened in hyperthyroidism and prolonged in hypothyroidism.[43] Isovolumic contraction time was also found to be shortened in hyperthyroid patients. Similar findings were present on the evaluation of PEP. That these changes were not related to the level of catecholamines was proved by the fact that the isovolumic contraction time of hyperthyroid subjects treated with reserpine remained unaltered.

EFFECT OF MISCELLANEOUS CONDITIONS ON SYSTOLIC TIME INTERVALS

During upright posture in normal individuals the PEP is prolonged, and the LVET and QS$_2$ are shortened.[44] Also a diurnal decrease in LVET and QS$_2$ without significant change in PEP occurs in normal subjects.[10,45] The isovolumic contraction time was found to lengthen from noon to 4:00 A.M. in patients with coronary artery disease studied by Aronow and coworkers.[46] No correlation was found by these authors between plasma catecholamine levels and systolic time intervals. These findings suggested a nocturnal decrease in left ventricular contractility in patients with coronary artery disease, the mechanism of which remains to be elucidated. In the adult population a slight increase in the PEP occurs with advancing age.[47] The LVET corrected for heart rate varies remarkably little with age.

Prolongation in left ventricular conduction results in lengthening of PEP. Results of some studies have indicated that prolongation is primarily in the electro-mechanical delay (QS_1); other studies have suggested that prolonged isovolumic contraction time is a major abnormality.[48,49] It is possible that both the delay in QS_1 and prolonged isovolumic contraction time account for the prolonged PEP in patients with left ventricular conduction defects.

LVET is probably the best approach for estimating the presence of diminished left ventricular performance in patients with conduction abnormalities. Right bundle branch block in the absence of left ventricular dysfunction does not appear to alter left ventricular STI.[9] Patients with right bundle branch block and left anterior hemiblock have prolonged STI similar to that observed in patients with complete left bundle branch block.[50]

In atrial fibrillation the LVET is directly related to the ratio of the R-R interval.[51] The PEP lengthens rather than shortens with shorter R-R intervals. This is in contrast to the usual response wherein the PEP is shortened with increasing heart rate. The lengthening of the PEP as well as the shortening of the LVET are more striking with R-R intervals of less than 0.8 second.[9] This presents certain difficulties in the interpretation of STIs in patients with atrial fibrillation, especially because there is a nonlinear relationship between cycle length and the PEP/LVET at the shorter R-R intervals. Premature ventricular contractions result in prolonged PEP and shortened LVET. The post extrasystolic beat shows a shorter PEP and longer LVET than normal beats.[9]

When atrial pacing is employed to increase heart rate the PEP does not shorten, and the QS_2 and LVET shorten less than with spontaneous increase in heart rate.[52]

The effects of exercise on STI are difficult to interpret because of the mechanical difficulties associated with measurement of STIs during exercise. Nevertheless, patients with angina may show relatively prolonged LVET following exercise.[53] An alternative method of evaluating STIs during exercise is the use of ear densitometry as a substitute for the carotid pulse tracing. The mechanical difficulties introduced by exercise are overcome by this method, and there is a good correlation between LVET obtained from direct aortic tracings and that obtained from densitometry tracings.[54]

Isometric hand grip can also be used as an alternative and simple cardiovascular stress test. Siegel and colleagues evaluated patients by this method and found that the isometric exercise had an inconsistent effect upon PEP, whereas the LVET index was significantly prolonged in patients with atherosclerotic heart disease, and the PEP/LVET was decreased, although not significantly.[55]

The STI has also been found helpful in patients with pericardial disease. In the presence of pericardial tamponade, marked respiratory variations in LVET can be demonstrated and probably represent the variations of the stroke volume that are responsible for pulsus paradoxus.[56] These changes appear to be more sensitive than the detection of pulsus paradoxus by the sphygmomanometer method. Another application of STIs in pericardial disease is in the detection of left ventricular dysfunction. In the presence of severe congestive heart failure the finding of normal LVET should lead one to suspect pericardial constriction as a possible cause of the congestive state.[9]

Hemodynamic alterations occurring during pregnancy have been known for several years; significant increase of cardiac output has been a consistent finding.[57] Burg and coworkers, on studying women throughout pregnancy, found abbreviation of the PEP in the first and second trimester and prolongation of PEP and PEP/LVET and shortening of LVET during the last trimester.[58] These changes are probably due to decreased left ventricular preload resulting from diminished venous return secondary to inferior vena caval obstruction by the gravid uterus.

Hooper and Whitcomb studied patients with chronic obstructive lung (COPD) disease and found prolonged PEP, shortened LVET and increased PEP/LVET ratio, despite the absence of cardiac symptomatology or clinical evidence of cardiac dysfunction.[59] These changes were more pronounced in patients with severe COPD. They speculated that the left ventricle, in addition to the right ventricle, is adversely affected by the increase in pulmonary vascular resistance present in patients with COPD.

LIMITATIONS OF THE TECHNIQUE

Changes in the duration of the STIs can be introduced by position and the time of the day when they are recorded. This is particularly important to recognize when one is doing serial studies on an individual patient. If there are only minimal or mild variations, this may not be evident if done in a different baseline state.

There is also need of excellent quality recordings to be able to recognize small STI variations. STI measurements may be difficult in patients with aortic valve disease when the dicrotic notch may be difficult to identify or in patients with emphysema or obesity in whom the initial high-frequency components of the second heart sound may not be recorded.

Adequate apexcardiograms can be obtained in about 90% of the patients without emphysema or obesity.

Patients with proven coronary artery disease may have normal STI. Patients with aortic valve disease may have increased and initially shortened PEP when congestive heart failure supervenes. If one performs the study at that particular moment without previous study, this information may be misleading.

The same considerations have to be made in the interpretation of systolic time intervals in patients receiving digitalis or other inotropic agents, since PEP that is prolonged in patients with congestive heart failure will become normal with the use of this agent. In this respect, one has to be aware of any medication that the patient is taking and also to recognize the possible influence of this drug on the STI. The limitation of this technique in the presence of simultaneous variables is well demonstrated in the different results that have been obtained in studying patients with acute myocardial infarction. Perloff and Reichek believed that the explanation for the discrepancy in observations on PEP and LVET in the presence of acute myocardial infarction lay in the number of variables such as heart rate, afterload, left ventricular end-diastolic pressure, inotropic state of the heart and aortic diastolic pressure.[60] It is obvious that the presence or absence of congestive heart failure or shock will significantly alter these measurements.

Similar problems may be expected in combined valvular lesions or associated left ventricular dysfunction in valvular heart disease.

SUMMARY

The evaluation of the different phases of ventricular systole can be conveniently done non-invasively by simultaneous recordings of the electrocardiogram, phonocardiogram, carotid pulse and apexcardiogram. The duration of each of the different phases of systole can be precisely determined by this technique, and the variation from normal can be assessed.

A decreased inotropic state of the heart will tend to prolong the IVCT and the PEP, and shorten the LVET. An opposite result will be found with enhanced inotropism. An increased preload will produce a shorter isovolumic phase and PEP and prolonged LVET. A decreased preload will produce opposite results.

Increased afterload produces variable responses in the isovolumic contraction and an increased ejection time. A decreased afterload will usually increase the ejection time and decrease the isovolumic contraction time and PEP.

Increased heart rate will shorten the isovolumic contraction time and the LVET.

By understanding these predictable changes in the phases of systole induced by alterations in ventricular chronotropism and inotropism, and the afterload and preload of the heart, one can predict the changes that will occur in the different phases of systole in the different pathologic processes that alter these variables.

When adequately obtained and interpreted STIs offer a conveniently derived and repeatable non-invasive method of evaluating patients with cardiovascular disorders.

REFERENCES

1. Hirschfeld, S., et al.: Measurement of right and left ventricular systolic time intervals by echocardiography. Circulation 51:304, 1975.
2. Marey, M. M.: De l'emploi du sphygmographe dans le diagnostic des affections valvulaires du coeur et des aneurismes des arteres; extrait d'une note de M. Marey. CR Acad. Sci. (D) 51:813, 1860.
3. Garrod, A. H.: On some points connected with the circulation of the blood arrived at from a study of the sphigmograph-trace. Proc. R. Soc. 23:140, 1874–1875.
4. Katz, L. N., and Feil, H. S.: Clinical observations on the dynamics of ventricular systole. I. Auricular fibrillation. Arch. Intern. Med. 32:672, 1923.
5. Lombard, W. P., and Cope, O. M.: The duration of systole of the left ventricle in man. Am. J. Physiol. 77:263, 1926.
6. Weissler, A. M., Harris, W. S., and Schoenfeld, C. D.: Systolic time intervals in heart failure in man. Circulation 37:149, 1968.
7. Weissler, A. M., Harris, W. S., and Schoenfeld, C. D.: Bedside technics for the evaluation of ventricular function in man. Am. J. Cardiol. 23:577, 1969.
8. Weissler, A. M., and Garrard, C. L., Jr.: Systolic time intervals in cardiac. disease. Mod. Conc. Cardiovasc. Dis. 40:1, 1970.
9. Weissler, A. M., Lewis, R. P., and Leighton, R. F.: The systolic time intervals as a measure of left ventricular performance in man. *In* Progress in Cardiology. Philadelphia, Lea and Febiger, 1972, vol. 1.
10. Weissler, A. M., et al.: The effect of deslano-side on the duration of the phases of ventricular systole in man. Am. J. Cardiol. 15:153, 1965.
11. Weissler, A. M., Harris, W. S., and Schoenfeld, C. D.: Systolic time intervals in heart failure in man. Circulation 38:149, 1968.
12. Weissler, A. M., Peeler, R. G., and Roehll, W. H., Jr.: Relationship between left ventricular ejection time, stroke volume and heart rate in normal individuals and patients with cardiovascular disease. Am. Heart J. 62:367, 1961.
13. Benchimol, A., and Dimond, E. G.: The apex cardiogram in ischemic heart disease. Br. Heart J. 24:581, 1962.
14. Wayne, H. H.: Non-invasive Technics in Cardiology. Chicago, Year Book Medical Publishers, 1973.
15. Fabian, J., Epstein, E. J., and Coulshed, H.: Duration of phases of left ventricular systole using indirect methods. I. Normal subjects. Br. Heart J. 34:874, 1972.
16. Spodick, D. H., and Kunar, S.: Isovolumic contraction period of the left ventricle; results in a normal series and comparison of methods of calculation by atraumatic technique. Am. Heart J. 76:498, 1968.
17. Stefadouros, M. A., and Withman, C. A.: Systolic time intervals by echocardiography. Circulation 51:114, 1975.
18. Vredevoe, L. A., Creekmore, S. P., and Schiller, N. B.: The measurement of systolic time intervals by echocardiography. J. Clin. Ultrasound 2:99, 1974.
19. Martin, C. E., et al.: Direct correlation of external systolic time intervals with indices of left ventricular function in man. Circulation 4:419, 1971.
20. Van De Werf, F., Piessen, J., Kestelos, T. H., and De Geest, H.: A comparison of systolic time intervals derived from the central aortic pressure and from the external carotid pulse tracing. Circulation 51:310, 1975.
21. Garrard, C. L., Jr., Weissler, A. M., and Dodge, H. T.: The relationship of alterations in systolic time intervals to ejection fraction in patients with cardiac disease. Circulation 42:455, 1970.
22. Benchimol, A., Diamond, E. G., and Shen, Y.: Ejection time in aortic stenosis and mitral stenosis. Am. J. Cardiol. 5:728, 1960.
23. Moskowitz, R. L., and Wechsler, B. M.: Left ventricular ejection time in aortic and mitral valve disease. Am. J. Cardiol. 15:809, 1965.
24. Wells, B. G.: The assessment of mitral stenosis by phonocardiography. Br. Heart J. 16:261, 1954.
25. Kelly, J. J., Jr.: Diagnostic value of phonocardiography in mitral stenosis. Am. J. Med. 19:862, 1955.
26. Surawicz, B., et al.: Role of the phonocardiogram in evaluation of the severity of mitral stenosis and detection of associated valvular lesions. Circulation 34:795, 1966.
27. Tavel, M. E.: Clinical Phonocardiography and External Pulse Recording, ed. 2. Chicago,

Year Book Medical Publishers, 1973, pp. 66, 67.
28. Oreshkov, V. I.: Isovolumic contraction time and isovolumic contraction time index in mitral stenosis. Br. Heart J. 34:533, 1972.
29. Benchimol, A., and Matusuo, S.: Ejection time before and after aortic valve replacement. Am. J. Cardiol. 27:244, 1971.
30. Wigle, E. D., Auger, P., and Marquis, Y.: Muscular subaortic stenosis. The direct relation between the intraventricular pressure difference and the left ventricular ejection time. Circulation 36:36, 1967.
31. Shah, P. M., and Slodki, S. J.: The A-II interval. A study of the second heart sound in normal adults and in systemic hypertension. Circulation 29:551, 1964.
32. Braunwald, E., Sarnoff, S. J., and Stainsby, W. N.: Determinants of duration and mean rate of ventricular ejection. Circ. Res. 6:319, 1958.
33. Spann, J. F., Jr., Buccino, R. A., Sonneblick, E. H., and Braunwald, E.: Contractile state of cardiac muscle obtained from cats with experimentally produced ventricular hypertrophy and heart failure. Circ. Res. 21:341, 1967.
34. Diamant, B., and Killip, T.: Indirect assessment of left ventricular performance in acute myocardial infarction. Circulation 42:579, 1970.
35. Lewis, R. P., Boudoulas, H., Forester, W. F., and Weissler, A.: Shortening of electromechanical systole or a manifestation of excessive adrenergic stimulation in acute myocardial infarction. Circulation 46:856, 1972.
36. Heikkila, J., Loumanmäki, K., and Pyorala, K.: Serial observations on left ventricular dysfunction in acute myocardial infarction. II. Systolic time intervals in power failure. Circulation 44:343, 1971.
37. Dowling, J. T., Sloman, G., and Urgulart, C.: Systolic time interval fluctuation produced by acute myocardial infarction. Br. Heart J. 33:765, 1971.
38. Hamosh, P., et al.: Systolic time intervals and left ventricular function in acute myocardial infarction. Circulation 45:375, 1972.
39. Harris, W. S., Schoenfeld, C. D., and Weissler, A. M.: Effects of adrenergic receptor activation and blockade on the systolic pre-ejection period, heart rate, and arterial pressure in man. J. Clin. Invest. 46:1704, 1967.
40. Markowitz, C., and Yater, W.: Response of explanted cardiac muscle to thyroxine. Am. J. Physiol. 100:162, 1932.
41. Yater, W. M.: Tachycardia, time factor, survival period, and seat of action of thyroxine in the perfused hearts and thyroxinized rabbits. Am. J. Physiol. 98:338, 1931.
42. Buccino, R. A., et al.: Influence of the thyroid state on the intrinsic contractile properties and energy stores and the myocardium. J. Clin. Invest. 46: 1969, 1967.
43. Morteza, A., et al.: Effect of the thyroid state on myocardial contractility and ventricular ejection rate in man. Circulation 38:229, 1968.
44. Stafford, R. W., Harris, W. S., and Weissler, A. M.: Left ventricular systolic time intervals as indices of postural circulatory stress in man. Circulation 41:485, 1970.
45. Wertheimer, L., Hassen, A. Z., and Delman, A. J.: The 24 hour (circadian) rhythm of the cardiovascular system. (Abstr.) Clin. Res. 20:404, 1972.
46. Aronow, W. L., Harding, P. R., and De-Orvattrov, I. M.: Diurnal variation of plasma catecholamines and systolic time intervals. Chest 63:722, 1973.
47. Harrison, T. R., et al.: Relation of age to the duration of contraction, ejection, and relaxation of the normal human heart. Am. Heart J. 67:189, 1964.
48. Adolph, R. J., Fowler, N. D., and Tanaka, K.: Prolongation of isovolumic contraction time in left bundle branch block. Am. Heart J. 78:585, 1969.
49. Bourassa, M. G., Birteau, G. M., and Allenstein, B. J.: Hemodynamic studies during intermittent left bundle branch block. Am. J. Cardiol. 10:792, 1962.
50. Baragan, J., et al.: Left ventricular dynamics in complete right bundle branch block with left axis deviation of QRS. Circulation 47:797, 1970.
51. Schoenfeld, C. D., et al.: Relationship between cycle length and left ventricular ejection time in atrial fibrillation (Abstr.) Clin. Res. 11:26, 1963.
52. Leighton, R. F., et al.: Effects of atrial pacing on left ventricular performance in patients with heart disease. Circulation 40:615, 1969.
53. Pouget, J. M., et al.: Abnormal responses of the systolic time intervals to exercise in patients with angina pectoris. Circulation 43:289, 1971.
54. Chirife, R., Forester, J. M., and Bing, O. H.: Left ventricular ejection time by densitometry in patients at rest and during exercise, atrial pacing and atrial fibrillation; comparison with central aortic pressure measurements. Circulation 50:1200, 1974.
55. Siegel, W., et al.: Use of isometric handgrip for the indirect assessment of left ventricular function in patients with coronary atherosclerotic heart disease. Am. J. Cardiol. 30:48, 1972.
56. Shabetai, R., Fowler, N. D., and Guntheroth, W. G.: The hemodynamics of cardiac tamponade and constrictive pericarditis. Am. J. Cardiol. 26:480, 1970.
57. Bader, R. A., Bader, M. E., Rome, D. J., and Braunwald, E.: Hemodynamics at rest and during exercise in normal pregnancy as studies by cardiac catheterization. J. Clin. Invest. 34:1524, 1955.
58. Burg, J. R., Dobek, A., Kloster, F. E., and Metcalfe, J.: Alterations of systolic time intervals during pregnancy. Circulation 44:560, 1974.
59. Hooper, R. G., and Whitcomb, M. E.: Systolic time intervals in chronic obstructive pulmonary disease. Circulation 50:1205, 1975.
60. Perloff, J. K., and Reichek, N.: Value and limitations of systolic time intervals (pre-ejection period and ejection time) in patients with acute myocardial infarction. Circulation 45:929, 1972.

Chapter 12

Ballistocardiography

WILLIAM DOCK

Definitions. A ballistocardiograph is defined as an apparatus for determining cardiac output by recording the movements of the body caused by contraction of the heart and ejection of blood into the aorta.

Since 1938 records of the shaking of the body in the head-foot axis have been called ballistocardiograms by physicians who believed that the motions during ventricular systole and early diastole were proportional to the volume of blood ejected into the aorta, or the force of left ventricular contraction.[1] The initial device, a platform mounted on stiff springs, had been called a cardiac seismograph.[2] This term, modified to seismocardiograph, is derived from *seismograph,* the word for apparatus used to measure and record the strength of tremors of the earth due to earthquakes or explosions. Others used the words dynamocardiograph, cardiohemodynamograph and vibrocardiograph for other devices used to sense motion of the trunk, thorax or entire body related to cardiac contraction and the blood flow in great vessels. Although it became evident by 1950 that none of these devices could be used to estimate left ventricular ejection or force of contraction, the name ballistocardiograph is still in wide use, and the notion that changes in the pattern reflect only left ventricular function still persists.[3]

The triaxial seismocardiograph (SCG) senses, in three axes perpendicular to each other, kinetic forces at the surface of the thorax, just as the vectorcardiograph senses the electrical potentials at the surface of the thorax. The electrical potentials are due to activation of the atria and ventricles and to repolarization of these chambers as contraction dies out. The seismocardiograph senses forces due to contraction of atria and ventricles and to the flow of blood into and out of these chambers.

INSTRUMENTATION

Ideally the electrocardiograph would be inscribed as the logarithm of the voltage, using direct current amplification and recording with a cathode beam, free of the inertia of our direct writing devices. This would accentuate the P waves and S-T elevations or depressions and prevent the flattening of low-frequency P and T waves due to condenser-coupled amplifiers. But we are accustomed to linear recording with direct writers and make allowances for their defects in the eyes of the physicist, who sees grave faults in all our phonocardiographs and seismographs.

Ideally the seismocardiogram would be recorded as the acceleration of bodies, weightless in orbiting satellites or in diving aircraft.[4] This ideal is approached by recording acceleration due to cardiohemic forces when the individual is suspended on a very light platform hung from a high ceiling. A less ideal method is to have the platform supported by a cushion of air.[5] None of these is of use to a clinician, who needs a device as simple as the direct-writing ECG that can be utilized with a patient lying on the examining table.

The Starr platform, modeled on that of Angenheister and Lau,[2] was the standard device used from 1938 to 1950.[1] The displacement of this platform, mounted on stiff springs, is proportional to the force acting on it, just as with bathroom scales, usually mounted on stiff springs. The patient's body, lying on such a platform, is not coupled firmly to it but acts through the shearing force exerted by the body. However, if the feet are firmly against a footplate vertical to the platform or if the patient stands on such a platform, coupling is adequate. As Bixby and Henderson showed, the motion of the shins of the patient lying on the platform yielded a similar pattern of forces.[6] This could be recorded with a standard ECG if a crosspiece with coils rested on the shins, and a magnet close to the coils was supported by a stand based on the table.[7] Such a device, recording voltage from the coils with the electrocardiographic galvanometer, became very popular. As a result, published papers in this field rose from an average of 3 per year prior to its use to a peak of 150 per year in 1955. The number of papers decreased and was less than 10 after 1970. The later papers in English dealt with triaxial recording or records made from platforms resting on bulky air cushions. There were only about a dozen such reports in 1971–1974. After 1970, head-foot ballistocardiography as a clinical tool was discarded except in the Soviet countries.

In 1954 I reported a simple system for recording from the thorax the forces in the transverse (right-left or X axis) and also in the back-front axis (Z). These were sensed by the magnet-coil pickup from a platform 18 in. square under the thorax of a supine subject. It was suspended from vertical springs for the lateral motion and rested on horizontal springs for up-and-down movement.[8] The Y axis was detected from the shins. After 1965 head-foot force was also recorded from the trunk, using an additional platform free to move in that axis. This was suspended from the frame that moved laterally.[9] All forces were detected by coils in the fields of horseshoe magnets and gave voltages proportional to velocity of motion. The output was integrated by a resistor-condenser circuit to record the displacement of each system.[10] This circuit filtered out 80% of slow-frequency motion due to respiration and 80% of the rapid oscillations due to tremor or heart sounds. The latter are most evident in records of bodily acceleration. The seismocardiographic forces lie between these extremes, and our system yields patterns similar to those recorded by magnifying and recording the actual motion of the platform with a photoelectric cell. The patient lies supine on a platform 18 in. wide and 25 in. long. It has a shoulder yoke and head rest, so the neck is $3\frac{1}{2}$ in., the occiput $5\frac{1}{2}$ in. above the platform. The patient's buttocks and legs rest on a firm mattress, 6 in. thick, 22 in. wide and 26 in. long. There is a 4-in. gap between the upper end of the mattress and the lower end of the recording platforms, which total 5 in. in height above the table on which platform and mattress rest (Fig. 12-1).

For many purposes the front-back platform alone would suffice; it is in this axis that the Russians monitor their astronauts, and it gives the most constant pattern from one normal subject to another or in inspiration and expiration. For recording respiratory variation in systolic force the sim-

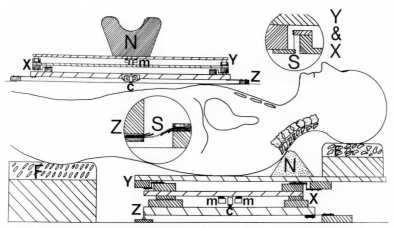

Figure 12-1. A device for recording the triaxial seismocardiogram from the thorax. The upper circle shows the suspension of the X and Y platforms from steel springs (*S*). The lower circle shows the horizontal cantilever springs supporting the cephalad end of the Z platform. To the left, *above,* is an end-on view of the device, with the neck yoke (*N*) on the Y platform, and showing the springs for the X and Z platforms and the coil (*C*) and magnet (*m*) to detect motion in the Y and Z axes. The large diagram shows a lateral view of the device, with the subject's neck wedged against the yoke (*N*). Note the springs permitting motion in the Y and Z axes and the coil (*C*) and magnet (*m*) to detect motion in the X axis. The buttocks and legs rest on a foam-rubber mattress (*F*). The base for the Z spring can either be cephalad to the platform, as in the side view, or lateral to it as in the end-on view.

ple head-foot record from the shins is ideal because the variation is greater below the hips than at the thorax. In our traces, upward motion indicates headward motion, rightward motion or backward motion. These three axes are inscribed simultaneously with any electrocardiographic lead showing a tall P wave and a sharp onset of QRS. Where only one galvanometer lead is available, the three axes can be inscribed seriatim with a superimposed R wave.[10]

With the various modifications of this device we have obtained consistent triaxial records on several thousand patients over the past 20 years. The information obtained seems clinically useful, as shown in the traces on which the following discussion is based. No colleague or house officer has been much interested in the method. Its production is so cheap that no firm has considered commercial production. This has neither surprised nor discouraged me—the same reception greeted the cathode-ray oscilloscope for electrocardiography, which I described in 1927.[11] Now

such oscilloscopes are used by the dozen in every hospital, but there was no interest in this device (except for vectorcardiography) for nearly 30 years. Should clinical interest in seismocardiography begin to increase, satisfactory triaxial devices could be constructed easily (as mine were) in the occupational therapy shop of any hospital. Similar but more elegant devices can be developed to achieve *clinically* useful seismocardiography in one or more axes.

ORIGIN OF THE CARDIOVASCULAR FORCES THAT SHAKE THE BODY

Kinetic force, the force required to set ventricular chambers and blood in motion or the force released when fluid in motion is decelerated, is the origin of the shaking of our bodies during each heart beat. When fluid is being set in motion the force of recoil is equal to the force imparted to the fluid. This "kick" is apparent to anyone who fires a gun or holds the nozzle of a hose. As Newton pointed out, and formulated into one of his laws, the force of recoil results in half of the energy of an explosive charge being "wasted"; it acts on the gun (or the jet engine) and not on the bullet, gas or fluid being ejected. Galabin, in 1875, ascribed the apex beat to the recoil of the ventricles from the ejection of blood into the pulmonary artery and aorta and noted that if the ventricles were not restrained by their attachments to the mediastinum and skeleton they would move in the opposite direction of the bloodstream and with a momentum equal to that imparted to the blood.

Physiologists calculate that because of the high pressure in the systemic circuit, the left ventricle uses only 10 to 15% of its force in imparting kinetic energy to blood entering the aorta; the rest is used for overcoming hydraulic pressure. The right ventricle uses over half its energy in accelerating blood, since pulmonic arterial pressure is one-fifth that in the aorta. Resistance to flow is much less in the lungs than in the body. During exercise these ratios change. Peripheral resistance falls, the kinetic fraction of left ventricular work rises, and that of the right ventricle falls, because both stroke volume and pulmonary arterial pressure rise with increased venous return. Systemic resistance falls during exercise. Except in patients with pulmonic hypertension, the right ventricle always has less resistance to overcome; both ventricles eject the same volume of blood per minute during the same total systolic time and hence impart the same kinetic energy to the blood. If they had the same axes of ejection they would contribute equally to the kinetic forces that shake the body. But the axes are not parallel, and it is probable that more than 60% of the head-foot IJ force, and an even larger fraction of the back-front force, is due to right ventricular ejection. Under all conditions the "Galabin force" causes the heart to tug on its attachments with kinetic energy equal to that of the ejected blood.

At any instant, this can be calculated in dynes by the formula, energy equals mass times the square of the velocity ($E = MV^2$). The seismocardiographic systolic force is thus related to the square of the velocity of the ejected streams of blood. Since the blood is not ejected into space, but into a system of branching tubes against hydraulic resistance, the ventricles also must stretch the tubes or accelerate the whole mass of blood in the tubes, so that the work of the ventricle can be calculated only from the rise in the intraventricular pressure and the surface area of the interior of the ventricle at the onset of systole. The force of ventricular systole can not be computed from triaxial SCGs and is not approximated by the force in any one axis.

THE SEISMOCARDIOGRAPHIC WAVES: NOMENCLATURE AND ORIGINS

As with the ECG waves, those of the SCG have been identified by letters. The atrial ECG waves are always P, and the repolarization waves, T, whether positive (upward on the trace) or negative. The ventricular depolarization waves at onset of systole are identified by time sequence and by direction. Q is always negative and is the initial wave only when it precedes R, a positive wave followed by S, a negative wave. But Q in one lead may be simultaneous with R in another, and S may be simultaneous with a late R in another lead. In the SCG, all waves are lettered in sequence but are always of the same polarity. The upward waves are H, J and L; the downward waves I, K and M. Waves due to atrial forces, evident in complete heart block or with P-R over 0.24 second, are in lower case—h, j and l upward; i, k and m downward. As in the ECG, where R in lead I may be synchronous with S in lead III, in the SCG I downward in the right-left axis may be synchronous with J headward. Just as Q or S may not be evident in one lead of the ECG, H, I or J may not be inscribed in one or more axes of the SCG. These facts must be borne in mind in all descriptions of the waves inscribed by seismocardiographs and by those who write or read about the cardiovascular forces that shake our bodies.

A ballistocardiographer might expect to see a force footward as the first effect of the tug of the left ventricle on its attachments. This would follow the Q wave of the electrocardiogram and begin with the rise in pressure in the aorta and the ejection of blood. What the seismocardiographer does see is quite unexpected, since the initial force produces the H wave, headward and backward, with a weaker force leftward or rightward. It begins to rise before blood is ejected into the aorta or pulmonary artery and as early as 0.02 second after Q. H is apparently due to pressing the atrioventricular valves and annulus headward during isometric rise in intraventricular pressure. The I deflection, which follows, is larger and is directed footward, frontward and rightward. It is the expected recoil from ejection of blood, and its rightward vector indicates that right ventricular force predominates, since the right ventricle ejects into the pulmonary artery, which points leftward as well as headward and backward. It does not persist throughout the ejection period or even to the peak of rise of pressure in the pulmonary artery or aorta. On the contrary, the IJ deflection begins 0.12 to 0.16 second after Q and at the peak of the carotid pulse. IJ is headward, leftward and backward. Its peak is 0.20 to 0.26 second after Q and precedes the incisura on the arterial pulse tracings. This means that the tug due to recoil from ejection is soon overcome by stronger forces due to the impact of blood on the pulmonary bifurcation and the arch of the aorta, structures more directly attached to the body than are the ventricles. The J wave, or the total force represented by the IJ deflection, is the largest seismocardio-

graphic feature in normal subjects and is very large in patients with high stroke volume of either or both ventricles. In patients with aortic insufficiency the stroke volume of the left ventricle may be 50 to 200% greater than that of the right ventricle. In such patients the IJ is rightward, but in most other subjects it is leftward, since the axis of ejection of the right ventricle is sharply leftward.

The K wave, which reaches its footward trough at the end of systole, seems to be due mainly to deceleration of blood in the descending aorta and impact on its bifurcation. It is small in the X and Z axes and may be absent in patients with coarctation of the aorta.[12] It decreases in size as patients go into shock. The L wave in early diastole is headward, rightward and backward and probably is due to recoil from the blood flowing from atria, superior vena cava and pulmonary veins into the ventricles.

The M wave, though small in normal subjects at rest, becomes very large in heart failure, A-V valvular reflux and constrictive pericarditis. It is ascribed to deceleration of blood flowing swiftly into the ventricles. Its vector is usually leftward, with smaller footward and frontward motion. There are presystolic headward, rightward and backward forces after the atrial P wave. With normal A-V conduction these may blend into the H wave of the ventricular complex, but with prolonged P-R intervals or in complete heart block, relatively large headward, rightward and backward waves are evident, with predominantly rightward vectors. These presumably are due to the recoil from blood ejected by the atria into the ventricles and may be as forceful in one or more axes as is the ventricular systolic force (Fig. 12-2). We can see how much the atrial forces modify the systolic ventricular complexes when atrial fibrillation reverts to sinus rhythm. In some patients the effect on the HIJ is striking (Fig. 12-3); in others it is minimal. When

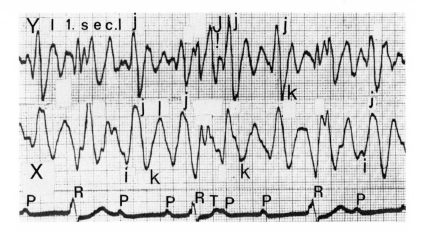

Figure 12-2. Record from a 62-year-old man with heart failure and complete A-V block. The atrial forces in both Y and X are stronger than the ventricular forces. In Y the ventricular force is reduced and altered when P-R is very brief (first and third ventricular complexes) and J is evident only in the second complex, when P-R is 0.36 second. In block without heart failure, atrial complexes in Y are usually small, although those in X and Z are large.[10]

the P-R interval is 0.12 to 0.24 second the atrial hij may be in phase with and augment ventricular HIJ or may be out of phase and thus decrease the ventricular waves.

This satisfactory schema, relating the shaking of the body by recoil from acceleration or impact of deceleration of blood entering or leaving the ventricles, is rudely shattered when we record ventricular ectopic beats[2] or runs of paced beats with left bundle branch block alternating with runs of sinus beats with normal QRS patterns.[9] For with aberrant activation of the ventricle the SCG forces may be very much smaller or very much larger than with normal activation. Worst of all, these forces may be large in very early ectopic beats with absence of second sounds and no systemic pulse wave. Here there is no ejection of blood from the ventricles, which have just begun to fill. Part of this force might be due to blood moving against the A-V valves, but in very early ectopic beats there are no first sounds and presumably no tensing of the A-V valves. Very early ectopic beats, with SCG waves larger in ectopic beats than in sinus beats, were commented on by Angenheister and Lau[2]

nearly 10 years before their American disciples concluded that SCG forces were proportional to left ventricular ejection.

When the atria of dogs are clamped off, systolic shaking of the body persists as the empty ventricles contract and flop back and forth vigorously.[14] Even larger forces are noted if the aorta and pulmonary artery are clamped off a few beats before the venae cavae are clamped, so that the ventricles and atria are distended with blood but none enters or leaves the heart.[14] These waves begin within 0.02 second after the Q wave, and they die out after the T wave. It must be assumed that some similar force due to ventricular displacement and the tug of the ventricles on the annulus contributes to the SCG patterns recorded from normal subjects and from people with heart disease. Presumably such forces are minimal with normal diastolic filling and ventricular activation. All this was ignored during the era of ballistocardiographic innocence when the systolic IJ was ascribed entirely to the velocity of the blood being ejected by the left ventricle. We had also ignored the fact that there is no rigid connection between the heart or great vessels and the skeleton, which is shaken from head to toe by each heart beat. The mediastinal fibers must be drawn taut before they pull on the sternum and vertebrae, so that force is stored during a tug and released when it ends. The amount of force lost depends on the length and elasticity of the fibers. The system also has a natural frequency of oscillation, and this leads to after-waves when a tug ceases. The importance of all this became evident only when we were confronted by the curious alterations respiration caused in the seismocardiogram.

THE RESPIRATORY VARIATION IN AMPLITUDE OF IJ

With the introduction of the 12-lead technique, electrocardiographers learned how much the patterns were influenced by the position of the heart in the chest. Normal people might have left or right axis deviation, depending on whether their hearts were more rotated or whether they were more vertical or horizontal than the average subject. The triaxial seismocardiogram taught us that people with vertical hearts had tall J waves in Y and shallow I in the X axis, while those with horizontal hearts had small J waves in Y and deep I waves in X. Some subjects show the electrocardiographic pattern of the vertical heart at the peak of inspiration but the horizontal heart's pattern of left axis deviation in expiration. Thus the ST pattern in lead III may reverse during each respiratory cycle (Figs. 12-4 and 12-5). The anatomic position has the same influence on the SCG during each respiratory cycle, but in addition there are changes due to the fact that right ventricular stroke volume rises and left stroke volume falls during inspiration. This may be associated with reversal of the IJ complex of the SCG (Figs. 12-4 and 12-5), or there may be marked variation in the ECG with little change in the SCG (Figs. 12-6 and 12-7). While the effects of any change in the anatomic position of the heart on the ECG and the SCG are similar, the alteration in the

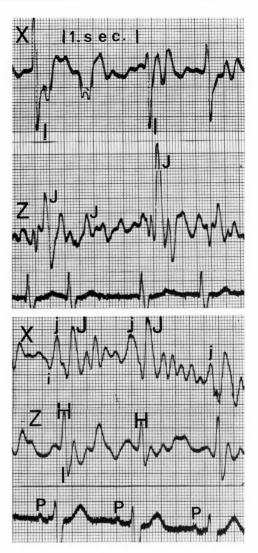

Figure 12-3. Record from an elderly man with atrial fibrillation (*above*) and sinus rhythm 3 weeks later (*below*). Bizarre and varying lateral (*X*) and backward (*Z*) forces with no presystolic waves during fibrillation but large atrial *IJ* presystolic waves laterally in sinus rhythm. More normal ventricular forces occur in both axes after treatment of arrhythmia.

ECG is often slow because of ventricular hypertrophy. The SCG can change its axis of ejection even from beat to beat as the stroke volumes of the two chambers vary with respiration. Right ventricular filling increases during inspiration as venous return is augmented by increased abdominal

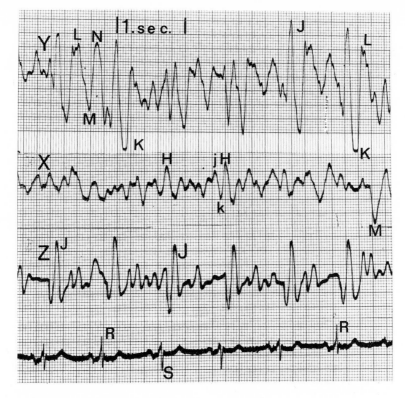

Figure 12-4. In a case of healed infarction with no symptoms, respiration reversed R and S amplitude in lead III but not in I or II. It also reversed SCG patterns in *Y* and *X* but not in *Z*.

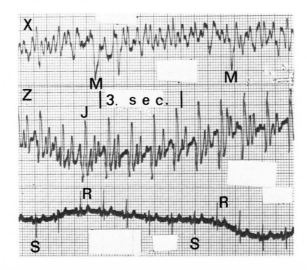

Figure 12-5. Same case, slow paper speed. Note deep M in *X* with tall R waves in lead III; no similar effect in *Z*.

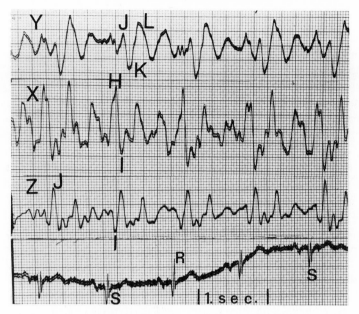

Figure 12-6. Record from a man with healed infarction, few symptoms, but the loud midsystolic click of mitral prolapse. While the ECG in lead III shows respiratory reversal of R and S amplitudes, there is minimal respiratory effect of breathing on the SCG, which is almost normal in Z. In Y and X the patterns are abnormal, with tall H in X, and notched, small H, I, J in Y.

and decreased intrathoracic pressure. The left ventricle slightly increases its stroke volume during expiration, but the change is much less and thus affects the SCG less than the decrease in right ventricular ejection. Many patients who show very little change in their ECG vectors during normal respiration have very large changes in the SCG.

The early ballistocardiographers noticed that the IJ wave decreased during the expiratory phase of respiration, and they were aware of the expiratory decrease in right ventricular stroke volume. But they

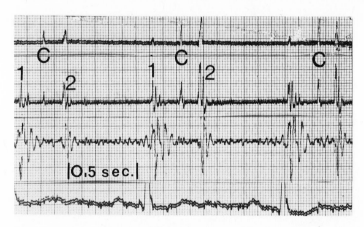

Figure 12-7. The same patient. Breathing alters intensity of the high-pitched click (*C*), best seen in upper trace (over 240 Hz.) and middle trace (80 to 240 Hz.), but not evident in lower trace (20 to 80 Hz.), where first sound is most evident. Lead II and lead I (not shown) were not affected by respiration. This case is unusual, since respiration usually alters the SCG far more than the ECG, and many patients with systolic click–mitral prolapse syndrome have normal SCGS.

were struck by the fact that the expiration decrease in IJ was much greater and involved more beats per cycle in older people and in younger subjects with angina or healed myocardial infarcts.[15] Normal subjects were found to have only one wave during expiration 40% smaller than the tallest wave during inspiration, and in most normal individuals the decrease was about 20%. Many anginal patients had one or two waves per cycle about 50% of the size of the largest wave (grade 1 abnormality), or several waves less than 40% as tall (grade 2), or only one or two waves about normal and most waves less than 30% as tall (grade 3 in Fig. 12-8). These patients had no respiratory variation in the height or rate of rise of the carotid pulse, and there were many patients with angina or healed infarcts who had normal patterns even with deep breathing. Since they recorded only the head-foot trace and ascribed the IJ force entirely to left ventricular ejection, the ballistocardiographers were forced to believe that some subtle change due to left ventricular disease had decreased the rate of rise in left ventricular pressure and that the resulting decrease in

the velocity of ejection caused the expiratory decrease—after all, halving velocity of ejection could cause a 75% decrease in kinetic force.

Some apparently normal subjects had rather large decreases in IJ amplitude during expiration, but in a 5-year follow-up these seemingly healthy individuals had had more episodes of heart "attacks" than controls with minimal expiratory decrease.[16] In each later decade of life a higher percentage of abnormal records was seen among normal people. Again, follow-ups at 10, 20 and 30 years at the University of Pennsylvania[17] and elsewhere[3] confirmed the rising incidence of heart attacks in these normal subjects. Thus, it was natural to accept abnormal respiratory variation in IJ as evidence of latent disease in the left ventricle. This gave added strength to the belief that head-foot motion of the body, recorded with simple devices, reflected normal or abnormal function of the heart. This was followed by the report that anginal attacks were fewer and milder in subjects whose IJ variation was decreased by elastic abdominal belts.[18]

Observation of the absence of respira-

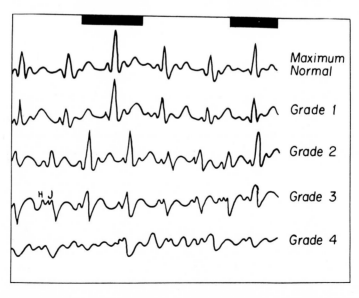

Figure 12-8. Grades of respiratory variation in the head-foot SCG from Starr ballistocardiograph. Black bar indicates inspiratory phase. Based on Brown, Hoffman and deLalla.[15]

tory variation in patients with constrictive pericarditis forced reexamination of the relation of IJ to left ventricular ejection. These patients had very marked *decrease* in systemic pulses during inspiration (paradoxical pulse), but no decrease in IJ was noted in patients studied at the University of Pennsylvania[19] or in those at Johns Hopkins[20] or in Brooklyn (Fig. 12-9). In these cases it was obvious that IJ amplitude was not related to left ventricular ejection and was due almost entirely to right ventricular stroke volume increasing as left ventricular ejection decreased during inspiration.

The final discredit to the assumption that left ventricular disease caused the grade 2 to 3 respiratory variation in IJ waves was the chance observation that normal young men, with 0 or grade 1 decrease during expiration when they had not smoked for an hour or two, had grade 2 to 3 after the first few deep "drags" on a cigarette.[21] In these cases, pulse rates and arterial pressures rose as they always do in all men or dogs when nicotine is administered. The pulse pressure also rose, and even during expiration this was higher than before smoking. The IJ of the SCG after smoking was usually as tall as or taller than before, but in those who showed grade 2 or 3 records even the first beat at onset of expiration was considerably decreased (Fig. 12-10). The assumption that IJ amplitude reflected left ventricular ejection had been badly shaken by the study of ectopic beats and cases of constrictive pericarditis. The era of ballistocardiographic innocence ended when the smoking tests of Brooklyn[21] were confirmed at the

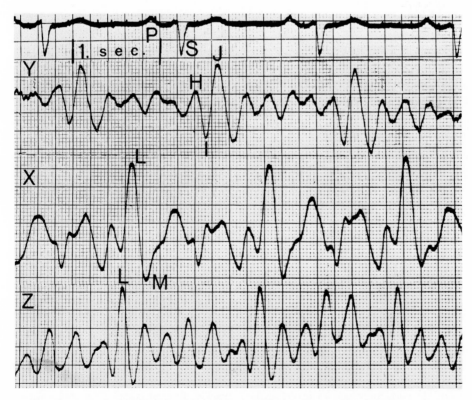

Figure 12-9. SCG from a 60-year-old man with constrictive pericarditis following occurrence of a tuberculous exudate 8 years before. The normal pattern in Y was constant although the systemic pulses faded away during inspiration. The large LM complexes in *X* and *Z* coincided with the apex thrust and third heart sound and also were constant during breathing.

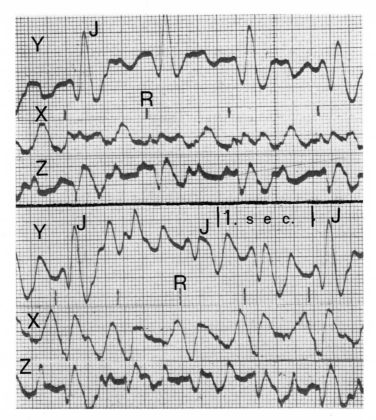

Figure 12-10. SCGS from a "normal," overweight, sedentary man 30 years old, who smoked more than 20 cigarettes a day, before (*above*) and after smoking a cigarette (*below*). Y is obtained from shins and shows a grade 3 pattern after smoking, when rate is faster, and SCG forces in X and Z show less decrease during inspiration and a larger presystolic wave than in controls.

University of Pennsylvania[22] and at Johns Hopkins Hospital.[23] A fresh approach to the significance and mechanism of respiratory variation in the systolic SCG was needed.

The shift in axis of ejection due to the rise and fall of the diaphragm contributes to the expiratory decrease in headward IJ, as does the physiologic fall in right ventricular stroke volume during expiration, if one accepts the evidence that 70% or more of the head-foot systolic forces are due to right ventricular ejection into the low-pressure pulmonic circuit. Changes in axis during expiration involve decreases in headward IJ with increases in force in the other axes of the SCG. But in grade 2 to 3 abnormality in the ballistocardiogram, whether spontaneous or due to smoking,

increases in IJ in the X and Z axes are minimal or absent. Such changes can only be due to a decrease in transmission of force from the generator to the skeletal structures and the recording system. During expiration, mediastinal tension decreases as the sternum falls and the diaphragm rises. The slack mediastinal sling transmits force less effectively than does the mediastinum tensed by diaphragmatic descent and elevation of the sternum. These changes in transmission of force are most marked in the sedentary, the obese and the potbellied. They are decreased in women wearing tight girdles or corsets and in men with elastic abdominal binders.[18] In sedentary people who have grade 1 even before smoking, there is often a striking change to grade 2 or 3 when they absorb nicotine.

This drug relaxes the mind and the voluntary muscles, and often the breathing becomes slower and more shallow than when the subject is tense and eagerly waiting to smoke.[23] In subjects who are in poor physical training but who do not smoke, marked increase in respiratory variation in head-foot Y may occur if they overbreathe rapidly for a minute, hold their breath in deep inspiration for 20 seconds and resume normal breathing. The fatigue of respiratory muscles due to this maneuver may be followed by grade 2 or 3 patterns during several cycles. In all these situations the relaxed mediastinal sling can take up the slack and allows recoil and impact to be partly absorbed and less effectively transmittd to the recording system.[24,25] As this affects transmission of head-foot forces to the hips and legs more than to the shoulders, records made from the shins (or the Starr table) show more variation than do the records from the thorax on the triaxial SCG. Hence the shin pickup is ideal for detecting grades of respiratory variation or their increase on smoking or decrease on application of an abdominal binder. Since the patients studied at Philadelphia, Baltimore and Rochester prior to 1951 were not asked to avoid smoking, it is probable that many of them gave more abnormal records than would be found in nonsmokers, but the prognostic value of such records is probably greater on that account.

The correlation of severity of respiratory variation with known heart disease, and with risk of future heart disease, seems to be accounted for by facts unrelated to impaired myocardial function. In the past those with cardiac diagnoses have often

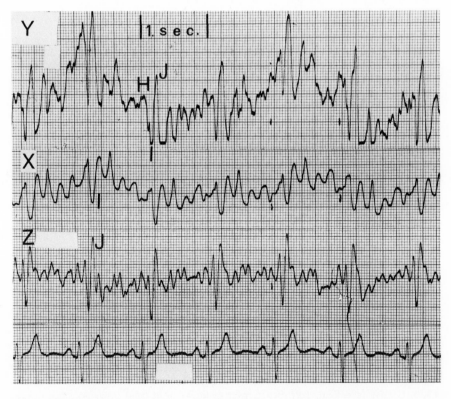

Figure 12-11. Record from a 64-year-old man with Q_1–T_1 pattern but no history of heart attack and many normal ECGs on previous annual records. He was lean and had never smoked; he has had no heart disease in ensuing 8 years. The heart sounds are those of a normal man of 20; the SCG is forceful, with normal pattern, and minimal decrease during expiration.

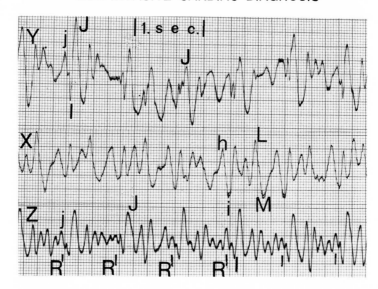

Figure 12-12. SCG from a 76-year-old man, 17 years after onset of angina. There have been transient ECG changes at rest, but negative 40-step test in recent years. The triaxial SCG shows presystolic forces, giving appearance of notched HI descent and grade 2 expiratory decrease in IJ in Y. These abnormalities have developed since normal traces were recorded 5 years ago but with no change in heart sounds or roentgenogram.

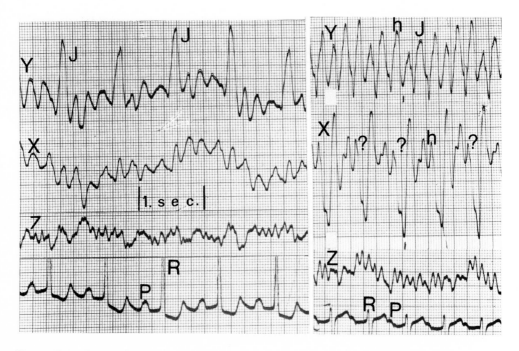

Figure 12-13. Case 1 (see text). *Left,* SCGs prior to insertion of Starr-Edwards valve in aortic site show strong headward systolic forces due to aortic insufficiency. Small chaotic waves in X and Z. *Right,* months after operation and relief of dyspnea, the forces in Z are feeble; in Y the J wave is reduced and the force in diastole greatly increased. The huge leftward wave (?) in X is due to summation of protodiastolic and presystolic forces.

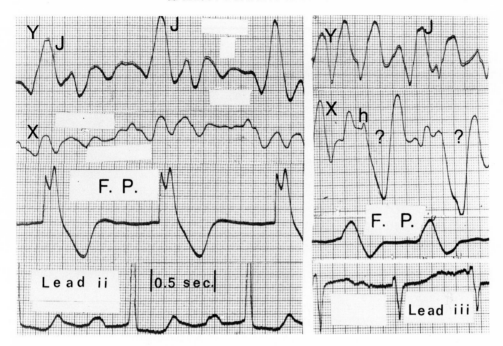

Figure 12-14. Case 1. The femoral pulse (*F.P.*), *left,* is typical of aortic reflux, and a loud sound was recorded with initial upstroke. *Right,* after operation, the femoral pulse of low cardiac output, although prosthesis function was normal. The changes in *Y* and *X* of SCG are as striking as those in the arterial pulses.

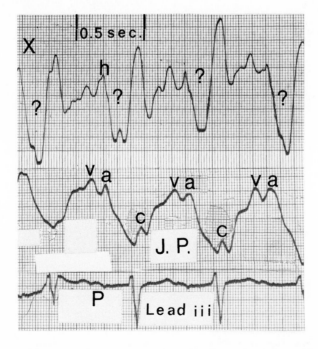

Figure 12-15. Case 1. The jugular pulse (*J.P.*) after operation shows the pattern of tricuspid reflux. The huge wave in *X* is due to right ventricular filling, with long P-R interval leading to summation of atrial ij wave with protodiastolic M, starting with atrial h wave and jugular a.

been urged to "take it easy" and avoid exercise, so that they became even more flabby. They often find it difficult to stop smoking, especially when waiting for test examinations. The sedentary, overweight

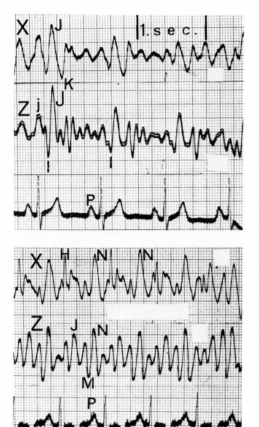

Figure 12-16. Case 2 (see text). Only *X* and *Z* of SCG are shown; *Y* was weak and chaotic. *Above,* the classical pattern of mitral stenosis, with small systolic and protodiastolic but large presystolic forces giving the premature notched HI descent, as atrial j overlaps ventricular H. *Below,* the pattern with tachycardia several months after insertion of the prosthesis in the mitral site. The sharp H, in *X,* coincides with the closing sound of the prosthesis; ventricular forces are small, but the protodiastolic M and N waves are large; atrial h coincides with N, making it the strongest force in both *X* and *Y.* The prosthetic sounds were normal, but this may occur when there is a leak around the ring and mitral reflux.

subjects, supposedly normal, often need nicotine to decrease hunger and relieve their emotional tension. These are all factors known to predispose to coronary disease. Also, they are most apt to have serious clinical episodes, not the trivial bouts of "acute indigestion" with positive electrocardiograms. On the opposite extreme are the lean, fit oldsters, with classical Q_1–T_1 or Q_3–T_3 patterns of healed infarction but no history of heart attack. These men usually have normal SCG patterns even after overbreathing and breath holding (Fig. 12-11). Nearly all such men have not smoked for decades and go for years with no clinical episodes of coronary disease. The grade 2 to 4 SCGs at rest, after the Valsalva maneuver or on smoking tell us what sort of patient or "normal" subject we have tested and what risk there is of future disease. Proper management, weight loss and exercise can favorably modify the prognosis and subsequent SCGs.

DIAGNOSTIC SIGNIFICANCE OF ABNORMAL PATTERNS OF THE SYSTOLIC SCG COMPLEX

The pioneer studies of the triaxial SCG of men weightless in diving aircraft showed that the average systolic force in the Z (back-front) axis is about 40% greater than in the Y (head-foot) axis and 15% greater than in the X (right-left) axis.[4] These ratios may vary from one subject to another with body build and cardiac position. The systolic complexes of the SCG may be normal in one or two axes when they are abnormal in another. This phenomenon is well recognized by electrocardiographers, since only one or two of 12 leads may be of diagnostic significance. In vectorcardiograms the systolic force in only one axis may be abnormal. Extracardiac factors play a larger role in modifying the amplitude and pattern of the SCG than of the ECG, as has been described in relation to respiratory change in anatomic axis. Large pericardial effusions attenuate the

ECG forces and may cause alternation of ECG and SCG patterns. Echocardiograms show that this is due to the alternate positions of the heart as it flops about from beat to beat.

Frequent and severe distortions of the SCG due to extracardiac factors are seen in the Y (head-foot) axis in cases of kyphosis or emphysema, where transmission to the body is impaired much more in the Y than in the Z (back-front) axis. Effects on the lateral axis are less than on Y but more than on Z. When there are normal patterns and minimal change during respiration in the Z axis, but small, chaotic head-foot waves in kyphotic or emphysematous subjects, there usually is no evidence of impaired cardiac function. Such traces explain the many "false positives" in ballisto-cardiograms obtained before 1955. When the aorta becomes tortuous with age, hypertension, valvular disease or mucinous degeneration, there may be small headward systolic waves but unusually large forces in the lateral axis.[8] Only when systolic forces are small for the heart rate in all axes should hypothyroidism be suspected, with low stroke volume and a slow pulse. Only when the forces are unusually large in at least two axes should the traces be taken as evidence for high stroke volume of both ventricles. Intracardiac shunts or reflux flow in systole or diastole can cause one ventricle to have a much higher output than the other and dominate the systolic pattern. Anemia, hyperthyroidism, peripheral arteriovenous shunts, Paget's osteitis, parkinsonian tremor and fever all increase

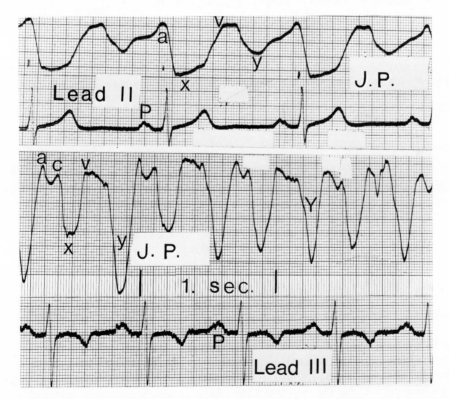

Figure 12-17. Case 2. *Upper panel,* before operation. The jugular pulse (*J.P.*) is that of pulmonic hypertension—a large a wave and a normal systolic x wave, excluding tricuspid reflux. *Lower panel,* months after operation. The deep jugular y wave is due to constrictive pericarditis. The systolic rise of tricuspid reflux is absent. The y wave begins only 0.04 second after the pulmonic second sound and 0.04 second before the opening sound of the mitral prosthetic valve.

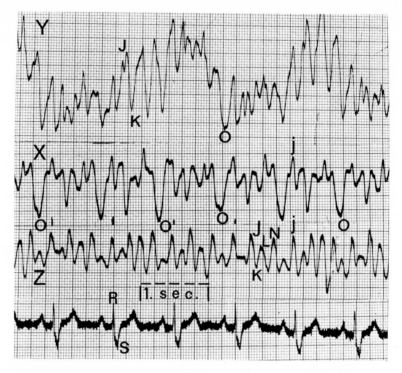

Figure 12-18. SCG from a man 49 years old, 24 years after right bundle branch block and right pleuropericardial rub had been recorded when he was in shock after chest trauma. There is now calcification over the right atrial area, but he is asymptomatic; there is no pulsus paradoxus. SCG shows notched J in Y, with deep O in some beats. In X, O is deep in all beats, starting 0.56 second after Q. There are tall atrial j waves, peak 0.20 second after Q, in all axes, but most striking in Z, where N is tall, but O is not seen.

cardiac output and the systolic amplitude of the SCG wave. The endless variety of changes in the systolic and diastolic complexes in heart disease were presented previously with triaxial records of patients with pericardial, myocardial or valvular disease.[26]

ALTERATIONS IN RELATIVE AMPLITUDE OF THE SYSTOLIC WAVES AND NOTCHING OF WAVES

Very early in the study of head-foot ballistocardiograms it was realized that H waves taller than J, or notches on H or J, and a shoulder on the HI descent were rarely observed in traces from normal subjects but were quite frequent in those with heart disease. Relatively tall H waves, sometimes premature and starting before Q,

were not uncommon with latent or obvious myocardial failure. Notched HI descent was described in patients with mitral stenosis, and notched J waves were observed in both congenital and acquired valvular disease and in coronary disease and heart failure.[27]

The notches and shoulders could easily be ascribed to asynchrony of closure of the A-V valve, which is delayed in mitral stenosis, or of onset of systole in cases of aberrant activation (bundle branch block or hemiblock in the left branch). But in many patients with marked right- or left-sided delay in activation, no notching of H or J was noted, although the first and second heart sounds were widely split. The "mitral notch" on the HI descent may be evident in all three traces of the SCG, or only in Y or Z; it occurs in both right and left bundle branch block and in septal hypertrophy with subaortic stenosis and in atrial myxoma. It may disappear with procedures that correct such lesions, or it may appear in septal hypertrophy only with procedures that increase mitral encroachment on the outflow tract. The H wave, starting up before ventricular systole (that is, before Q of the ECG), is obviously of atrial origin and disappears with atrial fibrillation or gives a bifid H when P-R is over 0.20 second. Often there is an associated fourth heart sound or the rumble of mitral stenosis, which also precedes Q and starts soon after P.

Notching of HI, as well as of J, may be a striking feature of the P and Z traces of men many years after their recovery from myocardial infarction and when they have otherwise normal traces, with strong systolic forces and little decrease in headward IJ during normal expiration (Fig. 12-12).

The I wave in X occurs with the J in other planes. It rarely is notched. J is often small or notched or both in Y, with little or no change in Z, in patients with fresh or healed infarction or during bouts of angina. Similar patterns may occur in acute and chronic myocardial disease, viral or rheumatic carditis, sarcoidosis, amyloidosis or cardiomyopathy of nutritional or trypanosomal origin (Chagas' disease). Many patients with abnormal wave forms in the HIJ complex in the Z axis have third or fourth sounds and abnormal ECGs and roentgenograms, so that the SCG abnormalities are useful only as evidence of the severity, not the nature, of the disease. Progressive abnormality is ominous. Regression toward normal is reassuring evidence of decreased embarrassment of the heart. In amyloidosis, aortic stenosis and other conditions of impaired ventricular compliance the HJ complex may be abnormal,

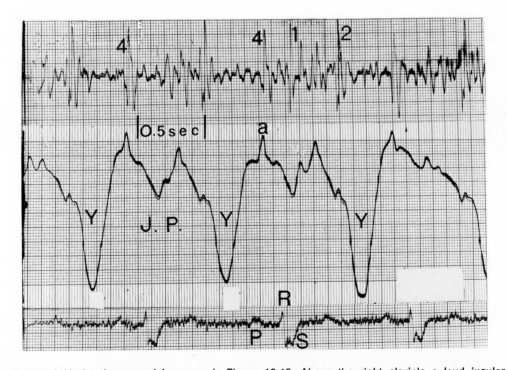

Figure 12-19. Another record from man in Figure 12-18. Above the right clavicle a loud jugular fourth sound is shown, synchronous with the sharp jugular a wave in the pulse curve (*J.P.*) at same site. The deep y wave begins 0.48 second after Q, and its deepest point is at 0.60 second, 0.04 second before the nadir of the O wave of the SCG.

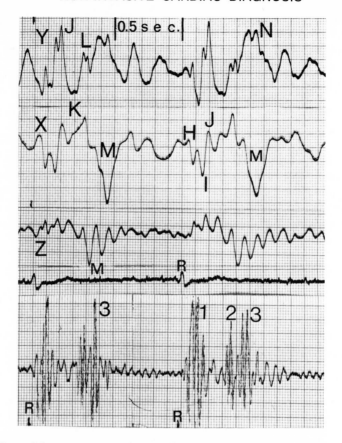

Figure 12-20. Record from a man, 54 years old, with atrial fibrillation and calcific pericardial plaques 16 months after myocardial infarction. There was no angina, but he had some dyspnea on exertion; there was no pulsus paradoxus. There is a tall notched J in Y, with broad N, synchronous with broad, deep M in X. Heart sounds at the apex indicate a loud third sound, 0.10 second after the second sound. Nadir of M is 0.56 second after Q.

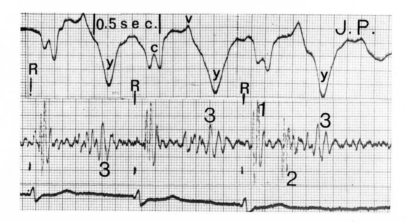

Figure 12-21. Another record from the man in Figure 12-20. The jugular pulse (*J.P*), with position of R waves indicated, is from a tracing made with the ECG. These R waves match those of lower traces, showing sounds over the jugular vein. There is a systolic rise in jugular pulse, due to tricuspid reflux, and a very deep y with matching jugular third heart sound. This is 0.22 second after second sound, much later than the apical third sound. The nadir of y is 0.58 second after Q.

without third or fourth heart sounds and with only small SCG waves in diastole.

ABNORMAL SCG WAVES IN DIASTOLE

The absence of the K wave in the Y axis is occasionally the first clue to the diagnosis of coarctation of the aorta,[12] but more often K is small or absent in shock. The intense renal and splanchnic vasoconstriction reduces flow in the abdominal aorta and thus the force imparted by deceleration. This is why a simple one-axis device under the pelvis could be used to monitor increasing or decreasing levels of shock.

Large SCG forces, in three axes, occur when high venous pressure in the systemic or pulmonic circuit causes blood to fill one or both ventricles faster in the protodiastolic period than it can be ejected in systole. This is most surprising when it is found in patients having routine follow-up after uneventful insertion of a prosthetic valve.

Case 1. Heart sounds, pulses and SCG were recorded in a 48-year-old man before and a few months after a Starr-Edwards valve had been inserted to replace an aortic valve with mucinous degeneration. This had caused months of intractable dyspnea; the operation relieved all his symptoms, correcting the carotid and femoral pulse of aortic insufficiency. But tricuspid reflux developed, presumably due to degeneration in the annulus and to the increased venous return after the aortic lesion was corrected. Huge diastolic SCG waves now dominate the triaxial records, and the jugular pulse is typical of tricuspid reflux (Figs. 12-13 to 12-15). More unusual is the development of tricuspid reflux after uneventful repair of mitral stenosis with a Starr-Edwards valve.

Case 2. For many years a 43-year-old man had had classical signs of mitral stenosis with few symptoms and no arrhythmia. Following operation for inguinal hernia he developed severe distress on exertion, which led to insertion of a mitral prosthesis. Symptoms persisted, and on reexamination several months later he had devel-

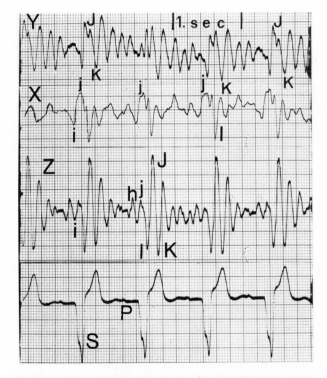

Figure 12-22. Case 3 (see text). In spite of the long P-R and QRS durations and a small apical ventricular aneurysm, there is a forceful, normal systolic complex in Z; notched J and tall I in Y and normal I in X. X and Z show the atrial hij waves expected when P-R exceeds 0.24 second. The atrial forces here are less than those often recorded in heart block.

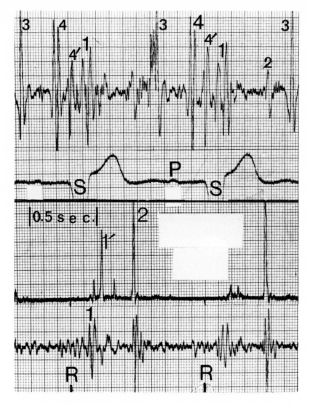

Figure 12-23. Case 3. Upper traces show the heart sounds (20 to 80 Hz.) at the apical area, with the third sound (*3*) louder than the reduplicated fourth sound (*4* and *4'*). The first sound is normally loud but not as loud as *3* or *4*. The lower trace is from the pulmonic area and shows the loud second sound (*2*). The first sound (*1*) is faint at 80 to 240 Hz., where *2* and the ejection sound (*1'*) are loud, but *1* is loud at 20 to 80 Hz. (*below*). The gallop sounds were loud only at the apex at low pitch, and disappeared near the sternum. This is an example of extreme auscultatory abnormality in old age, with strong systolic SCG forces and no myocardial failure.

oped huge diastolic SCG forces and a very deep dip in the jugular pulse (Figs. 12-16 and 12-17). These were impressive signs of postoperative constrictive pericarditis, although there was no pulsus paradoxus.

In these cases the changes in the SCG were the most striking evidence of deteriorating cardiac function in spite of uneventful correction of the initial lesion. In both cases the recording of jugular and hepatic pulses followed observation of the SCG and proved that the lesion causing rapid protodiastolic filling was not due to mitral reflux. Obviously the jugular pulse record is essential to distinguish mitral from tricuspid reflux as well as from the large MN waves noted in cases of constrictive pericarditis. As with other diastolic forces, these are usually much larger in the X axis than in Y or Z. This was first reported from Johns Hopkins Hospital[20] and is seen also in the forces evoked by atrial systole in patients with complete heart block or with P-R intervals over

0.24 second. In chronic pericardial disease the large protodiastolic M and N waves appear relatively early, before there are changes in the systemic pulse or the IJ forces in systole. Even late in the disease the systolic complexes are little affected and show no change during inspiration when the systemic pulse becomes very weak. In the mild cases, as well as in advanced disease, the large M waves are associated with a deep y in the jugular pulse (Figs. 12-18 to 12-21). Such patterns are frequently seen in patients who have no symptoms after successful valve implants or coronary revascularization since hemopericardium is frequent and heals with moderate pericardial and mediastinal fibrosis. This improves the transmission of the head-foot IJ, which may be much more "normal" after such operations even when revascularization has been unsuccessful.

Large protodiastolic M waves are usually present in patients with myocardial failure, ventricular aneurysm, or tricuspid insufficiency as well as in the rare cases of "pure" mitral reflux with huge left atria.[26] Nearly all of these patients have disabling symptoms, and many have loud third heart sounds. On the other hand, patients who have few or no symptoms but proved ventricular aneurysms or scars of large healed infarcts may have no large diastolic SCG waves and relatively normal systolic complexes.

Case 3. An unusual instance of this paradox was a 77-year-old woman who had no history of a heart attack and was free of symptoms after many years of untreated hypertension. In 1972 a routine ECG showed a very long P-R interval and left bundle branch block, with very loud and peculiar heart sounds. Apex pulsations were those of a small aneurysm, and at that area she had loud third sounds and loud duplicated fourth sounds (Figs. 12-22 and 12-23); the SCG showed large systolic forces, with normal pattern except in Y. At present, 3 years later, she has a pacemaker and is able to look after her ailing husband. Thus, when the ECG and heart sounds were most abnormal the good SCG indicated compensation and a good prognosis.

Elderly patients with hypertension, a pacemaker, bundle branch block or aortic insufficiency, but few or no symptoms, usually have large IJ waves, with minimal decrease in expiration, in one or two axes even when the pattern is abnormal in other axes (Figs. 12–24 and 12-25).

In mitral stenosis and in cardiopathies that stiffen the ventricular walls and decrease compliance, protodiastolic filling is slow, and there can be no large M waves, no third heart sounds. But as long as sinus rhythm is present, patients with mitral or tricuspid stenosis have large presystolic SCG waves. As in heart block without other lesions, presystolic forces mimic those of ventricular systole and may be even larger in the lateral axis (X). A large headward presystolic force in mitral or combined mitral and tricuspid stenosis occurs with the jugular a wave. Presumably this is the recoil from the high-velocity jets going to the ventricles. But only with prolonged P-R intervals are such waves clearly seen; with normal A-V conduction the atrial force blends into the H wave of the ventricular systolic complex (Fig. 12-26).

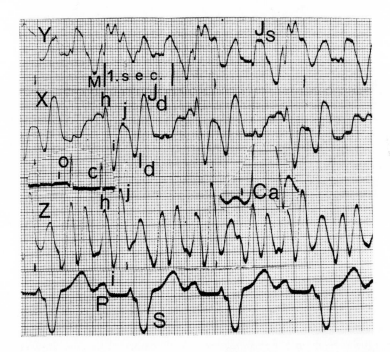

Figure 12-24. Record from a man 72 years old, 4 years after insertion of a Starr-Edwards aortic prosthesis. He has a slow pulse and no cardiac failure. The prolonged P-R and QRS were evident even before operation for aortic stenosis. The delayed left ventricular J wave (J_s) is evident only in Y. An early rightward J_d in X seems due to the right ventricle. Atrial forces are strong in X and Z, with distinct hij, but in Y there is a sustained, notched atrial thrust headward. The left insert between X and Z shows the high-pitched (>240 Hz.) prosthetic sounds, opening (O) and closing (C), at aortic area. A marker before O indicates end of S wave of ECG. The right insert shows the strong but delayed carotid upstroke and incisura, with end of S (indicated by marker) 0.12 second before upstroke.

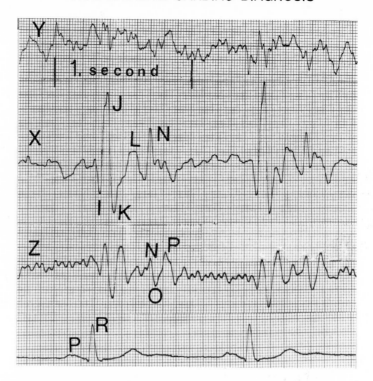

Figure 12-25. SCG of an 84-year-old hypertensive man, with a dilated, tortuous aorta but a slow pulse and no heart failure. As in many kyphotic old men the waves in Y are weak and chaotic. In X the forces are very strong, and the HIJK pattern is normal. In Z the systolic pattern is not unusual, but protodiastolic forces are relatively strong.

EVALUATION OF THE NORMAL AND ABNORMAL SEISMOCARDIOGRAM

A normal SCG with minimal respiratory variation in head-foot IJ waves is an important finding in all patients with established valvular or myocardial disease, because the prognosis in diagnosed organic disease is much better in those with normal SCGs than in controls of similar age and with similar diagnoses who have abnormal systolic, diastolic or respiratory patterns.[16,28,29] One reason practitioners abandoned the ballistocardiograph was the fact that it so often inscribed normal patterns in lean, fit, asymptomatic patients with obvious valvular or coronary disease. The other was that the head-foot traces showed abnormal decreases in systolic force during expiration in subjects who had no detect-

able change in pulses, electrocardiograms, heart sounds or roentgen shadows of the heart. This logic would have led doctors to abandon the electrocardiogram if only lead II had been used, because patients with valvular disease, frank heart failure or recent or healed infarction had normal QRS-T patterns, while other patients, symptomatic and with no other abnormal findings, had a QRS lasting twice as long as normal and even had inverted T waves. Possibly the most important fact about the triaxial seismocardiogram is that return toward a normal pattern shows that management is effective. This is true regardless whether return is gradual, due to diet and regular physical exercise, or rapid, due to spontaneous recovery, drug action or an operation. The serial seismocardiograms can also reveal deterioration in cardiac function due to progress of a disease or the

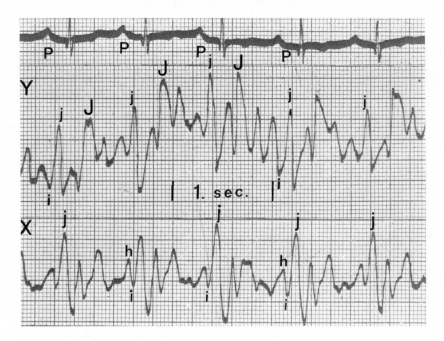

Figure 12-26. SCG from a man 46 years old with mitral and tricuspid stenosis, verified at valvulotomies. The long P-R interval brings out the powerful atrial thrust, due to jets of high velocity from the narrow orifices. These cause the tall j waves, as the body is shaken more forcefully than by the slightly subnormal ventricular ejections through normal outlets.

unfavorable effects of a drug or operation. The seismocardiogram thus can serve to give early warning. One exception to this rule is the improved IJ waves and decreased respiratory variation in these waves in patients in whom cardiotomy caused mediastinal fibrosis and better transmission of SCG forces even though stroke volume or velocity was not improved. Fortunately most patients with patent revascularizations show improved myocardial function, and seismocardiograms make them look even better.

The respiratory changes in head-foot systolic force are invaluable in revealing people at high risk of future coronary attacks, particularly when the trace deteriorates as they luxuriate in the relaxation afforded by a cigarette. But when they see this dramatic change, their minds may be "marvelously concentrated" on the hazards to the heart of dependence on nicotine. For the physician need not go into details of the extracardiac factors that account for a

grade 3 pattern in a patient after smoking half a cigarette; he need only compare it with the grade 1 pattern obtained when no cigarette had been smoked for an hour. The traces show the layman that tobacco has remarkable effects as an index of fitness and of the risk of developing symptomatic heart disease in the future.

SUMMARY

Records of the shaking of the body in the head-foot axis may be called ballistocardiograms even though this is not in accord with the dictionary definitions. They are of value only for demonstrating the expiratory decrease in apparent systolic force. This change is not correlated with a decrease in the force of the left ventricle, but it is correlated with poor physical fitness, obesity, cigarette smoking and future risk of heart attacks.

The triaxial seismocardiogram, like the vectorcardiogram, reveals the direction and amplitude of the vectors of force. When kinetic force is small in one axis, it may be large in one or both of the others.[26] The ratio of forces in the three axes at any phase of systole or diastole varies from one individual to another, both in normal subjects and in those with heart disease. Head-foot forces are most sensitive to extracardiac influences, of which the most significant is the reduced transmission of force from the cardiovascular to the skeletal structures and to the recording system during expiration.

Only in triaxial records, timed with the R wave of the ECG, can we evaluate the significance of the waves due to ventricular or atrial systole or to protodiastolic filling of the ventricles.

The triaxial SCG is the only simple device for indicating how the heart is functioning as a pump, whether the patient has a favorable or gloomy prognosis and whether he is deteriorating or improving. This index of physical fitness and of myocardial embarrassment may fall as a result of aging, nicotine absorption or disease, and it may rise in response to management. The index may be normal in the presence of compensated valvular or coronary disease or abnormal when all other tests of cardiovascular disease are negative.

REFERENCES

1. Starr, I., Rawson, A. J., and Schroeder, H. A.: Apparatus for recording the heart's recoil and the blood's impact in man (ballistocardiograph). Am. J. Physiol. 123:195, 1938.
2. Angenheister, G., and Lau, E.: Seismographische Aufnahmen der Herztätigkeit. Naturwissenschaften 16:513, 1928.
3. Lynn, T. N., and Wolf, S.: The prognostic significance of the ballistocardiogram in ischemic heart disease. Am. Heart J. 88:277, 1974.
4. Hixson, W. C., and Beischer, D. E.: Biotelemetry of the triaxial ballistocardiogram and electrocardiogram in a weightless environment, U.S. Naval School Aviation Med. Monograph 10, 1964.
5. Bancroft, W. H., Tucker, M., Jackson, D. H., and Eddleman, E. E., Jr.: Automatic computer processing of ultralow-frequency ballistocardiogram. *In* Ballistocardiography: Research and

Computer Diagnosis, edited by E. K. Francke. Basel, S. Karger, 1973.
6. Bixby, E. W., and Henderson, C. B.: A method of securing the direct body ballistocardiogram by means of a microscope giving a record easily calibrated. Circulation 8:578, 1953.
7. Dock, W., and Taubman, F.: Some technics for recording the ballistocardiogram directly from the body. Am. J. Med. 7:713, 1949.
8. Dock, W.: The value of lateral ballistocardiograms in differentiating aortic tortuosity from myocardial dysfunction. Am. J. Med. Sci. 228:125, 1954.
9. Dock, W.: A case with much larger ballistocardiographic forces evoked by beats of pacemaker than by those of sinus origin. Am. Heart J. 83:678, 1972.
10. Dock, W., Mandelbaum, H., and Mandelbaum, R. A.: The Application of Direct Ballistocardiography to Medical Practice. St. Louis, C. V. Mosby Co., 1953.
11. Dock, W.: Use of cathode ray oscillograph for electrocardiography. Proc. Soc. Exp. Biol. Med. 24:566, 1927.
12. Brown, H. R., Jr., and deLalla, V., Jr.: Ballistocardiogram in coarctation of the aorta. N. Engl. J. Med. 240:715, 1949.
13. Dock, W., and Grandell, F.: The significance of large lateral and small head-foot waves in the ballistocardiograms of ectopic beats. Am. Heart J. 53:641, 1957.
14. Thomas, H. D., et al.: The effects of occlusion of the venae cavae, aorta and pulmonary artery on the dog ballistocardiogram. Am. Heart J. 50:424, 1955.
15. Brown, H. R., Jr., Hoffman, M. J., and deLalla, V., Jr.: The ballistocardiographic findings in patients with symptoms of angina pectoris. Circulation 1:132, 1950.
16. Starr, I.: On the later development of heart disease in apparently normal people with abnormal ballistocardiograms eight to ten years after; histories of 90 people over 40 years old. Am. J. Med. Sci. 214:233, 1947.
17. Starr, I.: The prognostic value of ballistocardiograms. J.A.M.A. 187:511, 1964.
18. Brown, H. R., Jr., Hoffman, M. J., and de Lalla, V., Jr.: The use of abdominal supports in patients with angina pectoris, as selected by the ballistocardiograph. J. Clin. Invest. 29:799, 1950.
19. Wood, F. C., et al.: The diastolic heart beat. Trans. Assoc. Am. Physicians 64:95, 1951.
20. Scarborough, W. R., et al.: The ballistocardiogram in constrictive pericarditis before and after pericardiectomy. Bull. Johns Hopkins Hosp. 90:42, 1952.
21. Caccese, A., and Schrager, A.: The effects of cigarette smoking on the ballistocardiogram. Am. Heart J. 42:589, 1951.
22. Henderson, C. B.: Ballistocardiograms after cigarette smoking in health and in coronary heart disease. Br. Heart J. 15:278, 1953.
23. Davis, F. W., Jr., et al.: The effects of smok-

ing and exercise on the electrocardiograms and ballistocardiograms of normal subjects and patients with coronary disease. Am. Heart J. 46:529, 1953.

24. Dock, W.: Transmission of ballistocardiographic forces to platforms mounted on springs. Am. J. Med. Sci. 245:449, 1963.

25. Dock, W.: Effects of respiration on transmission of ballistocardiographic forces from the heart to the recording system. Am. Heart J. 58:102, 1959.

26. Dock, W.: The three plane ballistocardio-graph in heart failure. Am. J. Cardiol. 3:384, 1959.

27. Cossio, P., Berreta, J. A., Mosso, A. E., and Fustinoni, O.: El balistocardiograma antes y despues de la comisurotomia mitral. Prensa Med. Argent. 42:3881, 1955.

28. Baker, B. M.: The ballistocardiogram, predictor of coronary disease. Circulation 37:1, 1968.

29. Kiessling, C. E.: Preliminary appraisal of the ballistocardiogram. Trans. Assoc. Life Ins. Med. Dir. Am. 52:115, 1969.

Chapter 13

Non-Invasive Roentgenographic Studies in Cardiovascular Diseases

HEUN Y. YUNE AND EUGENE C. KLATTE

In spite of the development of many sophisticated techniques and procedures, the time-tested standard cardiac series and cardiac fluoroscopy retain an essential role in the diagnosis of cardiovascular abnormalities. Cardiac radiography is non-invasive, of moderate cost, and gives valuable anatomic information as to cardiac size, chamber configuration and determination of pulmonary blood flow, pulmonary vascular resistance and pulmonary venous pressure. When interpreted along with known clinical data and electrocardiographic findings, mistakes in diagnosis are rare.

NORMAL CARDIAC SERIES

The standard radiographic cardiac series consists of a posterior-anterior (PA), a lateral (LAT), a left anterior oblique (LAO) and a right anterior oblique (RAO) view. These radiographs are obtained with barium paste in the esophagus. A standard radiograph is a two-dimensional view of a three-dimensional structure. By utilizing the four views of the heart and great vessels, a three-dimensional mental image is obtained. Each view adds valuable information. While it is true that the majority of cardiac abnormalities may be diagnosed on a PA and lateral projection the oblique views add valuable data to the examination. It is important to analyze the appearance and spatial relationships of each of the cardiac chambers and the great vessels on each projection.

PA View (Figs. 13-1 and 13-2). The location of the cardiac chambers and the great vessels as seen on a PA chest radiograph are diagramed on Figure 13-2A. In a young individual the upper border of the right cardiac silhouette is formed by the superior vena cava. In older individuals the aorta may be elongated and be border forming. More inferiorly the superior vena cava blends with the right atrium, which forms almost all of the right cardiac border. The inferior vena cava may occasionally be visualized just above the diaphragm. This is particularly true in patients who have overexpanded lungs. The left cardiac border is made up from above downward of the aorta, pulmonary artery, left atrial appendage and left ventricle. A normal right ventricle is not border forming either to the right or left. In Figure 13-2A the position of aortic and mitral valves should be noted. The aortic valve is ap-

proximately in mid position and superimposed on the spine. The mitral valve is normally located approximately 1 to 2 cm. to the left of the spine, and 3 to 5 cm. above the left diaphragm.

Lateral (LAT) View (Figs. 13-1B and 2B). The lower half of the anterior surface of the cardiac silhouette is in contact with

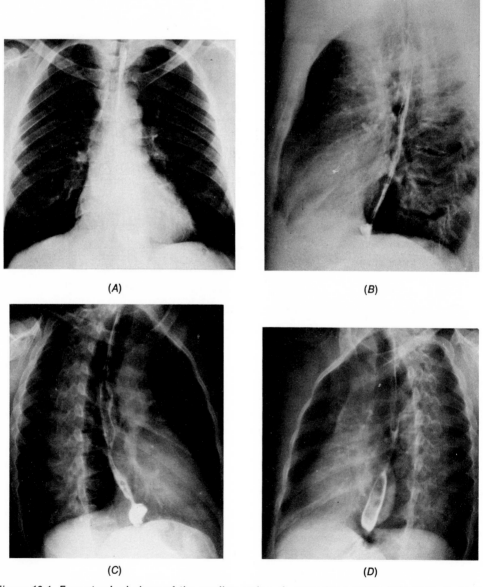

(A)

(B)

(C)

(D)

Figure 13-1. Four standard views of the cardiac series. *A*, posterior-anterior (PA) view; *B*, lateral (LAT) view; *C*, right anterior oblique (RAO) view; *D*, left anterior oblique (LAO) view. Refer to the text for explanation and compare to tracings on Figures 13-2A to D.

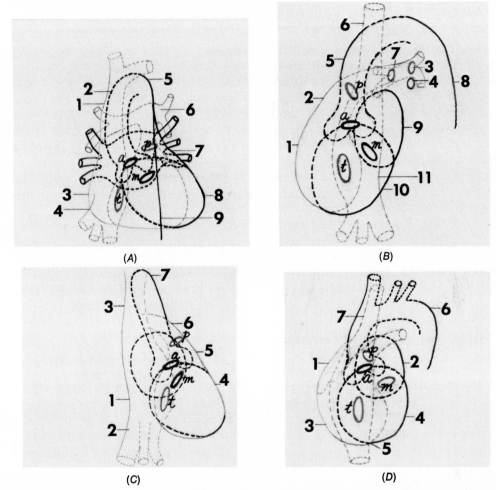

(A)

(B)

(C)

(D)

Figure 13-2A. Line tracings of Figure 13-1A (PA view): 1, right border of the superior vena cava; 2, right border of the ascending aorta; 3, right border of the right atrium; 4, point of confluence of the hepatic vein trunk and the inferior vena cava; 5, the aortic knob; 6, distal end of the main pulmonary artery (pulmonary conus); 7, the left auricular appendage; 8, left border of the left ventricle; 9, left lateral border of the descending thoracic aorta; p, pulmonary valve; a, aortic valve; m, mitral valve; t, tricuspid valve.

Figure 13-2B. Line tracings of Figure 13-1B (LAT view): 1, anterior surface of the right ventricle; 2, infundibular segment of the right ventricle; 3, left pulmonary artery at the left lung hilus; 4, end-on view of the left upper-lobe bronchus; 5, anterior surface of the distal ascending aorta; 6, imaginary line of the anterior surface of the superior vena cava; 7, position of the right pulmonary artery at the right lung hilus; 8, posterior surface of the proximal descending thoracic aorta; 9, posterior surface of the left atrium; 10, posterior

surface of the left ventricle; 11, posterior surface of the inferior right atrium; p, pulmonary valve; a, aortic valve; m, mitral valve; t, tricuspid valve.

Figure 13-2C. Line tracings of Figure 13-1C (RAO view): 1, Posterolateral surface of the right atrium; 2, Inferior vena cava; 3, Superior vena cava; 4, left anterior surface of the right ventricle (anterior interventricular groove); 5, pulmonary infundibulum of the right ventricle; 6, main pulmonary artery; 7, distal ascending and arch segments of the aorta; p, pulmonary valve; a, aortic valve; m, mitral valve; t, tricuspid valve.

Figure 13-2D. Line tracings of Figure 13-1D (LAO view): 1, right anterior surface of the right auricular appendage; 2, left posterior surface of the left atrium; 3, right anterior surface of the right ventricle; 4, left posterior surface of the left ventricle; 5, apex of the heart; 6, arch of the aorta; 7, an imaginary course of the anterior surface of the superior vena cava; p, pulmonary valve; a, aortic valve; m, mitral valve; t, tricuspid valve.

the posterior surface of the sternum. This border is formed by the right ventricle. Above, the right ventricle separates from the posterior surface of the sternum and continues backward toward the hilar arterial confluence. The main pulmonary artery is not well visualized on the lateral view because of surrounding vascular structures. The left pulmonary artery is a direct continuation of the main pulmonary artery and is clearly visualized on the lateral view. It has a specific comma-shaped configuration as it arches over the left upper lobe bronchus. The right pulmonary artery is approximately 1 to 2 cm. below the left pulmonary artery and is seen as a circular structure since it is projected "end on." The right and left pulmonary veins are inferior to their respective arteries. The ascending aorta may be visualized in older individuals; however, in younger people the border is indistinct. When the aorta becomes tortuous the ascending arch may elongate to the point where it may form a significant portion of the anterior upper cardiac silhouette. The transverse and descending thoracic aorta is readily visualized in older individuals because the left margins are surrounded by air-containing lung. In younger individuals the aorta may be difficult to visualize.

The upper half of the posterior surface of the cardiac silhouette is formed by the left atrium, and the lower half by the left ventricle. The midline posterior surface of the left atrium is within the mediastinum and can only be delineated by contrast material in the esophagus, since the anterior surface of the midthoracic esophagus is in direct contact with this surface. The lateral aspects of the left atrium may be visualized on a routine lateral chest radiograph since this portion of the atrium is in contact with the air-containing lung. This apparent border is in actual fact made up of the confluence of the pulmonary veins and left atrium, and since the left pulmonary vein is normally more posterior than the right,

in most individuals the posterior left portion of the left atrium is border forming. The right atrium is superimposed on the left ventricle. Either chamber may be border forming posteriorly. The left ventricle should not extend more than 2 cm. behind the posterior surface of the right atrium on a straight lateral chest radiograph. It is not uncommon for a lateral chest radiograph to be as much as 10 to 15 degrees rotated. This may significantly alter the appearance of the posterior cardiac silhouette and the apparent relationships of the left ventricle and right atrium. The inferior vena cava frequently may be visualized just above the right diaphragm and then blends with the right atrium.

Right Anterior Oblique (RAO) View (Figs. 13-1C and 2C). In this view the right ventricle and pulmonary artery form a consistent part of the mid-anterior cardiac border. The upper cardiac border is made up of the aorta, and the apex is made up of left ventricle. The posterior aspect of the cardiac silhouette is made up of the right and left atria. Because the arch of the aorta runs in a right-anterior to left-posterior direction, the ascending and descending segments of the thoracic aorta become superimposed and "closed" in the RAO view. This view is of specific help in that it gives a profile of the outflow tract of the right ventricle and the proximal pulmonary artery.

Left Anterior Oblique (LAO) View (Figs. 13-1D and 2D). In this view the four quadrants of the cardiac silhouette represent the four chambers of the heart. The top quadrants are the patient's right and left atria, and the lower right and left quadrants are the corresponding ventricles. The ascending, transverse and descending aorta is readily visualized in this view and the pulmonary arteries may be seen within the "aortic window."

Variations of Normal Heart (Figs. 13-3 to 5). The appearance of the cardiac silhouette may vary significantly in normal

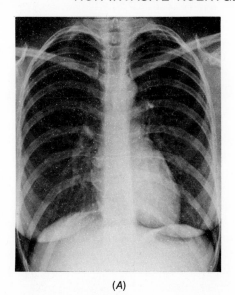
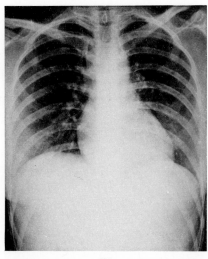

(A)   (B)

Figure 13-3. Variation of the normal. Difference in the appearance of the heart with deep in-spiration (A) and at the end of expiration (B). These two films were obtained only 5 minutes apart. With deep inspiration, the lower position of the diaphragms and maximum aeration of the lungs result in vertically oriented slender appearance of the heart. At the end of expiration, more horizontal orientation of the heart associated with elevated diaphragms and deflated lungs results in pseudocardiomegaly appearance.

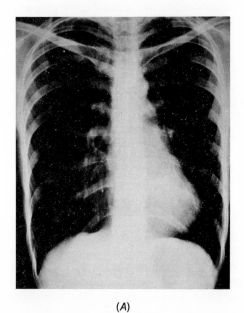
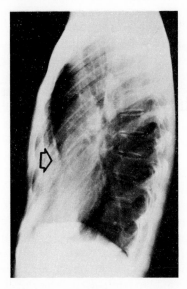

(A)   (B)

Figure 13-4. Variation of the normal—Pectus excavatum. Deeply concave midline anterior chest wall (*arrow*) has reduced the AP diameter of the thoracic cage, with the heart sandwiched be-tween the anterior chest wall and the spine. On the PA view, at a quick glance the cardiac silhouette simulates right ventricular enlargement with elevated cardiac apex.

individuals. Hyposthenic individuals frequently have a smaller appearing heart with a narrower transcardiac diameter. The hypersthenic stocky individual frequently has moderate elevation of the diaphragm, and the heart may appear somewhat larger in size. It is generally recognized that a conditioned athlete frequently has a larger heart than an average person. Without historical data, it is a common mistake to diagnose an enlarged heart in an athlete. Variations in the chest wall may also alter the appearance of the cardiac silhouette. A narrow anterior-posterior dimension or lack of the normal dorsal kyphosis may increase the transverse cardiac diameter. Individuals with pectus excavatum will also frequently have an abnormal appearing cardiac silhouette. In our experience, cardiac mensuration has limited value. It is true that the cardiothoracic ratio (widest diameter of the heart to the right of the spine plus widest diameter of the heart to the left of the spine divided by the transverse thoracic diameter at the level of the right diaphragm) is usually less than 0.5. Many individuals with abnormal hearts will have a normal cardiothoracic ratio. It is also not unusual for the cardiothoracic ratio to exceed 0.5, particularly in hypersthenic individuals or in individuals with poor inspiratory efforts. If there has been no change in geometry or degree of inspiration, the difference in serial transverse cardiac diameters is usually within 1 to 2 cm.; a change of cardiac diameter greater than 2 cm. usually denotes abnormality. It should be emphasized that both the transverse cardiac diameter and the cardiothoracic ratio are significantly increased if the radiograph is obtained in an anterior-posterior projection, rather than the routine 6-foot PA projection. A common mistake is to compare a 40-inch portable chest radiograph with a previous PA 6-foot radiograph of an individual and suspect a myocardial infarction. The portable radiograph is usually taken at 40 inches in an

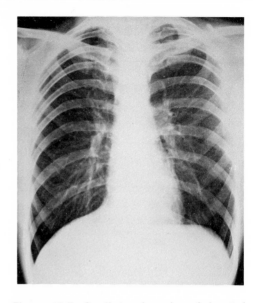

Figure 13-5. Small teardrop-shaped heart in a case of Addison's disease with dehydration and hypovolemia. The similar configuration of the heart and reduced transverse diameter of the heart in relation to the transverse diameter of the thoracic cage is a frequent observation in cases of diffuse pulmonary emphysema, in which hyperlucent lungs, splayed and stretched pulmonary vascular shadows, flattened diaphragms and increased AP diameter of the thoracic cage are characteristic associated findings.

AP projection. The apparent increase in cardiothoracic ratio and transcardiac diameter may be misdiagnosed as enlargement of the heart.

Pulmonary Vasculature (Figs. 13-1A, 1B, 2A, 2B, 6A to D). Pulmonary vasculature makes up the principal hilar structures. Because the left pulmonary artery arches over the left upper lobe bronchus, it is approximately 1.0 to 1.5 cm. superior to the right pulmonary artery. The branching linear shadows in the lungs are principally pulmonary vessels. The pulmonary arteries and pulmonary veins can usually be differentiated by their course. Because the pulmonary veins enter the left atrium at a lower level than the pulmonary arteries, the lower lobe pulmonary veins have a much more horizontal course than the corresponding pulmonary arteries. In the upper lobes the veins are in slightly more vertical position than the arteries; however, their differentiation is principally based on the ability to trace the veins as they converge into channels that cross the pulmonary artery. The upper lobe pulmonary veins usually cross the pulmonary arteries approximately at their point of division into lobar branches. In evaluating the pulmonary vasculature, one should attempt to determine: (a) pulmonary blood flow, (b) pulmonary vascular resistance and (c) pulmonary venous pressure. The right descending pulmonary artery is easily visualized along the right cardiac border. The pulmonary arteries can be traced through approximately third-order divisions, until they become imperceptible in the outer 1 to 2 cm. of the lung.

If pulmonary blood flow is significantly increased (at least two times normal) this is reflected by increase in size of proximal, intermediate and smaller distal pulmonary vessels. In our experience, increased pulmonary blood flow is usually best determined by an increase in size of the pulmonary arteries in the middle third of the lung. There is less variation in these vessels than there may be in the proximal pulmonary arteries. With increased flow, branches of the pulmonary arteries out to fifth-order divisions may become visible, and these can be traced almost to the pleural surface. If pulmonary blood flow is decreased, there is decrease in the size of the proximal and intermediate pulmonary arteries. This is readily determined not only on the PA but also on the oblique and lateral views of the chest. It is important to emphasize that we are considering pulmonary blood flow and not a gradient across the pulmonary valve. It is very common for an individual with mild to moderate pulmonary valvular stenosis to have perfectly normal pulmonary blood flow and therefore normal-appearing distal pulmonary vessels. It is only when there is a shunt of blood around the lungs, either

through atrial or ventricular communications, that pulmonary blood flow is significantly decreased.

Classically, increased pulmonary vascular resistance is radiographically manifested by an increase in size of the proximal pulmonary arteries and a decrease in size of the distal pulmonary vessels. This has been likened to a pruned tree. In individuals who have post-tricuspid shunts and increased pulmonary vascular resistance from birth, there is lack of normal maturation of the muscular and elastic pulmonary arteries. The elastic pulmonary arteries are those vessels greater than 1 mm. in diameter, and therefore these are the vessels that are seen on a radiograph. If maturation of the elastic pulmonary arteries does not occur, these vessels retain their fetal thick-walled, high-tensile strength characteristics, and as a result significant dilatation of the proximal vessels, either from increased pulmonary vascular resistance or increased pulmonary blood flow, may not occur. It is only when increased pulmonary vascular resistance arises in an individual who has had normal maturation of the pulmonary arteries that the classical appearance may be obtained. This is particularly seen in certain persons who have atrial septal defects and some patients with mitral valvular disease. It should be further emphasized that a significant number of adults with atrial septal defects may have marked dilatation of proximal pulmonary arteries with apparent disproportion between the proximal and distal vessels and yet not have measured increase in pulmonary vascular resistance.

The radiographic findings of pulmonary venous hypertension are accurate and frequently predate clinical signs and symptoms. In a normal chest radiograph the size of the pulmonary arteries and veins is larger in the lower lobes than in the upper lobes. This is because in the upright position approximately 80% of right ventricular output goes to the lower lobes. When

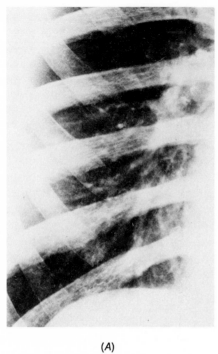

(A)

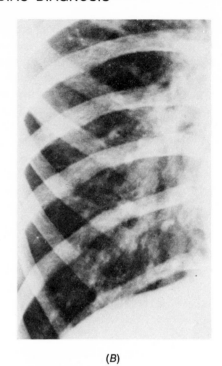

(B)

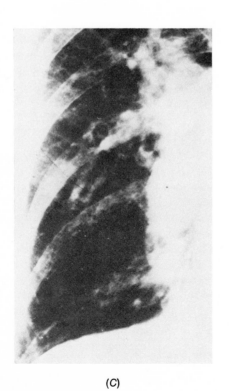

(C)

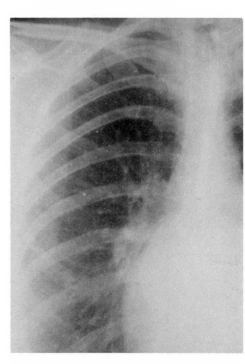

(D)

pulmonary venous pressure is increased, either from a failing left ventricle or a stenotic mitral valve, the increase in venous pressure is greater in the lower lobes than in the upper lobes. This is simply secondary to gravity. When pulmonary venous pressure in the lower lobes nears the oncotic pressure of the blood, fluid leaves the pulmonary capillaries and goes into the interstitial tissue of the lungs. This may compress the capillaries in the lower lung fields. At the same time, elevation of pulmonary venous pressure exceeds alveolar pressure in the upper lobes, and as a result there is a change of perfusion, with the majority of blood pumped by the right ventricle going into the upper lobes. The radiographic manifestations of pulmonary venous pressure may be initially seen as a change in perfusion, with dilatation of the upper-lobe vessels and a decrease in size of the lower-lobe vessels. This change of perfusion will usually occur at a left atrial pressure of about 18 mm.Hg. The increased fluid in the interstitial tissue of the lung may give the lungs a reticular appearance, and horizontal transverse lines going to the pleural surfaces may be noted in the lower lung fields. These are the so-called Kerley B lines, and presumably represent fluid between the secondary pulmonary lobules and dilatation of peripheral lymphatics. Kerley B lines are usually noted when left atrial pressure exceeds 20 mm. Hg. The increase in interstitial fluid also

may make the pulmonary arteries and veins indistinct.

As pulmonary venous pressure continues to rise, fluid collects in the alveoli, and pulmonary edema results. This is manifested by a rather homogeneous increase in density, which is most marked in the perihilar regions. It should be emphasized that one frequently may note atypical patterns of pulmonary edema in which the lungs have a reticular pattern or segmental involvement. This is particularly seen in individuals with underlying chronic obstructive pulmonary disease. It is also not uncommon for the right lung to be involved to a greater degree than the left lung. The reverse is quite rare. It is important to realize that the earliest radiographic manifestation of increased pulmonary venous pressure is dilatation of the upper-lobe vessels. This can only be evaluated on an upright chest radiograph. If a normal individual is filmed in a supine projection, dilatation of upper-lobe vessels is common. For this reason, portable chest radiographs on individuals with suspected cardiac failure should be obtained in the upright position if at all possible.

CARDIAC CHAMBERS AND GREAT VESSELS (FIGS. 13-7 TO 10)

Right Atrium. The right atrium forms the entire right cardiac border on the PA view. One might expect that if this chamber were to enlarge it would form a con-

---

Figure 13-6. Normal and abnormal pulmonary vasculature. *A,* Normal right pulmonary vasculature at hilar and basal area. Note that the right descending pulmonary artery supplying the right middle and lower lobes is easily visualized along the right cardiac border. A few lobar pulmonary veins are noted to cross the right descending pulmonary artery to enter the left atrium.
Figure 13-6B. Increased pulmonary blood flow in a patient with atrial septal defect. Pulmonary arteries are markedly dilated and can be traced toward the lung periphery in third- and fourth-order branches.

Figure 13-6C. Increased pulmonary resistance in a patient with large patent ductus arteriosus. The perihilar pulmonary arterial trunks are enormously dilated and rapidly taper toward the periphery (pruned-tree appearance), which is characteristic of pulmonary hypertension.
Figure 13-6D. Pulmonary venous congestion. The vasculature in the upper right lung and perihilar region is noted to be more prominent than in the lower lung field. The right descending pulmonary artery is rather small. The upper lobe pulmonary veins are readily visible.

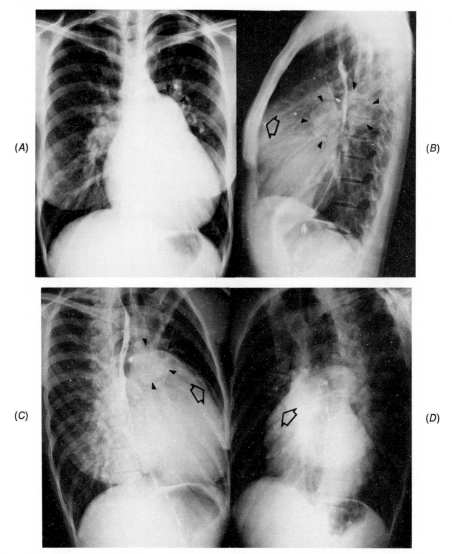

Figure 13-7. Right atrial enlargement. The patient has an untreated large atrial septal defect with markedly increased pulmonary blood flow. Enlargement of the right atrium (*arrow* on *D*) and the right ventricle (*arrow* on *B* and *C*), as well as markedly enlarged pulmonary artery (*arrowheads* on *A*, *B*, and *C*) are noted. Typical findings of pulmonary hypertension are heavily dilated pulmonary arteries in the hilar region that rapidly taper toward the periphery of the lung. Note: The giant right atrium associated with squared superior right heart border on LAO view is seen also on Figure 13-12A.

Atrial septal defect. Secondary to a communication between the atria, blood flows from the higher pressured left atrium to the lower pressured right atrium, which also receives blood from the venae cavae. As a result, blood flow through the right atrium, right ventricle and pulmonary vessels may increase severalfold, causing dilatation of these structures. The thicker-walled left atrium acts simply as a conduit for blood to the thinner-walled right atrium and usually remains normal in size, as do the left ventricle and aorta, which are not directly involved in the shunt.

spicuous bulge to the right. In actual fact, this is rarely true unless there is massive dilatation of the right atrium, as may be seen in certain patients with tricuspid regurgitation. When the right atrium enlarges, it is more inclined to enlarge anteriorly. In the left anterior oblique view the right atrium normally forms the upper one third to one half of the right cardiac border. The right atrium, along with the right ventricle, forms a smooth concentric curve. When the right atrium is enlarged, it usually will form the entire right cardiac border, and the right cardiac border will be "squared." An enlarged right atrial appendage may also be border forming anteriorly and square the anterior aspect of the heart, when viewed in lateral projection. Occasionally the right atrium will enlarge posteriorly and overlap the esophagus in the lateral or right anterior oblique view. In our experience, posterior enlargement of the right atrium is uncommon unless this chamber is massively enlarged. The point of differential pulsation of right atrium and right ventricle can be discerned fluoroscopically. The patient is positioned in the left anterior oblique projection, and the point of differential pulsation is determined. If the right atrium forms more than one half of the right cardiac border in this projection, right atrial enlargement may be assumed.

Right Ventricle. In general, right ventricular hypertrophy is difficult, if not impossible, to determine, and it is only when ventricular dilatation occurs that specific configurations become apparent. In the normal individual the right ventricle is not border forming on the PA projection. When the right ventricle hypertrophies and dilates there is clockwise rotation of the heart, and the right ventricle may form a significant portion of the left cardiac border. The left cardiac border may then be straightened, or the upper left cardiac border may form a convex curve. When the right ventricle dilates, it also dilates anteriorly and may encroach on the retro-

sternal space. In our experience the most valid view for right ventricular enlargement is the right anterior oblique view. The outflow tract of the right ventricle is usually the first portion to dilate, and when this occurs a convex bulge of the right ventricular outflow tract is readily noted in the right anterior oblique projection.

Left Atrium. When the left atrium dilates, it enlarges posteriorly and displaces the esophagus and left lower lobe bronchus posteriorly. The left atrial appendage may also enlarge with left atrial dilatation. This may form a convex bulge just below the pulmonary artery. If the left atrium dilates, its portion of the cardiac silhouette will be thicker than the remainder of the heart and on the PA projection will have increased density. If the left atrium dilates to the point where it is surrounded by air-containing lung, a "double density" may be noted. With massive left atrial enlargement there may be splaying of the carina and elevation of the left main-stem bronchus. On rare occasions the left atrium may be so dilated that it may form both left and right cardiac borders.

Left Ventricle. The left ventricle forms the apex and the posterior inferior aspect of the heart. With left ventricular dilatation the apex of the heart moves downward and to the left. The posterior border also enlarges, and the left ventricle extends prominently behind the inferior vena cava as seen in the lateral view. Left ventricular hypertrophy without left ventricular dilatation may be difficult to discern. In certain individuals there is concentric rounding of the apex; however, any experienced individual has seen many cases of left ventricular hypertrophy with a normal cardiac silhouette.

Aorta. The aorta is an important clue to the diagnosis of cardiac disease. It maintains a fairly constant relationship with cardiac size until middle age. Beyond that point, aortic elongation and dilatation may be seen secondary to degenerative changes

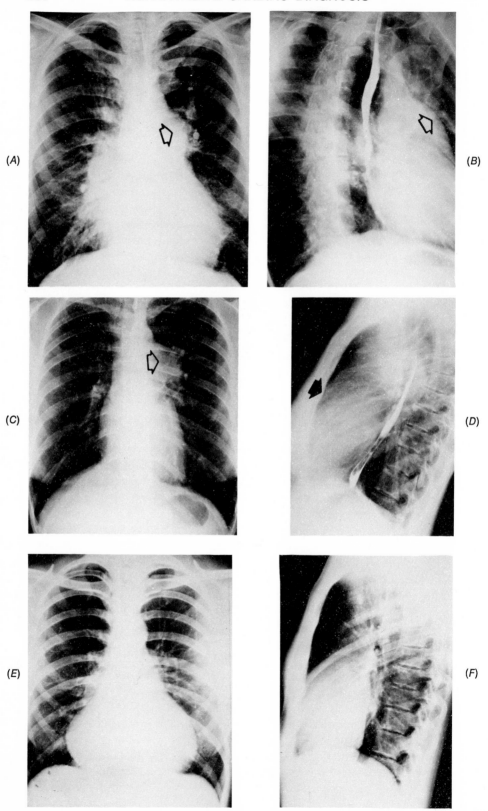

in the aortic wall. If one takes this into consideration, aortic size may be correlated with cardiac output and systemic pressure. The majority of individuals with systemic hypertension will have moderate diffuse dilatation of the thoracic aorta. Individuals with chronic low-output states, such as chronic myocardial disease, will have smaller aortas. Certain individuals with increased blood flow through the aorta, as in patent ductus arteriosus, may have dilatation of the ascending and transverse aorta over to the point of origin of the ductus arteriosus. Individuals with aortic valvular stenosis will have dilatation of the ascending aorta to the point of origin of the innominate artery. The aortic knob will be normal in size. A right aortic arch may be a clue to the diagnosis, since this condition occurs primarily in tetralogy of Fallot, tricuspid atresia and truncus arteriosus and sometimes in transposition of the great vessels.

Pulmonary Arteries. The main and proximal pulmonary arteries are dilated in most individuals with increased pulmonary blood flow. They also may be dilated in patients with increased pulmonary vascular resistance. Dilatation of the main pulmonary artery and left pulmonary artery is frequently noted in pulmonary valvular stenosis. The disproportion in size of the left and right pulmonary arteries is almost pathognomonic of this anomaly.

CARDIAC FLUOROSCOPY

Cardiac fluoroscopy adds significant information to the radiographic examination of the heart. It is our routine to intially ob-

---

Figure 13-8. Right ventricular enlargement (see also Figure 13-7). A and B, Large uncorrected ventricular septal defect with severe pulmonary hypertension. Note markedly dilated pulmonary infundibulum of the right ventricle and the main pulmonary artery (*arrows*). Aneurysmally dilated perihilar pulmonary arteries from severe pulmonary hypertension have obscured the upper right heart border on PA view.

Ventricular septal defect. A ventricular septal defect may occur either in the muscular portion of the ventricle where it is usually small or in the membranous portion where the defect tends to be larger. During ventricular contraction a certain amount of blood will be shunted from the higher-pressured left ventricle into the right ventricle, then through the pulmonary circulation, left atrium and left ventricle. Depending on the size of this defect, pulmonary blood flow may increase to a volume several times normal. Dilated cardiac chambers are therefore the right ventricle, left atrium and left ventricle. The radiographic manifestation of increased pulmonary blood flow is noted only if this flow is at least two times normal.

Figure 13-8 C and D). Markedly dilated left pulmonary artery (*arrow* on C), without right pulmonary artery dilatation, in association with right ventricular hypertrophy (*arrow* on D) is typical of pulmonary valvular stenosis with poststenotic dilatation extending into the left pulmonary artery but not into the right pulmonary artery. Note that there is no feature of pulmonary hypertension or congestion in the lung fields.

Pulmonary valvular stenosis. Isolated pulmonary valvular stenosis is almost always a congenital lesion. Rheumatic endocarditis seldom involves the pulmonary valve directly. In pulmonary valvular stenosis, unless the opening is extremely narrow, the pulmonary blood flow is not reduced. Right lung vasculature usually appears normal. Frequently the pulmonary arterial shadow is quite large at the left lung hilus secondary to the jet-and-eddy-current in the main pulmonary artery above the stenotic orifice of the pulmonary valve. The jet flow will reach the left but not the right pulmonary artery, because the latter makes a right-angle turn off the axis of the main pulmonary·artery.

Figure 13-8 E and F. Isolated enlargement of the right ventricle. This conspicuous localized bulge of the lower right heart border on PA view was contiguous to the right ventricle, as confirmed on other projections. Ordinarily this type of density if proven to be outside the cardiac chambers is characteristic of pericardial cyst. In this case it turned out to be a benign mesenchymoma on the wall of the right ventricle. Note that there is no abnormal pulmonary vasculature. There is no sign of generalized dilatation of the right ventricle or any fullness in the pulmonary outflow tract. Ordinarily a fairly well circumscribed density would be seen superimposed on the anterior heart shadow on the lateral view if this were a pericardial cyst.

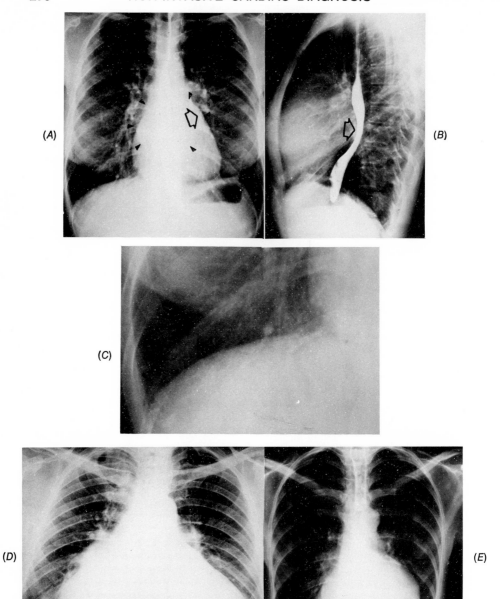

Figure 13-9. Left atrial enlargement. PA and lateral views of the cardiac series (*A* and *B*) and enlarged view of right lung base (*C*) in a patient with moderately symptomatic rheumatic mitral valvular stenosis. Typical findings of left atrial enlargement are noted on PA and lateral views. Note "double density" created by enlarged left atrium (*arrowheads* on *A*), fullness in the region of the left auricular appendage (*arrow* on *A*), indentation on the anterior wall of the barium-filled esophagus (*arrow* on *B*) and engorged interlobular lymphatics in the peripheral lung fields (*arrowheads* on *C*).

Mitral valvular stenosis. Stenosis of the mitral valve elevates left atrial pressure, causing dilatation of this chamber. Pulmonary venous

tain the four standard cardiac views with barium paste in the esophagus. These are first studied, and then fluoroscopy is utilized to determine or confirm suspected abnormalities. There is no indication for "prolonged sightseeing" with a fluoroscope. Specific information gained is (1) generalized or localized contractility of the myocardium, (2) pulsation of the aorta, (3) pulsation of the pulmonary arteries, (4) determination and localization of intracardiac calcifications.

By far the most important aspect of the fluoroscopic examination is discernment of cardiac contractility. The poor contractions of an individual with myocardial failure, in contradistinction to the increased contractions of an individual with aortic valvular insufficiency, help determine the cause of cardiac dilatation. Localized abnormalities of contractility are frequently seen in individuals with coronary artery disease. The splinting of diastolic dilatation in individuals with constrictive pericarditis may be dramatic.

Aortic pulsation correlates closely with stroke volume. Aortic pulsations are increased in individuals with aortic insufficiency. These increased pulsations involve both the ascending and descending aorta. Aortic pulsations are usually decreased in individuals with low cardiac output. Increased pulsations limited to the ascending aorta may be noted in some individuals with aortic valvular stenosis.

Pulsations of the main and proximal pulmonary arteries may be helpful in determining the status of the pulmonary vasculature. Individuals with significantly increased pulmonary blood flow usually have increased pulsations of not only the main and proximal but also secondary and tertiary branches of the pulmonary arteries. Individuals with increased pulmonary vascular resistance may show increased pulsation of the main and proximal pulmonary arteries. Pulmonary valvular stenosis may be associated with increased pulsation of the main pulmonary artery. This increased pulsation also frequently extends into the left pulmonary artery, and there is a difference in pulsation between the left and right pulmonary arteries. This difference in pulsation may be secondary to increased blood flow to the left lung from the jet of blood being directed into the left pulmonary artery.

As previously mentioned, cardiac fluoro-

---

congestion is always present in varying degree. Rising pulmonary venous pressure is quickly reflected in the pulmonary capillary, arterial and right ventricular pressures. On the radiograph, pulmonary venous congestion is manifested by a change in pulmonary perfusion. More blood will circulate through the upper lobes than normal, and upper lobe pulmonary veins will dilate conspicuously. Fluid may leave the pulmonary veins and enter interstitial tissue with resultant engorgement of the pulmonary lymphatics and interlobular edema. These are seen as subpleural horizontal transverse lines in the lung bases on the chest radiograph. Right ventricular hypertrophy and, later, dilatation may occur. When the right ventricle becomes decompensated, even tricuspid insufficiency with right atrial enlargement may develop (see Figure 13-12A).

Figure 13-9D. Gigantic left atrial enlargement presenting to the right of the original right heart border. This is a patient with long-neglected mitral insufficiency. A left atrium of this magnitude is seldom if ever seen in pure mitral valvular stenosis.

Figure 13-9E. Giant left atrium presenting more prominently to the left side, squaring the upper left heart border in the region of the auricular appendage.

Mitral insufficiency. Rheumatic mitral valvular disease is usually a combination of stenosis and insufficiency. One may predominate the other. In mitral valvular insufficiency the left ventricle is required to compensate for the loss of blood, which has regurgitated back into the left atrium through incompetent valves. The left ventricle is forced to accommodate more blood and will begin to dilate. Regurgitating blood from the left ventricle will raise left atrial pressure. Hemodynamic changes in pulmonary circulation similar to those found in mitral stenosis will then follow. An additional prominent radiographic feature in mitral insufficiency, in contradistinction to mitral stenosis, is left vetricular dilatation.

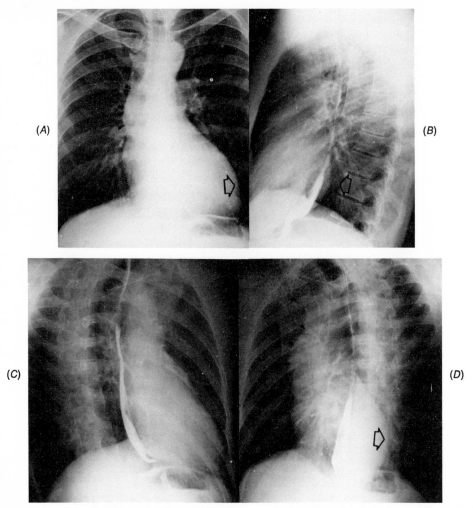

Figure 13-10. A to D. Enlarged left ventricle. Aortic valvular stenosis. Note hypertrophy of the left ventricle (*arrow* on *A, B* and *D*) and prominent dilatation of the proximal ascending aorta (*arrowheads* on *A* and *D*). The dilatation of the aorta does not extend into the arch or the descending segment. Although it may be significantly enlarged, the left ventricle is hidden by the right ventricle on RAO view (*C*), and, therefore, unless the ventricle is extremely large, RAO view is not helpful at all.

Aortic valvular stenosis. When the aortic valve is stenosed, the left ventricle must pump harder to overcome this resistance and supply adequate blood to the systemic circulation. As a result, left ventricular pressure increases, causing hypertrophy of muscle fibers and eventually thickening of the wall. Significant cardiac enlargement does not always occur; the only manifestation may be concentric rounding of the cardiac apex. Left ventricular failure may cause dilatation of the chamber, displacing the cardiac apex to the left. Dilatation of the ascending aorta often occurs secondary to the jet of blood through the stenotic orifice of the aortic valve and the lateral turbulence (eddy current) it causes. Since blood volume entering the systemic circulation is not increased, dilatation of the aorta does not extend beyond the ascending segment. The force of this jet-flow-and-eddy current is nullified as it makes the turn in the arch.

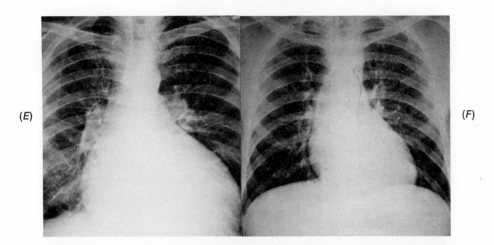

(E)   (F)

Figure 13-10E. Marked left ventricular enlargement in a patient with severe aortic insufficiency. Note that there is relatively less conspicuous dilatation of the ascending aorta. On the PA view alone, this configuration suggests diffuse cardiomegaly that is compatible with either pericardial effusion or myocardopathy, but other views of the cardiac series confirmed that this enlargement was primarily due to left ventricular dilatation.

Aortic Valvular Insufficiency. Rheumatic aortic valvular disease is also usually a combination of stenosis and insufficiency. Again, one usually predominates over the other. Aortic valvular insufficiency is also frequently associated with luetic aortitis and dissecting aneurysm of the ascending aorta in cystic medial necrosis. A portion of the blood that has entered the aorta during ventricular systole will regurgitate back into the left ventricle during diastole simultaneously with blood flowing into the left ventricle from the left atrium. This increased blood volume in the left ventricle at the end of diastole is ejected into the aorta, increasing its stroke volume, and is again regurgitated into the left ventricle during the next cycle of ventricular diastole. The end result on the aorta is increased amplitude of pulsation, not only in the ascending, but also in the arch and descending, segments.

Figure 13-10F. Coarctation of the aorta. Note notched left lateral wall of the coarcted segment of proximal descending aorta seen between the posterior left fifth and sixth rib shadows (outline slightly retouched). The rib notchings *(arrowheads),* left ventricular hypertrophy and dilatation of the ascending aorta are readily appreciated.

Coarctation of the aorta. Coarctation of the aorta may be seen in early infancy with severe left heart failure. The noninfantile type of coarctation is usually located just beyond the origin of the left subclavian artery and may go undetected until well after puberty. In this condition because of reduced blood flow to the trunk and lower extremities, collateral circulation routes are established, ordinarily through the internal mammary artery and intercostal arteries. Prominently dilated intercostal arteries may produce notching on the under surface of the upper ribs. Dilated internal mammary arteries may be seen as undulating shadows on the posterior surface of the sternum on lateral chest radiograph. The aorta immediately distal to the coarctation is frequently dilated because of the jet stream and lateral turbulence of blood flowing through the coarctation (poststenotic dilatation). This dilatation enables localization of the coarctation. If the coarctation is very severe and the opening extremely small, poststenotic dilatation may not be present. To counter the resistance of the coarctation the left ventricle hypertrophies.

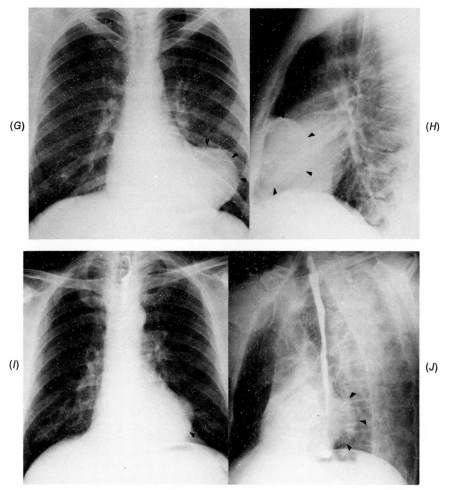

Figure 13-10G and H. Giant aneurysm (*arrowheads*) on the anterior wall of the left ventricle following myocardial infarction. Fluoroscopically this aneurysm demonstrated typical paradoxical pulsation in relation to the left ventricular pulsation. Note normal-appearing aorta and no evidence of left atrial enlargement.

Figure 13-10 I and J. Left ventricular aneurysm on its posterior wall (*arrowheads*). Because of its location, it is best demonstrated on LAO view (*J*). The aneurysm also demonstrated paradoxical pulsation.

A left ventricular aneurysm with significant left ventricular dysfunction can progress to failure. However, the aneurysm may remain localized without significant morphologic changes of the outflow or inflow tracts of the left ventricle.

A myocardial infarction with or without a left ventricular aneurysm may involve the papillary muscle, and dysfunction occurs. As a result, acute mitral valvular insufficiency may develop with rapidly progressing left heart failure. If infarction of the ventricular septum occurs, it may perforate acutely, with resultant hemodynamic changes of ventricular septal defect. In this situation the the ischemic and weakened left ventricle frequently cannot cope with tthe additional burden, and fatal heart failure may develop rapidly.

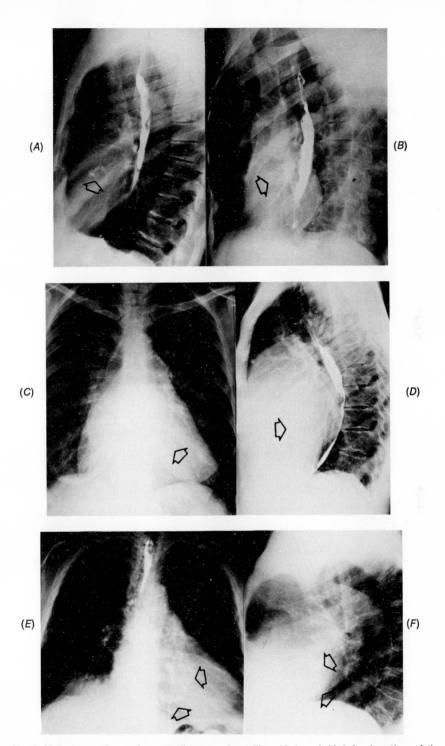

Figure 13-11. Valvular and annulus calcifications (see Figs 13-1 and 13-2 for location of the various valves on different projections). *A* and *B.* Calcific aortic valves (*arrows*)—aortic stenosis. On straight PA projection, the aortic valve is superimposed over the lower dorsal spine shadow, and therefore its calcification cannot be detected on PA view.

Figure 13-11C and D. Chronic mitral stenosis and insufficiency with calcification (*arrows*). Note large left atrium and right ventricle.

Figure 13-11E and F. Heavily calcified mitral annulus (*arrows*). Extensive calcification of the mitral annulus can occur without valvular disease and therefore without much clinical symptomatology.

scopy may be very helpful in determining right atrial size. The fluoroscopic sign of right atrial enlargement is atrial-type pulsations along the entire right cardiac border in the left anterior oblique view.

Cardiac fluoroscopy plays an essential role in determining the location and type of intracardiac calcifications. This is particularly helpful in the diagnosis of valvular calcifications.

Our cardiac fluoroscopy routine is to initially observe the patient in the PA projection. Myocardial contractility is determined, as is pulsation of the aorta and the pulmonary vessels. The patient is then turned to a right anterior oblique position, and a careful search is made for intracardiac calcifications. The patient is then turned to a left anterior oblique position, and cardiac contractility and aortic pulsations are again discerned. Right atrial size is determined. If calcifications were noted in the right anterior oblique view, their locations are reconfirmed in this view.

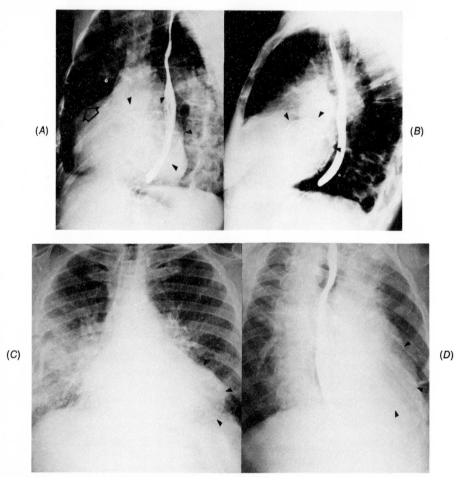

Figure 13-12A and B. Calcification of the chambers. LAO and lateral views of heavily calcified left atrial walls. This is a patient with known chronic mitral valvular disease (mitral stenosis and insufficiency). Note rimlike calcification on all walls of the left atrium (*arrowheads*). Note also markedly dilated right atrium, which is best demonstrated on LAO view as a "squared" upper segment of the right heart border (*arrow* on A).

Figure 13-12C and D. Extensive rimlike calcification of the left ventricular wall (*arrowheads*), demonstrated on PA and RAO projections. This is a giant anterior left ventricular wall aneurysm. Note marked cardiomegaly and chronic pulmonary congestion.

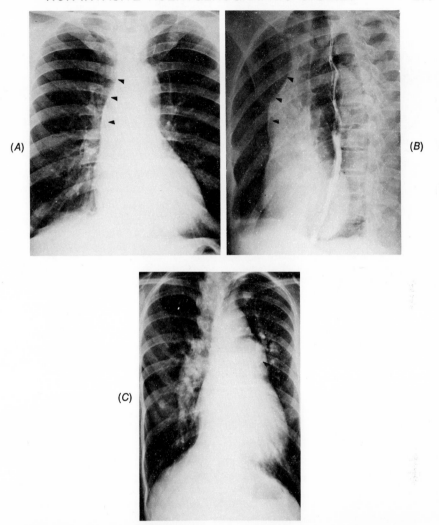

Figure 13-13A and B. Calcification of great vessels. Extensive calcification of the walls and dilatation of the ascending aorta (*arrowheads*), associated with moderate left ventricular hypertrophy. This is a patient with known syphilitic aortitis and aortic insufficiency; *C,* Rimlike calcification surrounding enormously enlarged main pulmonary artery (*arrowheads*). This is a case of untreated large atrial septal defect. Note typical findings of pulmonary hypertension. Similar calcification may be seen in neglected cases of large patent ductus arteriosus.

CARDIAC CALCIFICATIONS (FIGS. 13-11 TO 15)

Calcification may be seen in many parts of the heart. Calcifications are usually secondary to dystrophic or necrotic changes of any layer of the heart or walls of vascular structures.

Valvular calcifications may be important in determining the diagnosis. Aortic valvular calcifications are seen in approximately 90% of individuals with aortic valvular stenosis. Mitral valvular calcifications that are radiographically visible are much less common. Valvular calcifications are very rarely noted in the right side of the heart. Calcifications of the annulus of the heart are common in elderly people. The

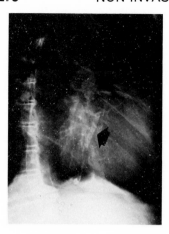

Figure 13-14. Coronary artery calcification. An overpenetrated RAO view of the heart with extensive tubular calcification of the anterior descending (*top arrow*) and the left circumflex coronary artery (*bottom arrow*). Note their typical location and configuration.

spatial relationships between the aortic and mitral valves are such that the aortic valve is anterior, superior and slightly to the right of the mitral valve. In the PA chest radiograph, the aortic valve is almost always in the midline, while the mitral valve is just to the left of the spine.

Intraluminal calcifications may result from a calcified thrombus or calcification of an intraluminal neoplasm, such as myxoma. Statistically, both of the lesions are most frequently found in the left atrium.

Postnecrotic calcifications of the myocardial wall are seen almost exclusively in the left heart. Calcification of the wall of the left atrium is a rare complication, usually of long-standing mitral valvular disease. Calcification of the wall of the left ventricle is usually the result of myocardial infarction. The most frequently observed location of such postinfarct scarring is on the anterolateral wall of the left ventricle. Calcification of the wall of the aorta is common. When this calcification is limited to the ascending aorta, specific luetic inflammatory disease should be strongly considered.

Calcifications of the pulmonary arteries are almost always associated with increased pulmonary blood flow and increased pulmonary vascular resistance. Calcification in the pulmonary vessels is extremely rare in patients under 20 years of age. The ductus arteriosus not uncommonly may calcify in adult patients.

Coronary artery calcifications are very

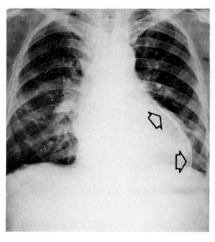
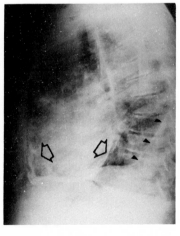

(A)　　　　　　　　　　　　(B)

Figure 13-15. Calcification of the pericardium. Extensively calcified pericardial husk surrounds the heart (*arrows*) in a patient with chronic constrictive pericarditis. Note pulmonary congestion associated with pleural effusion (*arrowheads*).

common. The amount of calcification in the coronary arteries may not parallel the severity of the coronary occlusive disease.

Calcification of the pericardium is becoming progressively less common. This is usually associated with constrictive pericarditis.

SUMMARY

The non-invasive roentgenologic examination of the heart consists of the standard cardiac series and cardiac fluoroscopy. This technique is essential in the diagnosis of all cardiovascular abnormalities. It has many advantages over invasive techniques widely in use at the present time.

For a proper roentgenologic analysis of the heart, one must have a working knowledge of the relative size and location of each cardiac chamber and of great vessels in the normal person. Detailed outlines of the cardiac silhouette and the great vessels in each of the four standard views of the cardiac series are given. Cardiac fluoroscopy provides additional information concerning myocardial contractility, abnormal hemodynamics manifested in altered pulsations of various chambers and great vessels and localization of intracardiac calcifications.

Examples of variations of the normal heart are cited to emphasize the fact that altered size or shape of the heart per se does not indicate the presence of heart disease.

In the evaluation of the hemodynamic status of a given heart the appearance of the pulmonary vasculature is probably the single most important source of information. For this reason a more detailed discussion of analysis of the pulmonary vasculature is presented.

The positive roentgenologic signs of abnormal cardiac chambers and great vessels are reviewed in conjunction with illustrative cases that correlate and highlight altered hemodynamics with various heart diseases.

REFERENCES

1. Bjork, L.: Roentgen diagnosis of left ventricular aneurysm. Am. J. Roentgenol. 97:338, 1966.
2. Blount, S. G., Jr., McCord, M. C., Komesu, S., and Lanier, R.: Roentgen aspects of isolated valvular pulmonic stenosis. Radiology 62:337, 1954.
3. Brean, H. P., Marks, J. H., Sosman, M. C., and Schlesinger, M. J.: Massive calcification in the infarcted myocardium. Radiology 54:33, 1950.
4. Burch, G. E., de Pasquale, N. P., and Phillips, J. H.: The syndrome of papillary muscle dysfunction. Am. Heart J. 75:399, 1968.
5. Chen, J. T. T., et al.: Correlation of roentgen findings with hemodynamic data in pure mitral stenosis. Am. J. Roentgenol. 102:280, 1968.
6. Davis, G., Kincaid, O., and Hallerman, F.: Roentgen aspects of cardiac tumors. Semin. Roentgenol. 4:384, 1969.
7. Dubnow, M. H., Burchell, H. B., and Titus, J. L.: Post-infarction ventricular aneurysm: A clinical, morphologic and electrocardiographic study of eighty cases. Am. Heart J. 70:753, 1965.
8. Eliot, R. S., and Mork, J. N.: Aortic regurgitation past 50. Geriatrics 22:90, 1967.
9. Fouche, R. F., Beck, W., and Schrire, V.: The roentgenologic assessment of the degree of left to right shunt in secundum type atrial septal defect. Am. J. Roentgenol. 89:254, 1963.
10. Glancy, D. L., Freed, T. A., O'Brien, K. T., and Epstein, S. E.: Calcium in the aortic valve. Ann. Intern. Med. 71:245, 1969.
11. Granger, R. G.: Interstitial pulmonary edema and its radiological diagnosis: A sign of pulmonary venous and capillary hypertension. Br. J. Radiol. 31:201, 1958.
12. Hoffman, R. B., and Rigler, L. G.: Evaluation of left ventricular enlargement in the lateral projection of the chest. Radiology 85:93, 1965.
13. Hublitz, U. F., and Shapiro, J. H.: Atypical pulmonary patterns of congestive failure in chronic lung disease: Influence of pre-existing disease on the appearance and distribution of pulmonary edema. Radiology 93:995, 1969.
14. Klatte, E. C., Campbell, J. A., and Lurie, P. R.: Aortic configuration in congenital heart disease. Radiology 74:555, 1960.
15. Klatte, E. C., Tampas, J. P., and Campbell, J. A.: Evaluation of right atrial size. Radiology 81:48, 1963.
16. Levy, M. J., and Edwards, J. E.: Anatomy of mitral insufficiency. Prog. Cardiovasc. Dis. 5:2 (Sept.), 1962.
17. Lieber, A., Rosenbaum, H. D., Hanson, D. J., and Kwaan, H. M.: Accuracy of predicting pulmonary blood flow, pulmonary arterial resistance, and pulmonary venous pressure from chest roentgenograms. Am. J. Roentgenol. 103:577, 1968.
18. Logue, R. B., Rogers, J. V., and Gay, B. B.,

Jr.: Subtle roentgenographic signs of left heart failure. Am. Heart J. 65:464, 1963.

19. Nice, C. M., Jr.: Cardiovascular Roentgenology: A Validated Program. New York, Harper & Row, 1967.

20. Rider, D. G., Feldt, R. H., Weideman, W. H., and Dushane, J. W.: Ventricular septal defect. Circulation 32:43, 1965.

21. Warburton, R. K., Tampas, J. P., Soule, A. B., and Taylor, H. E., III: Coronary artery calcification: Its relationship to coronary artery stenosis and myocardial infarction. Radiology 91:109, 1968.

22. Yune, H. Y., and Klatte, E. C.: Roentgenographic diagnosis of heart disease. Postgrad. Med. 55:159, 1974.

Chapter 14

Serum Digitalis Level Determination

FRANK I. MARCUS

If the proper aim in digitalis therapy is to provide the maximum dose consistent with a wide margin of safety, knowing the blood level eases the physician's ever-present burden of reaching actionable decisions from insufficient premises.[1]

EVALUATION OF SERUM DIGOXIN LEVELS

The level of digoxin in the serum is determined by the dose of the drug, its bioavailability, distribution within the various compartments of the body, metabolism and excretion. The physician's estimate of the serum digoxin concentration is at best a guess. Computer predictions of the serum digoxin concentration based on a system that corrects for dose, height, weight, sex, age and serum creatinine or blood urea nitrogen explain only 18% of the total variants for serum digoxin concentrations and, in fact, are not significantly different from predictions of the serum digoxin levels by physicians who regulate digoxin therapy unassisted by a computer.[2] Thus, prediction of digoxin levels is not an adequate substitute for measurement of serum digoxin levels. The question whether measurement of digoxin in serum levels improves patient therapy is still to be verified; however, the frequent use of serum digoxin assays in clinical practice has been reported to decrease the frequency of adverse reactions to digoxin.[3]

ACCURACY AND REPRODUCIBILITY OF TEST RESULTS

Prior to consideration of interpretation of serum digoxin levels in the management of patients with heart disease, the physician must be informed as to the accuracy and reproducibility of the test results. A survey conducted in 1972 by the College of American Pathologists indicated that samples of plasma, all containing the same amount of digoxin, were assayed as containing a mean of 1.94 nanograms (ng.) digoxin per ml. by tritium assay and 4.10 ng. per ml. by an iodinated method.[4] Surveys conducted by the same organization in 1974 showed a considerable decrease in the variation of assay of serum digoxin by laboratories using different methods. Nevertheless, if one receives a report of digoxin assayed by one laboratory as compared to another, mean differences of nearly 1 ng. per ml. may be reported if the sample contains approximately 2 ng. digoxin per ml. or differences of 0.5 ng. per ml. if the sample contains 0.7 ng. per ml.

Why is it so difficult to decrease further

the variation of the immunoassay? To appreciate the problems of the digoxin immunoassay it is necessary to understand the basis of this procedure. The assay described by Smith and coworkers is performed as follows:[5] A constant amount of tritium-labeled digoxin is added to a tube containing patient serum or plasma. Antidigoxin antibody, obtained after immunization of an animal (rabbit or sheep) with a digoxin-protein conjugate, is then added to the tube and the mixture is incubated. The nonradioactive digoxin and the tritium-labeled digoxin compete to bind to the antiserum. The greater the concentration of nonradioactive digoxin, the greater the chance that the nonradioactive digoxin will bind to the antidigoxin antibody. Dextran-coated charcoal is then added to the tube, which selectively adsorbs the digoxin unbound to antibody. The supernatant fluid containing the digoxin bound to antibody is then counted in a liquid scintillation counter. The number of counts in the supernate is then compared to counts in a series of control tubes containing standard amounts of digoxin. High counts mean low digoxin values; low counts mean high values. This appears to be a straightforward assay procedure. It is sensitive to 0.2 ng. per ml. (a nanogram is 10^{-9} gm.).

SPECIFICITY OF DIGOXIN ANTISERUM

There are several factors that can alter the accuracy of the assay other than the obvious necessity for meticulous care in pipetting or diluting of solutions. First, one cannot assume that the antidigoxin antibody has the required degree of specificity for digoxin. The antidigoxin antibody described by Smith and coworkers was rigorously evaluated and was found not to interact appreciably with steroid compounds, such as cholesterol, cortisol, progesterone and testosterone, even in concentrations in excess of physiologic levels.[5] Also, sera from patients not receiving digoxin all gave results within 2% of the "zero" value. These analyses imply a high degree of specificity of the antidigoxin antibody. However, other investigators using their antiserum, or antiserum provided commercially, have reported assay values as high as 4 ng. per ml. in patients taking spironolactone but not digoxin or in women in the third trimester of pregnancy.[6-8] This implies a degree of specificity of the antidigoxin antibody that is not suitable for assay of digoxin. Presently there are no standards for specificity that manufacturers of digoxin assay kits must meet, and the specificity of the antiserum is generally not stated or obtainable from the manufacturers.

Most hospital or commercial laboratories now utilize a ^{125}I derivative of digoxin as an isotope for the assay instead of tritium-labeled digoxin. ^{125}I may be counted in a gamma counter, a less expensive and more widely available instrument than that required for scintillation counting. The substitution of the ^{125}I derivatives of digoxin has not been without problems. ^{125}I cannot be incorporated directly into the digoxin molecule. The ^{125}I derivative of digoxin usually consists of ^{125}I tyrosine attached to digoxigenin (digoxigenin is digoxin devoid of the three digitoxose sugars). 3-0 Succinyldigoxigenin-(^{125}I) tyrosine is an iodine-containing tracer frequently used for this purpose. This compound does not have the same affinity for binding to antidigoxin antibody as does digoxin and cannot compete for the antibody in equimolar amounts. Thus, dissociation of this isotope from the antibody is more likely to occur as compared to dissociation of the nonisotopic digoxin or tritium-labeled digoxin from the antidigoxin antibody. This dissociation may occur, for example, in the process of separation of the free from the bound digoxin with dextran-coated charcoal. Digoxin and ^{125}I digoxigenin derivative could dissociate from the antibody at different rates because of the lesser affinity for binding of the ^{125}I digoxigenin derivative. Avoidance of this problem requires strict control of exposure times of patient sample and standards to charcoal. Recently a ^{125}I derivative of digoxin (^{125}I tyrosine-methyl esther of digoxin [not digoxigenin]) has become available. This ^{125}I digoxin derivative appears more stable and has been reported to yield less variability in results using different batches of isotopes.[9]

The antidigoxin antibody has been called digoxin-specific antiserum. However, digitoxin will bind to antidigoxin antibody. One has to be cautious in interpreting an assay result if one is not certain of the digitalis preparation that the patient is receiving. For example, if a patient is taking digitoxin and has a serum digitoxin level of 20 to 25 ng. per ml. the sample will yield a serum "digoxin" level between 1 and 1.5 ng. per ml.

SUBSTANCES THAT INTERFERE WITH THE ASSAY

There are other problems identified with the assay that may produce spurious results. Liquid scintillation counting of plasma containing digoxin may produce falsely high values if the serum is hemolyzed or if hyperbilirubineamia is present,[10] because these pigments cause quenching (a process of diminution of light transmission due to chemicals or color in the liquid scintillation fluid). Relatively small amounts of quenching can be corrected by addition of an internal standard, but accurate quench correction is not possible with severely hemolyzed samples or serum from severely jaundiced patients. Samples of serum from patients who are uremic also may alter the accuracy of counting by means of the tritium assay since they cause chemoluminescence of the scintillation fluid, causing falsely low values.[10] If the patient has received ^{125}I isotopes within a day or two of withdrawal of the blood sample for assay the results may be spuriously low.

Finally, there are "plasma factors" not yet clearly identified that result in different assay findings when the same concentration of digoxin is added to plasma from different patients.[11,12] The same amount of digoxin added to plasma may yield results as high as 27% above and 13% below the true value. One of the plasma factors may be hypoalbuminemia. Hypoalbuminemia enhances the binding of the ^{125}I derivative to the antibody and may result in a value as much as threefold low.[13] Knowledge that standard curves may vary if the known standards of digoxin are added to different sera is of practical importance in the assay. For example, one immunoassay kit was provided with the recommendation that horse serum should be used to obtain standard curves. When standard concentrations of digoxin were added to digoxin-free human plasma rather than horse serum different standard curves resulted and individual plasma assay results were different.[14] Ideally the patient's serum should be assayed with standards made from the patient's serum before digoxin is administered, but this is obviously not possible under clinical situations.

COMPARISON OF DIFFERENT ASSAY TECHNIQUES

It is indeed surprising that assays of patient samples of digoxin by different methods yield comparable results since there are many unsolved problems in obtaining accurate serum digoxin measurements. Comparison of patient samples using a tritium digoxin isotope and using a ^{125}I digoxin derivative as an isotope showed excellent correlation with a correlation coefficient of 0.967.[15] Similar, but lower, correlation ($r = 0.832$) has been demonstrated with patient samples containing digoxin assayed by radioimmunoassay and by the ^{86}Rb uptake method.[16] Correlation between immunoassay using ^{3}H digoxin and the ^{125}I derivatives of digoxigenin has ranged from poor to excellent.[17-19] A comparison of digoxin samples assayed by different commercial kits was recently reported.[20] It was found that a patient sample analyzed as containing 0.1 ng. per ml. by one kit was assayed as 0.8 ng. per ml. by another kit.

Knowledge of the factors that may cause either falsely high or low values should alert the physician to factors that may cause a spurious value. He may then request that the assay be repeated in another laboratory using a different method or he may be forced to disregard the data and rely on his clinical judgment.

CORRELATION OF SERUM DIGOXIN LEVELS WITH DIGITALIS TOXICITY

Can plasma levels of digoxin be used to verify or predict the presence of digitalis intoxication? Beller and associates found that serum drug concentrations were significantly higher in toxic than in nontoxic patients.[21] The mean serum digoxin concentration in toxic patients was 2.3 ± 1.6 ng. per ml. (± 1 standard deviation), whereas the mean level in nontoxic patients was 1 ± 5 ng. per ml. Considerable overlap occurred even though the difference between the two groups was highly significant. They found a significantly greater prevalence of advanced heart disease, atrial fibrillation, anorexia, acute or chronic pulmonary disease and renal failure in toxic than in nontoxic patients. With two exceptions,[22,23] a large number of articles have verified these results.[24]

As experience with digoxin assay accumulates, some patients have been found to be intoxicated who have serum digoxin levels well below 2 ng. per ml. This could have been predicted from animal experiments. Smaller doses of digoxin caused toxic arrhythmias in hypokalemic dogs than in normokalemic controls.[25,26]

At the beginning of toxicity the plasma concentration and the myocardial concentrations in the hypokalemic animals were well below the controls.[26] These experiments document digitalis sensitivity during acute hypokalemia, a well-recognized clinical entity. Other conditions in which the patients are sensitive to the toxic effects of digitalis are anoxia due to chronic pulmonary disease or advanced heart disease. Enhanced sympathetic activity appears to sensitize the individual to digitalis-induced arrhythmias[27,28] and may contribute to the sensitivity seen in patients with cor pulmonale and with advanced heart disease. In experimentally induced digitalis intoxication, sympathetic nerve activity is substantially augmented and high-intensity activity is temporally correlated with ventricular arrhythmias. Spinal cord section prevents all these effects and increases the dose of ouabain required to produce ventricular arrhythmias.

An informative study correlating tolerance to acetylstrophanthidin and plasma digoxin concentrations was recently reported.[29] Acetylstrophanthidin titration tests were performed on 133 patients with diverse cardiac disorders. All patients were receiving maintenance doses of digoxin. The sensitivity and tolerance to a dose of 1.0 mg. acetylstrophanthidin were associated with a wide range of serum digoxin values. The selected dose of acetylstrophanthidin 1 mg., was based on the observation that patients with atrial fibrillation who have well-controlled ventricular rates while taking maintenance doses of digitalis tolerate this dose without adverse effect and that patients who develop ventricular arrhythmias with 0.6 mg. or less of acetylstrophanthidin are close to or at digitalis intoxication. The data presented in Table 14-1 were derived from this report. It shows that there is an inverse relationship between the serum digoxin levels and the percent of patients who could tolerate 1 mg. of acetylstrophonthidin. The authors found that 22% of patients who had serum digoxin levels of 0.7 ng. per ml. or less could not tolerate 0.6 mg. of acetylstrophanthidin and were thought to be exquisitely sensitive to digitalis. These same investigators reported that 30% of patients who had serum digoxin levels between 2.2 and 2.8 ng. per ml. could tolerate a 1-mg. dose of acetylstrophanthidin without adverse effects. These data illustrate that the serum digoxin level is at best a guide to digoxin tolerance and that some patients who have serum levels of 2 ng. per ml. or greater may tolerate further digitalis given cautiously. Resistance to the toxic effects of digitalis is illustrated in children who can usually tolerate plasma levels of digoxin of 2 to 3 ng. per ml. without evidence of toxicity.[30],[31] The explanation for digitalis resistance under these circumstances probably lies in the differing responsiveness of Purkinje tissue to digitalis in the young as compared with the adult.[32]

The major clinical use of the serum digoxin assay is to verify the suspicion of digitalis intoxication. A serum digoxin level above 2 ng. per ml. in a patient with suspected toxicity enhances the diagnostic possibility of digitalis toxicity, but one should require evidence that the arrhythmia decreases in frequency or is abolished within the anticipated half-life of the cardiac glycoside used. It has been found that only 10% of patients who have ventricular premature beats and a serum digoxin level in excess of 2 ng. per ml. will show a decrease in the frequency of the premature ventricular beats within days after digoxin is discontinued.[33] The diagnosis of digitalis intoxication is still presumptive even if premature beats disappear within the anticipated half-life of digoxin and if the serum digoxin level is above 2 ng. per ml. Many patients will show a decrease or disappearance of the arrhythmia with bed rest, treatment of congestive heart failure or removal from a stressful environment.

Other indications for obtaining serum concentrations of digoxin are to verify drug compliance. Regulation of the dose of digoxin in patients with changing renal function, such as patients with severe congestive heart failure or after cardiac surgery,

TABLE 14-1

Comparison of Acetyl Strophanthidin Tolerance with Serum Digoxin Levels

Range of serum digoxin concentration ng./ml.	% patients tolerant to 1.0 mg. acetylstrophanthidin	% patients with arrhythmias induced by less than 0.6 mg. acetylstrophanthidin
0.0–0.7	60	22
0.8–1.4	40	32
1.5–2.1	28	45
2.2–2.8	30	58
>2.8	1	80

may be aided by determination of serum concentrations.

STUDY OF DIGOXIN PHARMACOKINETICS WITH THE USE OF DIGOXIN ASSAY

The ability to measure plasma digoxin concentration has contributed greatly to the study of the pharmacokinetics of the cardiac glycosides. It is doubtful if the differences in the bioavailability of the various tablets of digoxin would have been recognized without the capability to measure digoxin in plasma and in urine.[34]

DIGOXIN BIOAVAILABILITY AND DRUG-DRUG INTERACTION

The documentation that tablet formulation influences bioavailability was soon followed by the observation that in-vitro dissolution of digoxin was correlated directly with bioavailability.[35] This led to the U.S. Food and Drug Administration requirement for dissolution of digoxin tablets.[36] Among factors that influence the bioavailability of digoxin are the formulation of the tablet, the particle size and the excipients.[37] Changes in formulation of tablets have been undertaken previously by manufacturers without knowledge that these changes would have an effect on bioavailability. One example is that which occurred in England when the Wellcome Company changed its manufacturing equipment in 1969. This change was reversed in 1972, but tablets manufactured from 1969 to 1972 had a greatly decreased bioavailability and caused a decrease in serum digoxin concentrations in many patients.[38] Tablets manufactured after 1972 had a bioavailability equal to those manufactured before 1969. There was a subsequent increase in the serum digoxin level in many, but not all, patients. Those patients who had the lower levels with the lesser bioavailable product seem to have the greatest percent increase when given tablets with the higher bioavailability.

The measurement of serum digoxin levels has permitted a comparison of digoxin bioavailability in normal subjects given an intravenous infusion, digoxin elixir and digoxin in tablet form.[39] The magnitude of interdrug differences appears most accurately determined by the steady-state serum concentrations or steady-state urinary digoxin excretion.[40] Measurement of the area under the serum concentration curve after single-dose administration or 24-hour urinary excretion of digoxin after administration of a single dose of drug is exaggerated when a slowly absorbed drug product is compared with a rapidly absorbed one.[40] The pediatric elixir and lanoxin tablets are equally well absorbed in normal volunteers. These preparations have a bioavailability of about 70% of a 1-hour intravenous infusion of digoxin.[39] This indicates that 0.17 mg. of digoxin given intravenously is the equivalent of 0.25 mg. digoxin orally, but considerable individual variation exists even in normal subjects. Ingestion of digoxin tablets after food does not alter the steady-state serum digoxin levels.[41]

The problem of drugs interacting with cardiac glycosides has recently been reviewed.[42] The major drug interactions with digoxin are concerned with those agents that adsorb digoxin, thereby interfering with digoxin absorption. Included are non-absorbed substances, such as cholestyramine,[43] Colestipol, kaolin and pectin (Kaopectate), and nonabsorbable antacids.[44] Neomycin[45] and salicylazosulfapyridine[46] (used to treat patients with regional enteritis) have also been shown to interfere with digoxin absorption. The ingredient in antacid preparations that appears to adsorb digoxin is magnesium trisilicate, which is contained in Gelusil.[47] Antacids containing magnesium hydroxide, such as Maalox, do not adsorb digoxin or alter the dissolution of digoxin. Malabsorption states, especially those associated with a decrease in D-xylose absorption, appear to interfere with the absorption of digoxin from tablets.[48] The absorption of digoxin may be normal under these conditions when the elixir is given.[48,49] Since a small fraction of digoxin undergoes biotransformation, the drug is not susceptible to hepatic enzyme induction that alters the metabolism of cardiac glycosides. The enterohepatic circulation of digoxin is not an important determinant of the half-life of this drug since attempts to shorten the half-life by chronic administration of either activated charcoal[50] or cholestyramine[51] do not influence the serum level of the drug.

DIGOXIN EXCRETION

Since digoxin is eliminated predominantly by renal excretion, differences in renal function are a major source of individual variation in the disposition of digoxin. Prior to the development of the digoxin immunoassay, a positive correlation between creatinine clearance and digoxin clearance was appreciated.[52] This relation suggested that glomerular filtration is the dominant mechanism in the renal excretion of digoxin and that the decreased glomerular filtration rate is associated with a prolonged digoxin half-life in patients with chronic impairment of renal function such as patients with glomerulonephritis[53,54] or the elderly.[55] Subsequently it has been demonstrated that digoxin is also eliminated by renal tubular secretion.[56,57] Indeed, drugs such as spironolactone can interfere with the renal tubular secretion of digoxin and can cause an increase in steady-state serum digoxin concentrations.[57] Tubular secretion of digoxin may account for the poor correlation between creatinine clearance and digoxin half-life[58] (Fig. 14-1). This poor correlation precludes the quantitative use of creatinine clearance to adjust digoxin dose but does not negate the general principle that a marked increase of serum creatinine (>3.0 mg. per 100 ml.) is associated with an increased half-life of digoxin. Patients with this degree of diminution in renal function should be given a smaller than usual maintenance dose. Alterations in the extrarenal excretion of digoxin may also be a factor that determines the serum half-life of digoxin in patients with renal failure.[59] The finding that there is a decreased volume of distribution of digoxin in severe renal failure suggests that the loading dose of digoxin should be reduced under these circumstances.[60] This may be due to decreased tissue uptake, possibly due to a diminished affinity for binding of digoxin to membrane ATPase in severe renal diseases.[61] The lack of a strict relation of digoxin half-life with serum creatinine and the variability in the volume of distribution of digoxin make the determination of the serum concentration of digoxin a most useful guide to therapy in patients with severe renal diseases.

SUMMARY

It is important that the physician understand the principles of digoxin immunoassay and its pitfalls in order to properly evaluate the data obtained. Low serum digoxin levels help explain a lack of therapeutic effect. A level above 2 ng. per ml. indicates that the chances of digoxin intoxication are increased as compared with a lower level, but does not necessarily preclude the administration of further doses of digoxin if clinically indicated. Therefore, serum di-

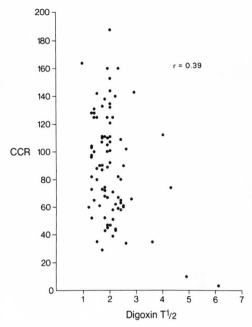

Figure 14-1. A plot of creatinine clearance and serum digoxin half-life in days. There is a poor correlation (r = 0.39) between these two parameters.[58]

goxin levels are an aid in the regulation of digoxin dose in selected patients. There are indications that frequent use of the serum digoxin assay in clinical practice decreases the frequency of adverse reactions to digoxin.

The serum digoxin assay has been instrumental in obtaining information regarding digoxin bioavailability and drug-drug interaction.

REFERENCES

1. Lown, B.: Foreword in Digitalis by T. W. Smith and E. Haber. Boston, Little, Brown & Co., 1974.
2. Peck, C. C., et al.: Computer-assisted digoxin therapy. N. Engl. J. Med. 289:441, 1973.
3. Duhme, D. W., Greenblatt, D. J., and Koch-Weser J.: Reduction of digoxin toxicity associated with measurement of serum levels. Ann. Intern. Med. 80:516, 1974.
4. Ewy, G. A., et al.: Digitalis intoxication, management and prevention. Cardiovascular Drug Therapy, Philadelphia, F. A. Davis Co., 1974.
5. Smith, T. W., Butler, V. P., and Haber, E.: Determination of therapeutic and toxic serum

digoxin concentrations by radioimmunoassay, N. Engl. J. Med. 281:1212, 1969.

6. Zeegers, J. J. W., et al.: The radioimmunoassay of plasma-digoxin. Clin. Chim. Acta 44:109, 1973.

7. Falch, D.: Determination of digoxin in plasma by radioimmunoassay. J. Oslo City Hosp. 23:35, 1973.

8. Phillips, A. P.: The improvement of specificity in radioimmunoassays. Clin. Chim Acta 44:333, 1973.

9. Drewes, P. A., and Pileggi V. J., Jr: Faster and easier radioimmunoassay of digoxin. Clin. Chem. 20:343, 1974.

10. Butler, V. P., Jr: Assays of digitalis in the blood. Prog. Cardiovasc. Dis. 14:571, 1972.

11. Anggard, E. E., Chew, L. F., and Kalman, S. M.: A source of error in digoxin radioimmunoassay. N. Engl. J. Med. 237:935, 1972.

12. Burnett, G. H., et al.: Variability of standard curves in radioimmunoassay of plasma digoxin. Clin. Chem. 19:725, 1973.

13. Holtzman, J. L., Shafer, R. B., and Erickson R. R.: Methodological causes of discrepancies in radioimmunoassay for digoxin in human serum. Clin. Chem. 20:1194, 1974.

14. Kostenbauder, H. B., Foster, T. S., and McGovren, J. P.: Radioimmunoassay in pharmacy in practice. Am. J. Hosp. Pharm. 31:763, 1974.

15. Pippen, S. L., and Marcus F. I.: Comparison of digoxin immunoassay using tritiated digoxin and ^{125}I tyrosine-methyl-ester of digoxin. Unpublished data.

16. Lader, S., Bye, A., and Marsden, P.: The measurement of plasma digoxin concentration of two methods. Eur. J. Clin. Pharmacol. 5:22, 1972.

17. Hogan, E. D., and Riley, W. J.: Radioimmunossay of plasma digoxin with use of iodinated tracer. Clin. Chem. 19:187, 1973.

18. Burnett, G. H., et al.: Variability of standard curves in radioimmunoassay of plasma digoxin. Clin. Chem. 19:725, 1973.

19. Gutcho, S., McCarter, H., and Rapun, R.: Radioimmunoassay of digoxin: An intercomparison of results with these methods. Clin. Chem. 19:1058, 1973.

20. Kubasik, N. P., Schauseil, S., and Sine, H. E.: Comparison of commercial kits for radioimmunoassay. Clin. Biochem. 7:206, 1974.

21. Beller, G. A., et al.: Digitalis intoxication. N. Engl. J. Med. 234:989, 1971.

22. Fogelman, A. M., et al.: Fallibility of plasma digoxin in differentiating toxic from nontoxic patients. Lancet 2:727, 1971.

23. Howard, D., et al.: A prospective survey of the incidence of cardiac intoxication with digitalis in patients being admitted to hospital and correlation of serum digoxin levels. Aust. N.Z. J. Med. 3:279, 1973.

24. Smith, T. W.: Digitalis toxicity: Epidemiology and clinical use of serum concentration measurements. Am. J. Med. 58:470, 1975.

25. Lown, B., et al.: Effects of alterations of body potassium on digitalis toxicity. J. Clin. Invest. 31:648, 1952.

26. Marcus, F. I., et al.: The effect of acute hypokalemia on the myocardial concentration and body distribution of tritiated digoxin in the dog. J. Pharmacol. Exp. Ther. 178:271, 1971.

27. Gillis, R. A.: Cardiac sympathetic nerve activity: Changes induced by Oubain and propranolol. Science 166:508, 1969.

28. Gillis, R. A., et al.: Neuroexcitatory effects of digitalis and their role in the development of cardiac arrhythmias. J. Pharmacol. Exp. Ther. 183:154, 1972.

29. Klein, M. D., et al.: Comparison of serum digoxin level measurement with acetyl strophanthidin tolerance testing. Circulation 49:1053, 1974.

30. O'Malley, K., et al.: Plasma digoxin levels in infants. Arch. Dis. Child. 48:55, 1973.

31. Rogers, M. C, et al.: Serum digoxin concentrations in the human fetus, neonate and infant. N. Engl. J. Med. 237:1010, 1972.

32. Hordof, A., Hodess, A., and Rosen M. R.: Developmental changes in cardiac action potential characteristics and their modification by Ouabain (Abstr.) Am. J. Cardiol. 35:145, 1975.

33. Hedger, J. H., and Wittenberg, S. M.: Low incidence of digoxin induced ventricular premature depolarizations in hospitalized adults with elevated serum digoxin levels (Abstr.). Circulation 48 (Suppl. 4):18, 1973.

34. Lindenbaum, J., et al.: Variation in biological availability of digoxin from four preparations. N. Engl. J. Med. 235:1344, 1971.

35. Lindenbaum, J., et al.: Correlation of digoxin-tablet dissolution-rate with biological availability. Lancet 1:1215, 1973.

36. Food and Drug Association Drug Bulletin, January, 1974.

37. Shaw, T. R. D., and Carless, J. E.: The effect of particle size in the absorption of digoxin. Eur. J. Clin. Pharmacol. 7:269, 1974.

38. Johnson, B. F., et al.: Biological availability of digoxin from Lanoxin produced in the United Kingdom. Br. Med. J. 4:323, 1973.

39. Greenblatt, D. J., et al.: Equivalent bioavailability from digoxin elixer and rapid dissolution tablets. JAMA 229:1774, 1974.

40. Prebisz, J. J., Butler, V. P., Jr., and Lindenbaum, J.: Digoxin tablet bioavailability: Single-dose and steady-state assessment. Ann. Intern. Med. 81:469, 1974.

41. White, R. J., et al.: Plasma concentrations of digoxin after oral administration in the fasting and postprandial state. Br. Med. J. 1:380, 1971.

42. Bigger, T. J., Jr., and Strauss, H. C.: Digitalis toxicity: Drug interactions promoting toxicity and the management of toxicity. Semin. Drug Treat. 2:147, 1972.

43. Smith, T. W.: New approaches to the management of digitalis intoxication. *In* Symposium on Digitalis. Oslo, Gyldendal Norsk Forlag, 1973, p. 312.

44. Binnion, P. F.: Absorption of different commercial preparations of digoxin in normal human subjects and the influence of antacids, antidiarrheal and ion-exchange agents. *In* Symposium on Digitalis. Oslo, Gyldendal Norsk Forlag, 1973, p. 216.

45. Lindenbaum, J., et al.: Impairment of digoxin absorption by neomycin (Abstr.). Clin. Res. 20:410, 1972.

46. Juhl, R., et al.: Diminished urinary digoxin excretion after salicylazosulfapyridine (Abstr.) Fed. Proc. 34:916, 1975.

47. Khalil, S. A. H.: Bioavailability of digoxin in presence of antacids. J. Pharm. Sci. 63:1641, 1974.

48. Heizer, W. D., Smith, T. W., and Goldfinger, S. E.: Absorption of digoxin in patients with malabsorption syndromes. N. Engl. J. Med. 285:257, 1971.

49. Jusko, W. J., et al.: Digoxin absorption from tablet and elixir. The effect of radiation-induced malabsorption. J.A.M.A. 230:1554, 1974.

50. Belz, G. G.: Plasma concentrations of intravenous β-methyl digoxin with and without oral charcoal. Klin. Wochenschr. 52:749, 1974.

51. Bazzano, G., and Bazzano, G. S.: Effect of digitalis-binding resins on cardiac glycoside plasma levels (Abstr.). Clin. Res. 20:241, 1972.

52. Bloom, P. M., and Nelp, W. B.: Relationship of the excretion of tritiated digoxin to renal function. Am. J. Med. Sci. 44:133, 1966.

53. Doherty, J. E., Perkins, W. H., and Wilson, M. C.: Studies with tritiated digoxin in renal failure. Am. J. Med. 37:536, 1964.

54. Marcus, F. I., et al.: The metabolism of tritiated digoxin in renal insufficiency in dogs and man. J. Pharmacol. Exp. Ther. 152:372, 1966.

55. Ewy, G. A., et al.: Digoxin metabolism in the elderly. Circulation 39:449, 1969.

56. Marcus, F. I.: Metabolic factors determining digitalis dosage in man. *In* Basic and Clinical Pharmacology of Digitalis. Springfield, Ill., Charles C Thomas, 1974.

57. Steiness E.: Renal tubular secretion of digoxin. Circulation 50:103, 1974.

58. Doherty, J. E., and Marcus, F. I.: Unpublished observations.

59. Reidenberg, M. M., and Katz, M. A.: Slow extrarenal excretion of digoxin. N. Engl. J. Med. 289:1148, 1973.

60. Reuning, R. H., Sams, R. A., and Notari, R. E.: Role of pharmacokinetics in drug dosage adjustment. I. Pharmacologic effects. Kinetics and apparent volume of distribution of digoxin. J. Clin. Pharmacol. 13:127, 1973.

61. Jusko, W. J., and Weintraub, M.: Myocardial distribution of digoxin and renal function. Clin. Pharmacol. Ther. 16:449, 1974.

Chapter 15

Interpretation of Antiarrhythmic Drug Levels[*]

J. THOMAS BIGGER, JR., AND ELSA-GRACE V. GIARDINA

The intensity of antiarrhythmic drug action, like that of many drugs, is best related to the concentration of the drug at its site of action. When one is treating ventricular arrhythmias one can estimate the intensity of drug action at the arrhythmic site by observing the graded effect on frequency of ventricular premature depolarizations (VPDs) and, with procainamide or quinidine, the change in coupling interval of VPDs.[1,2] Also, the intensity of digitalis effect on the A-V node can be assessed by careful measurement of ventricular rate under standard conditions.[3] Many studies support the concept that the cardiac sites of antiarrhythmic drug action are in equilibrium with the plasma drug concentration in the steady state and that, when plasma drug concentration is changing, the heart concentration of drug changes rapidly to reach a new equilibrium with plasma. These relationships, determined when intensity of action is clearly evident, can be used to guide therapy when intensity of action cannot be assessed, e.g., when drugs are employed to *prevent* arrhythmias rather than to *control* an existing arrhythmia. In addition "nonspecific" cardiac or extracardiac effects may provide clues to plasma concentration.[4,5] The intensity of drug action is usually a sigmoid function of the serum concentration plotted on a log scale. There are many factors that alter the cardiac action of a given plasma antiarrhythmic drug concentration. However, when a factor alters the drug concentration–effect relationship it often does so in a reasonably predictable manner. Therefore, awareness of the plasma drug concentration and knowledge of the nature and intensity of the modifying factor allow a good estimate of the intensity of cardiac effect. It is our purpose to discuss factors that influence the relationship between dose and antiarrhythmic plasma drug concentration and the relationship between plasma drug concentration and cardiac antiarrhythmic effect.

* Supported in part by HL 12738, HL 70204 and the Chernow Foundation.

ANTIARRHYTHMIC DRUG DOSE AND PLASMA DRUG CONCENTRATION

Considering the many ways in which antiarrhythmic effect may vary as a function of antiarrhythmic drug plasma concentration, the range of plasma concentrations that produce antiarrhythmic effect is remarkably narrow. There is much greater variation in the *drug dose* and antiarrhythmic response than in the *drug plasma concentration* and antiarrhythmic response. There is relatively large variability in plasma drug concentration among individuals treated with the same drug-dosing regimen (amount of drug and frequency of dosing). Some of the factors that influence the relationship between plasma concentration and drug dose are listed in Table 15-1. The use of "standard" dosing regimens without adjusting dose to each individual patient is responsible for much of the enormous variability in plasma drug concentration between individuals in the population. For example, some of the variability in the dose-plasma concentration relationship can be eliminated by adjusting drug doses on the basis of body weight since the apparent volume of distribution usually varies as a function of body weight. This is not invariably the case. Digoxin is a reasonably polar molecule, and much of the body stores is found in skeletal muscle and relatively little in fat. Therefore, when obese subjects lose a large amount of fat, their body weight drops, but their digoxin dose should remain approximately constant.[6] When ventricular failure or hypotension occurs, the changes in regional blood flow that ensue may be very important in altering the plasma concentration of antiarrhythmic drug after a given dose. Reducing flow to skeletal muscle will reduce the apparent volume of distribution of antiarrhythmic drugs or greatly delay the equilibration of drug in the plasma and its storage sites in skeletal muscle or both.

The plasma protein (albumin) binding of antiarrhythmic drugs varies widely among different individuals and may vary in a single individual when the physiologic state changes or other drugs are given. This is important since it is the free drug in plasma that is thought to be in equilibrium with the arrhythmic site and that is available for glomerular filtration. Thus, a decrease in plasma protein binding of a drug that is eliminated largely by glomerular filtration, without renal tubular reabsorption or secretion, may *increase* its rate of excretion.

The situation is quite different for drugs that are eliminated by either hepatic metabolism or renal tubular secretion. In this instance, if the elimination process for a drug is efficient, the binding to plasma albumin merely serves to *enhance* the elimination of the drugs, i.e., albumin serves

TABLE 15-1

Factors Influencing the Relationship between Drug Dose and Drug Plasma Concentration

A. Apparent volume of distribution
   1. Tissues to which the drug distributes
   2. Mass of each tissue to which drug distributes
   3. Blood flow to each tissue to which drug distributes
   4. Partition coefficient for drug between plasma and each tissue to which drug distributes
B. Plasma protein binding
C. Absorption
   1. Extent
   2. Rate
D. Rate of elimination
   1. Excretion of unchanged drug
      a. Urine
         Filtration and/or secretion or reabsorption
      b. Bile
         Enterohepatic recycling
   2. Metabolism
      a. Rate of delivery of drug to metabolizing site
      b. Extraction of drug by the metabolizing organ
      c. Rate of metabolism
      d. Competition of other molecules for either extraction or metabolism
      e. Plasma drug concentration at which the metabolizing mechanism saturates

to transport the drug to the eliminating sites. The liver extracts a very large fraction (about 70%) of the lidocaine or propranolol that passes through the hepatic sinusoids either from hepatic arterial blood or the portal vein. Decreasing plasma protein binding of either of these two drugs without any other change would only tend to decrease its elimination rate. However, changes that alter plasma protein binding of drugs may be associated with other changes that produce unexpected results. For example, several groups have noted that diphenylhydantoin (DPH) binding to serum proteins is reduced in uremia.[7,8] Reidenberg and coworkers found about 7.5% unbound DPH in the serum of a small group of normal persons and 10 to 25% unbound serum DPH in patients with uremia;[9] the percentage of unbound DPH was inversely correlated with the creatinine clearance. This effect alone would be expected to reduce the rate of DPH elimination. However, Letteri and associates found that the steady–state DPH plasma concentration was reduced in uremia;[8] after 2 weeks of a dose of 300 mg. a day, normal subjects had an average plasma concentration of 12.9 μg./ml. while plasma DPH concentration averaged 4.4 μg./ml. in a group of uremic patients. It is not yet clear if the low DPH plasma concentration in uremia is due to an increased apparent volume of distribution or increased rate of hepatic metabolism or both, but it is difficult to attribute to the changes in protein binding alone.

Absorption is usually not a significant problem with the antiarrhythmic drugs except for digoxin. However, changes in rate or extent of absorption do occur and may not be considered because their occurrence is not common. Orally administered quinidine and procainamide are not absorbed at all from the stomach at the usual pH of the gastric juice (<1.5) because only the un-ionized form of these drugs is absorbed, and these substances are organic bases. Therefore, there is a lag between an oral dose of quinidine or procainamide and its appearance in the blood; the duration of this lag is dependent on the gastric emptying time. The absorption of DPH from the gastrointestinal tract is delayed and erratic; the peak plasma concentration after an oral dose may occur as late as 8 to 10 hours. Usually DPH is fully bioavailable when either the preparation of the original manufacturer or the generic form is administered orally.[10] Occasionally one encounters a patient who does not completely absorb orally administered DPH. Much remains to be learned about drug interaction causing incomplete or delayed absorption of DPH from the gastrointestinal tract. A special problem exists with oral administration of lidocaine or propranolol. When either of these two drugs is absorbed, a large fraction enters portal vein blood and passes through the liver, which takes up and metabolizes much of the drug presented to it—the so-called *first-pass effect*.[11,12] In the case of lidocaine, oral administration not only produces low plasma concentrations but also is accompanied by nausea and dizziness.[13] One of the metabolites of lidocaine, monoethylglycinexylidide, is suspected of causing these symptoms.[14] The first-pass effect is prominent with propranolol as initial, small doses are given. However, the situation with chronic dosing schedules or after larger doses of propranolol is not so clear. It is thought that a smaller fraction of the total dose is extracted from portal blood by the liver under these conditions.[15] Absorption of most antiarrhythmic drugs from sites of intramuscular injection is good. Quinidine, procainamide and lidocaine are all well absorbed after intramuscular injection. Plasma concentrations peak more rapidly after intramuscular injection than after oral dosing because absorption begins immediately. Effective plasma concentrations of lidocaine are obtained 5 to 15 minutes after injection of 4 mg./kg. into the deltoid muscle. The intramuscular route is often used for speed and convenience or when chronic oral therapy is interrupted because the patient's condition requires that he be given nothing by mouth, e.g., for surgical operations. Intramuscular therapy with DPH is quite another matter. Plasma concentrations drop sharply when intramuscular therapy is substituted for oral therapy; only about 50% of an intramuscular dose is absorbed.[16] Digoxin is also poorly absorbed from intramuscular injection sites. Information is not available on absorption of propranolol after intramuscular injection.

One of the most important factors influencing the relationship between drug dosing and plasma concentration of antiarrhythmic drugs is the variability of drug elimination among groups of patients. The rates of elimination given in Table 15-2 represent typical figures and not ranges. For example, time for the elimination ($t\frac{1}{2}$e) of quinidine is listed as 6 to 8 hours in Table 15-2, but Kessler and associates studied a small group of patients and found the elimination $t\frac{1}{2}$e of quinidine to vary from 3 to 19 hours.[17] The range of quinidine $t\frac{1}{2}$e was 3 to 16 hours in their nine patients who lacked ventricular fail-

ure, hepatic dysfunction or renal dysfunction (the median $t\frac{1}{2}$e was 7.2 hours). The extremes of the $t\frac{1}{2}$e are just as striking for the other antiarrhythmic drugs: procainamide 1.8 to 10 hours, propranolol 1.5 to 8 hours, DPH 6 to 60 hours and lidocaine 1 to 8 hours. Perhaps this very wide variability in range should be emphasized more. All else being equal, the almost tenfold range of $t\frac{1}{2}$e for any given antiarrhythmic drug means that there should be a tenfold variation in the steady-state peak concentration in a population treated with an identical dosing schedule. This expectation is realized and provides a strong rationale for monitoring plasma drug concentrations during antiarrhythmic therapy. Usually clues to departures from the median $t\frac{1}{2}$e values of antiarrhythmic drugs can be found in the history, physical examination or standard laboratory procedures. Estimates of $t\frac{1}{2}$e can be made on this basis, and dosing regimens can then be refined according to actual measurement of plasma concentration.

When to Measure Plasma Concentrations. Usually a dosing regimen is based on the "idealized" median values for the drug's kinetic parameters (Table 15-2). Then one observes the patient for the anti-

TABLE 15-2

Absorption, Distribution, Elimination of Antiarrhythmic Drugs

	Quinidine	Procainamide	Propranolol	Lidocaine	Diphenyl-hydantoin
Fraction Absorbed	0.9–1.0	0.9–1.0	0.8–1.0*	0.8–1.0*	0.8–1.0†
Volume of Distribution (L./kg.)	2.0–3.0	1.8–2.5	2.5–4.0	1.25–2.0	0.6–0.9
Half-Time for Elimination (hr.)	6–8	3–5	2–5	1–2	10–30‡
Effective Plasma Concentration	2–5 μg./ml.	3–10 μg./ml.	20–200 ng./ml.	1–5 μg./ml.	5–20 μg./ml.
Percent Bound to Plasma Protein	80	20	90	10–20	90
Metabolite(s)	Hydroxy-quinidine; dihydroxy-quinidine	N-Acetylpro-cainamide	4-Hydroxypro-pranolol; isopropyl-amine	Monoethylgly-cinexylidide; glycine-xylidide	5-(p-Hydroxy-phenyl) 5-phenyl-hydantoin

* Prominent "first-pass" effect
† Absorption rate variable
‡ Michaelis—Menten kinetics

arrhythmic action or toxic manifestations as a function of time after therapy is initiated. The more the physician understands about the pharmacodynamics (the biologic actions) and pharmacokinetics (the change of concentration in various body compartments as a function of time and dose) of a drug, the more selective and effective he can be in his evaluation of a drug regimen for its efficacy and safety. It is particularly useful to know when a drug regimen will achieve its steady state. When this point in therapy is reached, one will expect no further therapeutic benefit or new concentration–dependent toxic manifestations to arise unless the dosing or physiologic state of the patient changes. Also, this is a very useful time to measure the plasma drug concentration when an antiarrhythmic drug is being used prophylactically, e.g., to *prevent* atrial or ventricular fibrillation.

When is steady state achieved? One very useful rule of thumb is that 90% of steady state is achieved after 3.3 elimination half-times have elapsed. This rule works for: (1) intermittent, slow intravenous injections, (2) repeated intramuscular injections, (3) constant-rate intravenous infusions and (4) multiple oral dosing regimens. For example, if the $t\frac{1}{2}e$ for procainamide is 4 hours, then a constant-rate infusion will achieve 90% of steady state at 13.2 hours. If a constant dose of procainamide were being administered intramuscularly or orally every 4 or every 6 hours, the plasma concentration would also reach 90% of steady state at 13.2 hours. In the case of constant infusion the plasma concentration would be nearly stable after 13.2 hours; in the intermittent dosing cases, the plasma concentration would fluctuate between nearly constant limits after 13.2 hours. If the half-time for elimination of DPH is 2 days in a patient treated with 400 mg. DPH a day, 90% of steady state will not be reached for 6.6 days.[18]

If intermittent doses are given every elimination half-time, e.g., every 4 hours

for procainamide or every 7 hours for quinidine, the minimum plasma concentration will be almost precisely half the maximum concentration. If the drug is given at longer intervals, the fluctuation will be even greater. A significant goal of antiarrhythmic therapy is to maintain the plasma concentration above some minimum effective concentration with a reasonable interval between doses, e.g., at least 6 to 8 hours. For drugs like procainamide or quinidine, this usually means that the peak concentration may approach toxic values, or the minimum concentration may dip below the minimum therapeutic range. Therefore it is good practice to search for toxicity 1 to 2 hours after oral doses and for recurrence of the arrhythmia just before the next dose. If clinical and electrocardiographic observations are equivocal, determination of drug plasma concentrations at these same times is very useful. It is very important to draw the sample for drug determination in a precise relationship to dosing in order to answer the specific question being asked.

After the steady–state plasma drug concentration has been determined, changes in drug doses usually produce entirely predictable changes in plasma drug concentration. DPH is a notable exception to this rule, however. This drug has concentration–dependent elimination kinetics—at higher plasma concentrations, elimination slows. This can be explained in the following way: DPH is metabolized by a hepatic hydroxylase that can become saturated by doses in the therapeutic range—usually at doses between 300 and 600 mg./day. Once the enzyme becomes saturated, only a constant amount of DPH can be eliminated per unit time, i.e., first-order kinetics change to zero-order kinetics.[19,20] This has a practically important result. A small increase in dose, e.g., from 400 to 500 mg./day, may saturate the hydroxylase and cause an unexpectedly large increase in plasma DPH concentration and toxicity.

Excellent control of antiarrhythmic drug

dosing can usually be achieved by careful clinical observation and application of pharmacokinetic principles. However, one should consider measuring plasma drug concentrations when any of the conditions in Table 15-3 exists. The first two conditions are the classic indications for measuring plasma concentrations—unexpected lack of effectiveness or toxicity. The third condition is important and commonly encountered. When the dosing schedule seems unlikely to produce antiarrhythmic drug concentrations, e.g., 250 mg. of procainamide every 8 hours or 200 mg. of quinidine every 12 hours, but the arrhythmia seems controlled, several possible explanations should be considered. The patient's volume of distribution may be small, his drug elimination rate very slow, or both, or, more likely, the arrhythmia that was being treated has disappeared. If the plasma concentration is measured and found to be low, as expected, then, depending on the natural history of the condition being treated, the physician can decide either to increase the dose to achieve effective plasma levels as prophylaxis against an intermittent arrhythmic condition or to discontinue therapy. The last three indications for measuring plasma drug concentrations (Table 15-3) are used in the attempt to carefully regulate therapy in the presence of events that are likely to influence the relationship between drug dosing and plasma concentration. Obtaining plasma concentrations under these three circumstances anticipates potential problems rather than waiting for clinical evidence of antiarrhythmic drug concentrations that are too high or too low.

SPECIFICITY OF THE DRUG ASSAY

Important considerations in interpreting laboratory reports of antiarrhythmic plasma concentrations are: (1) Is the test specific for the parent drug? (2) Are metabolites of the parent drug measured by the assay? (3) Are extraneous compounds measured in the test? Drug metabolism studies are often performed with radiolabeled compounds in a small number of subjects, but large-scale measurement of drug plasma or urine concentrations depends on methods that can detect nonradioactive drug. The measurement of most antiarrhythmic drugs is a two-step process. The first step is extraction to separate the drug of interest from other compounds that might be detected in the assay. The second step is quantitation of the extracted compound by spectrophotometry, spectrophotofluorometry or gas chromatography by means of standard curves of the substance or internal standards (gas chromatography). Table 15-4 lists common methods currently used to assay antiarrhythmic drugs.

It is not our purpose here to discuss the technical details of these assays, but a few points are useful to put the values reported by the laboratory into perspective. With any extraction procedure the possibility exists for loss of drug. With gas chromatographic methods this can be controlled by adding the internal standard prior to extraction; this maneuver assumes that the internal standard has extraction characteristics that are nearly identical to the drug being measured. The fluorometric assays for quinidine, procainamide and propranolol are critically dependent on the ex-

TABLE 15-3

Indications for Measuring Plasma Concentrations of Antiarrhythmic Drugs

1. When the arrhythmia does not respond to treatment as expected
2. When symptoms arise that suggest drug toxicity
3. When the dosing regimen seems unlikely to produce antiarrhythmic plasma concentrations, but the arrhythmia *seems* controlled
4. After a change in physiologic state that may alter the drug's absorption, distribution or elimination
5. To evaluate compliance or abuse of the drug
6. After the patient has been prescribed other drugs that are suspected of interacting with the antiarrhythmic drug

TABLE 15-4

Methods and Specificity of Assays for Antiarrhythmic Drugs

Drug	Method of Assay	Measures Metabolites	Metabolites Active
Quinidine	a. Protein precipitation; fluorometry	Yes	
	b. Extraction; fluorometry	No	No(?)
Procainamide	a. Extraction, Bratton-Marshall reaction; spectrophotometry	No*	
	b. Extraction; fluorometry	No*	Yes
	c. Extraction; gas chromatography	No	
Propranolol	a. Extraction; fluorometry	No*	
	b. Extraction; gas-liquid chromatography	No	Yes
Lidocaine	a. Extraction; gas-liquid chromatography	No	Yes
Diphenylhydantoin	a. Extraction; gas-liquid chromatography	No	
	b. Extraction; high-performance liquid chromatography	No	No(?)

* Under some circumstances a variable amount of the metabolite may be measured.

traction step to separate the drug from chemicals that fluoresce in a manner similar to the drug being measured. It has been shown that the popular protein-precipitation method for quinidine measures fluorescence other than that of quinidine, particularly the inactive metabolites of quinidine; there is much less interference when the double-extraction method is used.[21] Recently Kessler and colleagues suggested that erroneous conclusions about quinidine dosing in renal failure were attributable to this difference in methods.[17] Similarly the Bratton-Marshall reaction, used for measuring procainamide, will measure any primary amine, e.g., many sulfonamides, and the specificity of this assay depends on the double extraction. The major metabolite of procainamide, N-acetylprocainamide, is not measured in the usual assay for the parent drug but may partially decompose to procainamide when plasma or the extract is allowed to stand at room temperature.[22] Also, under some circumstances the fluorometric assay for procainamide gives values that are somewhat higher than the Bratton-Marshall reaction;[22,23] this may be due to interfering fluorescent substances. Radioimmunoassays are being developed for several of the antiarrhythmic drugs and should have the advantage of high specificity. Two problems may arise with radioimmunoassays: (1) interference from other radioactive substances and (2) active metabolites that may not be detected by the highly specific assay.

Another important aspect of specificity of assay relates to the metabolic products of antiarrhythmic drugs. There is some information available on the antiarrhythmic action and other biologic effects of the antiarrhythmic drugs, but there are large gaps in our knowledge of this subject. All of the antiarrhythmic drugs are metabolized to a significant extent. There is less information available about quinidine than the other drugs, but at least half of a quinidine dose appears to be metabolized.[24] About half of a dose of procainamide is acetylated;[25] this is quite variable and strongly influenced by genetic factors.[26] Ninety percent or more of DPH,[27-29] propranolol[12] and lidocaine[30,31] doses are metabolized. In most of the assays, metabolites are not measured (Table 15-4). The fact that metabolites are not measured by the drug assays is ideal if the metabolites are inert. However, if the metabolites partially account for the antiarrhythmic activity or the undesirable effects seen during therapy, then measurement of the plasma concentration of the parent drug may not give a complete picture or may even be misleading.

Are the Metabolites of Antiarrhythmic Drugs Biologically Active? It is very important to know about the pharmacodynamics of the metabolites of antiarrhythmic drugs. Are the metabolites antiarrhythmic in their own right? Are their toxic effects qualitatively or quantitatively different from the parent molecules? How rapidly are the metabolites of antiarrhythmic drugs eliminated? If the metabolites are inert or much less active than their parent molecules and tend to accumulate, do the metabolites compete for cardiac sites that bind antiarrhythmic drugs and interfere with the binding and action of the parent molecule? The answers to these and other similar questions would be very useful to the physician using these drugs therapeutically. Unfortunately much of the information we need is not yet available.

The study of quinidine metabolism in man has been neglected so that the following statements come from a small data base. The fraction of the quinidine dose that is metabolized before excretion is very variable in man. Studies in a small number of human subjects indicate that quinidine is hydroxylated in man.[24,32] Most of the metabolites found in human urine are hydroxylated at one site, either on the quinidine or on the quinuclidine ring. A small quantity of dihydroxy derivatives of quinidine is found in the urine of some individuals. It has been stated that the hydroxy metabolites are much less antiarrhythmic than quinidine,[33] but the evidence for this statement has not been presented in detail. This is an important question to resolve since the hydroxy metabolites accumulate in renal insufficiency, often producing high concentrations.[17]

Procainamide is metabolized to a variable but significant extent in man by acetylation of the aromatic nitrogen. Procainamide is acetylated by the same type of N-acetyltransferase that metabolizes sulfamethazine, isoniazid and hydralazine. This suggests that much of the variability in metabolism of procainamide is due to genetic influences, i.e., whether or not an individual is a rapid or slow acetylator. When renal function is reduced the plasma level of N-acetylprocainamide (NAPA) is often as high as or higher than the procainamide concentration. Studies in mice suggested that NAPA was about 70% as effective as procainamide itself.[34,35] Inference from human studies during procainamide therapy suggests that NAPA is nearly as active an antiarrhythmic agent as procainamide.[35,36] If clinical trials bear this out, NAPA might be preferable to procainamide for antiarrhythmic therapy since it may not be as likely to produce the lupus erythematosus–like syndrome in slow acetylators.

Propranolol has a number of metabolites, the two most important seem to be 4-hydroxypropranolol and isopropylamine.[12] The 4-hydroxy metabolite has about the same degree of beta receptor–blocking activity as propranolol itself. This may account for the fact that the extent of beta-adrenergic blockade is greater for a given plasma propranolol concentration after an oral dose than after an intravenous dose. At present there is no reliable "cold" method for measuring 4-hydroxypropranolol, although methods using high-performance liquid chromatography (HPLC) look very promising. When this active metabolite can be measured along with propranolol itself, much of the current difficulty in relating plasma drug concentration to clinical activity should be overcome. Isopropylamine and naphthoxylactic acid are produced by a one-step N-deisopropylation of propranolol.[38] There is no evidence yet that napthoxylactic acid has pharmacologic activity.[12] Isopropylamine is excreted in the urine unconjugated, which indicates that the tissues must be exposed to this molecule. Dogs treated with 0.1 to 30 mg./kg. intravenous doses of isopropylamine showed a dose-dependent increase in arterial pressure and heart rate.[38] Isopropylamine given intra-arterially in doses of 0.3 to 10 mg. produces a dose-dependent decrease in hind-leg vascular resistance.[38] To our knowledge there have been no measurements of plasma isopropylamine concentrations in man; we expect that the concentration is low since only a small amount of this metabolic product is found in the urine after a dose of propranolol.

Diphenylhydantoin is extensively metabolized by a hepatic hydroxylase to 5-phenyl-5-parahydroxyphenylhydantoin (HPPH). After an intravenous dose of DPH, about 75% of the dose can be recovered in the urine as HPPH-glucuronide.[8] As mentioned previously the hydroxylase saturates at fairly low plasma DPH concentrations. Hydroxylation in individuals varies tremendously.[29] Since HPPH is only 55% protein bound, it is cleared more rapidly by the kidney than DPH itself; the renal clearance of HPPH (about 300 ml./min.) greatly exceeds the glomerular filtration rate, indicating that this molecule is secreted by the tubule.[39] There is some evidence that HPPH is significantly less active as an anticovulsant than DPH. Studies of HPPH's antiarrhythmic activity have not been performed, but the antiarrhythmic activity of HPPH might also be expected to be less than that of DPH.

Lidocaine is metabolized by the deethylation occurring in its aliphatic side chain to produce, first, monoethylglycinexylidide (MEGX) and, then, glycinexylidide (GX). Significant plasma concentrations of MEGX or GX are found in the plasma of a small fraction of the patients receiving infusions of lidocaine to treat arrhythmias.[31] Animal studies suggest that MEGX is about 80% as antiarrhythmic as lidocaine and GX about 10%. No clinical

studies have been reported in which either MEGX or GX was used as an antiarrhythmic. The convulsive actions of MEGX and GX have also been compared experimentally (in rats) to that of lidocaine.[42] MEGX seems to be 80 to 100% as prone to produce convulsions as lidocaine itself; GX has only about 10% the convulsive potency of lidocaine.

The next few years should bring a great deal of new information on the biologic effects of antiarrhythmic drug metabolites that will allow better control of antiarrhythmic therapy.

Factors That Alter the Cardiac Effect of a Given Plasma Drug Concentration. Factors that alter the relationship between dose and plasma concentration were discussed above. Although plasma concentration correlates much better with antiarrhythmic effect than dose, there are factors that alter the concentration-effect relationship. Some of these are listed in Table 15-5.

Many antiarrhythmic drugs accumulate in the heart, i.e., the concentration in the heart is higher than in plasma. For example, the heart: plasma ratio for digoxin or quinidine is about 20:1. Equilibrium between heart and plasma is established rather rapidly. The heart: plasma ratio for

TABLE 15-5

Factors Influencing the Relationship between Plasma Drug Concentration and Drug Effect

1. Differences in extent and rate of transfer of drug to its site of action
2. Differences in affinity of site of action for the drug molecule
3. Competition with other drugs or molecules for the site of action
4. Differences in intensity of effect following drug binding at the site of action
5. The nature of cellular alterations and geometry responsible for the arrhythmia
6. Interaction with intracellular or extracellular ions, e.g., K^+, Ca^{++}, Mg^{++}, H^+, HCO_3^-
7. Nature and extent of heart disease
8. Active metabolites that are not measured in the assay

any drug varies from individual to individual, and this may influence an individual's response to a drug. However, it should be remembered that measurement of tissue drug concentration is only a crude estimation of the drug concentration at its site of action because much of the drug in tissue may be bound to sites that do not participate in drug action. It is known that much of digitalis bound to the heart is not bound to Na^+-K^+-ATPase, the cardiac "digitalis receptor." In ischemic heart disease focal areas of the heart are temporarily underperfused. Such areas are thought to participate in the arrhythmias that are common in ischemic hearts. Antiarrhythmic drugs may have difficulty in reaching the ischemic zones because of the reduced perfusion. Cardiac hypertrophy may present a similar hindrance to the distribution of drug molecules to their site of action. Drug action may be altered by competition with other molecules of similar structure that compete for binding at the site of action. The major clinical antiarrhythmic action of propranolol stems from its beta-adrenergic blocking action. This blockade is competitive so that increasing the concentration of catecholamines in the vicinity of the beta receptor partially reverses this action. It is possible that metabolites of antiarrhythmic drugs compete for binding sites in a similar fashion. If this is so, then accumulation of metabolites in patients with renal insufficiency might cause a decrease in effect of a given concentration of parent drug. Such an effect has not been demonstrated, but this problem has received very little attention from investigators. Also, it is possible that, because of alterations in the myocardial cells or their environment in disease states, the linkage between drug binding at site of action with its effects on gating in membrane ion channels is altered.

We still know very little about the alteration of molecular interactions between antiarrhythmic drugs and components of cardiac cells and the way in which disease states alter these interactions. However, several important factors are known that alter the effect of a given plasma antiarrhythmic drug concentration on the heart, even if their mechanism is poorly understood. One of the best known is the interaction between K^+ and antiarrhythmic drugs. It is well known that reduced plasma K^+ concentrations tend to *augment* the "electrical effects" of digitalis on the heart. On the other hand, reducing plasma K^+ concentration tends to *reduce* the antiarrhythmic effect of quinidine, procainamide, lidocaine or diphenylhydantoin. Raising the plasma K^+ concentration increases the effect of a given plasma concentration of any of these drugs. Increasing plasma-free Ca^{++} concentration tends to promote the action of digitalis but reduce the action of other antiarrhythmic drugs. Other ions interact with the antiarrhythmic drugs but have not been studied as extensively. Although we do not know the molecular mechanism, heart disease and heart failure seem to alter the response of the heart and vasculature to a given plasma concentration of an antiarrhythmic drug.

Other drugs may interact with the effects of an antiarrhythmic drug. Quinidine has an alpha-adrenergic blocking action. When nitroglycerin or antihypertensive drugs that interfere with adrenergic neural activity are given together with quinidine, profound hypotension may occur, particularly after exercise. Obviously if a patient takes two drugs with similar cardiac effects simultaneously, e.g., quinidine and procainamide therapy, the total effect will be magnified. This may inadvertently occur in a mobile society where patients change physicians often or see physicians during the course of traveling.

SUMMARY

There are many factors that alter the relationship between drug doses and plasma drug concentrations. Many of the factors that influence the dose-response relationship can be predicted and therapy adjusted accordingly. However, under many circumstances it is quite useful to actually measure the plasma drug concentrations as a guide to therapy. It should be kept in mind that the assays used by the laboratory may or may not measure metabolites of the drug being administered. Even if all the relevant active compounds derived from the drug *are* measured, one has to keep in mind the various factors that may alter the relationships between plasma drug concentration and cardiac effects of the drug.

REFERENCES

1. Bigger, J. T. Jr., and Heissenbuttel, R. H.: The use of procainamide and lidocaine in the treatment of cardiac arrhythmias. Prog. Cardiovasc. Dis. 11:515, 1969.
2. Giardina, E.-G. V., and Bigger, J. T. Jr.: Procainamide against re-entrant ventricular arrhythmias. Circulation 48:959, 1973.
3. Gold, H., et al.: Clinical pharmacology of digoxin. J. Pharmacol. Exp. Ther. 109:45, 1953.
4. Bigger, J. T. Jr.: Arrhythmias and antiarrhythmic drugs. Adv. Intern. Med. 18:251, 1972.
5. Heissenbuttel, R. H., and Bigger, J. T. Jr.: The effect of oral quinidine on intraventricular conduction in man: Correlation of plasma quinidine with changes in intraventricular conduction time. Am. Heart J. 80:453, 1970.
6. Ewy, G. A., et al.: Digoxin metabolism in obesity. Circulation 44:810, 1971.
7. Odar-Cederlof, I., Lunde, P., and Sjoqvist, F.: Abnormal pharmacokinetics of phenytoin in a patient with uremia. Lancet 2:831, 1970.
8. Letteri, J. M., et al.: Diphenyhydantoin metabolism in uremia. N. Engl. J. Med. 285:648, 1971.
9. Reidenberg, M. M., et al.: Protein binding of diphenyldantoin and desmethyimipramine in plasma from patients with poor renal function. N. Engl. J. Med. 285:264, 1971.
10. Albert, K. S., et al.: Bioavailability of diphenylhydantoin. Clin. Pharmacol. Ther. 16:727, 1974.
11. Shand, D. G., and Rangno, R. E.: The disposition of propranolol. I. Elimination during oral absorption in man. Pharmacology 7:159, 1972.
12. Dollery, C. T., and George, C.: Propranolol: Ten years from introduction. *In* Cardiovascular Drug Therapy, edited by K. L. Melmon. Philadelphia, F. A. Davis Co., 1974.
13. Scott, D. B., Jebson, P. J., Godman, M. J., and Julian, D. G.: Oral lidocaine. Lancet 1:93, 1970.
14. Smith, E. R., and Duce, B. R.: The acute antiarrhythmic and toxic effects in mice and dogs of 2-ethylamino-2,6-aceto-xylidine (L-86), a metabolite of lidocaine. J. Pharmacol. Exp. Ther. 179:580, 1971.
15. Evans, G. H., and Shand, D. G.: Disposition of propranolol. V. Drug accumulation and steady-state concentrations during chronic oral administration in man. Clin. Pharmacol. Ther. 14:487, 1973.
16. Wilder, B. J., Serrano, E. E., Ramsey, E., and Buchanan, R. A.: A method for shifting from oral to intramuscular diphenylhydantoin administration. Clin. Pharmacol. Ther. 16:507, 1974.
17. Kessler, K. M., et al.: Quinidine elimination in patients with congestive heart failure or poor renal function. N. Engl. J. Med. 290:706, 1974.
18. Bigger, J. T. Jr.: Pharmacologic and clinical control of antiarrhythmic drugs. Am. J. Med. 58:479, 1975.
19. Gerber, N., and Wagner, J. G.: Explanation of dose dependent decline of diphenylhydantoin plasma levels by fitting to the integrated form of the Michaelis-Menten equation. Res. Commun. Chem. Pathol. Pharmacol. 3:455, 1972.
20. Atkinson, A. J. Jr., and Shaw, J. M.: Pharmacokinetic study of a patient with diphenylhydantoin toxicity. Clin. Pharmacol. Ther. 14:521, 1973.
21. Cramer, G., and Isaksson, B.: Quantitative determination of quinidine in plasma. Scand. J. Clin. Lab. Invest. 15:553, 1963.
22. Gibson, T. P., Lowenthal, D. T., Nelson, H. A., and Briggs, W. A.: Elimination of procainamide in end stage renal failure. Clin. Pharmacol. Ther. 17:321, 1975.
23. Koch-Weser, J., and Klein, S. W.: Procainamide dosage schedules, plasma concentrations, and clinical effects. J.A.M.A. 215:1454, 1971.
24. Palmer, K. H., Martin, B., Baggett, B., and Wall, M. E.: The metabolic fate of orally administered quinidine gluconate in humans. Biochem. Pharmacol. 18:1845, 1969.
25. Dreyfuss, J., Bigger, J. T. Jr., Cohen, A. I., and Schreiber, E. C.: Metabolism of procainamide in rhesus monkey and man. Clin. Pharmacol. Ther. 13:366, 1972.
26. Stein, R. M., et al.: The acetylation of procainamide. Is procainamide N-acetyltransferase a type 1 enzyme? Clin. Res. 34:385a, 1975.
27. Noach, E. L., Woodbury, D. M., and Goodman, L. S.: Studies on the absorption, distribution, fate and excretion of 4-^{14}C-labeled diphenylhydantoin. J. Pharmacol. Exp. Ther. 122:301, 1958.
28. Glazko, A. J., et al.: Metabolic disposition of DPH in normal human subjects following intravenous administration. Clin. Pharmacol. Ther. 10:498, 1969.
29. Kutt, H.: Biochemical and genetic factors regulating Dilantin metabolism in man. Ann. N.Y. Acad. Sci. 179:704, 1971.
30. Strong, J. M., and Atkinson, A. J.: Simultaneous measurement of plasma concentration of lidocaine and its de-ethylated metabolite by mass fragmentography. Anal. Chem. 44:2287, 1972.

31. Strong, J. M., Parker, M., and Atkinson, A. J. Jr.: Identification of glycinexylidide in patients treated with intravenous lidocaine. Clin. Pharmacol. Ther. 14:67, 1973.

Metabolic products of the cinchona alkaloids in 32. Brody, B. B., Baer, J. E., and Craig, L. C.: human urine. J. Biol. Chem. 188:567, 1951.

33. Conn, H. K. Jr.: Quinidine as an antiarrhythmic agent: Basic and clinical consideration. *In* Advances in Cardiopulmonary Diseases, edited by A. I. Bangai and B. L. Gordon. Chicago, Year Book Publishers, 1964, vol. 11.

34. Drayer, D. E., and Reidenberg, M. M.: N-acetylprocainamide—An active metabolite of procainamide. Proc. Soc. Exp. Biol. Med. 146:358, 1974.

35. Elson, J., Strong, J. M., Lee, W.-K., and Atkinson, A. J., Jr.: Antiarrhythmic potency of N-acetylprocainamide. Clin. Pharmacol. Ther. 17:134, 1975.

36. Giardina, E.-G. V., Heissenbuttel, R. H., and Bigger, J. T. Jr.: Intermittent intravenous procaine amide to treat ventricular arrhythmias. Ann. Intern. Med. 78:183, 1973.

37. Fitzgerald, J. D., and O'Donnell, S. R.: Pharmacology of 4-hydroxy propranolol, a metabolite of propranolol. Br. J. Pharmacol. 43:222, 1971.

38. Walle, T., Ishizaki, T., and Gaffney, T. E.: Isopropylamine, a biologically active deamination product of propranolol in dogs: Identification of deuterated and unlabeled isopropylamine by gas chromotography-mass spectrometry. J. Pharmacol. Exp. Ther. 183:508, 1972.

39. Bochner, F., et al.: The renal handling of diphenylhydantoin and 5-(p-hydroxyphenyl)-5-phenylhydantoin. Clin. Pharmacol. Ther. 14:791, 1973.

40. Burney, R., et al.: Antiarrhythmic effects of lidocaine metabolites. Am. Heart J. 88:765, 1974.

41. Strong, J. M., et al.: Pharmacological activity, metabolism and pharmacokinetics of glycinexylidide. Clin. Pharmacol. Ther. 17:184, 1975.

42. Blumer, J., Strong, J. M., and Atkinson, A. J.: The convulsant potency of lidocaine and its N-dealkylated metabolites. J. Pharmacol. Exp. Ther. 186:31, 1973.

Chapter 16

Laboratory Studies in Cardiovascular Diseases

CALVIN L. WEISBERGER, MARUN S. HADDAD AND EDWARD K. CHUNG

The purpose of this chapter is to survey some of the clinical laboratory tests that may aid in cardiac diagnosis. While it is true that drawing blood from a peripheral vein or artery is invasive testing, we certainly do not consider this technique in the same light as cardiac catheterization or angiography. Although a wide range of testing is available we intend to discuss only common laboratory tests that are clinically valuable for the diagnosis of various cardiac disorders. Certain laboratory tests considered to be extremely valuable in the diagnosis of common heart diseases will be discussed in detail.

COMPLETE BLOOD COUNT

The simplicity and accuracy of hemoglobin and hematocrit determinations make them the screening tests of choice for anemia. Anemia may play a significant role as a causative or precipitating factor in cardiovascular disease. High-output heart failure and coronary insufficiency are examples of this. Cyanosis may not be evident in spite of marked anemia since a minimum of 5 gm. of reduced hemoglobin is required for the clinical picture of cyanosis.

Hemoglobin and hematocrit can be mildly reduced because of hemodilution in congestive heart failure. Varying degrees of hemolytic anemia due to red blood cell trauma and intravascular hemolysis may be observed following insertion of a prosthetic valve—especially one with a paraprosthetic leak.[1] There may be absence of the spleen in cyanotic infants in whom a peripheral smear shows numerous nucleated red blood cells and Howell-Jolly bodies; serious cardiac anomalies may be associated.[2] Advanced polycythemia, whether primary or secondary, can result in thrombotic and hemorrhagic episodes by virtue of its effect on blood viscosity and peripheral sludging.

The prognostic significance of the hematocrit in patients with acute myocardial infarction is controversial.[3,4] Leukocytosis has been reported to be a risk factor in myocardial infarction.[5] However, the degree to which cigarette smoking may contribute to these findings remains unclear. Leukocytosis—i.e., in the range of 12,000 to 15,000 leukocytes—occurs almost invariably with acute myocardial infarction, sometimes as early as 2 hours after the onset of chest pain, and may last from 5 to 7 days. This is associated with neutrophilia and a slight shift to the left. Persistence of the leukocytosis beyond a week, or an extremely high white count, suggests the development of a complicating factor such as pulmonary embolism, pneumonia or postinfarction pericarditis.

ERYTHROCYTE SEDIMENTATION RATE

An increased tendency toward sedimentation of erythrocytes in shed blood has long been recognized in certain pathologic conditions, particularly inflammation. The sedimentation rate is a rough measure of abnormal concentration of fibrinogen and plasma globulins. It is increased in many conditions—infectious diseases; neoplastic diseases; connective tissue diseases, including rheumatic fever; and localized acute inflammation. Its determination is useful in the follow-up of acute rheumatic fever, as is C-reactive protein determination. It may remain increased during the acute phase of rheumatic fever despite severe cardiac decompensation. The sedimentation rate is almost always accelerated following acute myocardial infarction; acceleration starts a few hours to 2 to 3 days after the infarction and persists for several weeks. The sedimentation rate cannot, however, be used as a guide to the healing of myocardial infarction. An increase in the sedimentation rate is a useful sign in the diagnosis of post-myocardial infarction and post-thoracotomy syndrome.

SEROLOGY

Most patients with group A streptococcal infection show an *antibody response to streptolysin.*[6] This is a hemolytic substance produced by most strains of group A streptococci and a few strains of groups C and G. The serum antistreptolysin O level (ASO titer) has become widely used in the detection of a recent streptococcal infection and is particularly useful in the diag-

nosis of acute rheumatic fever. Other streptococcal antibodies that have been studied in this disease are antihyaluronidase, antistreptokinase, DNase and antistreptococcal M protein. A single determination is of little significance, but a rise in titer or persistent elevation of serum titer over several weeks may be of considerable diagnostic value. A titer equal to or greater than 250 Todd units is considered to be abnormally high. A repeated low titer usually signifies that the patient is free of active rheumatic fever.

An *antihyaluronidase titer* (AHT) 1:256 or higher is considered to be elevated; again, more than one measurement is needed for meaningful interpretation. Since as many as 20% of group A streptococcal infections do not demonstrate elevation of ASO titer, AHT is extremely valuable as an adjunct to it. The accuracy of AHT in detecting group A streptococcal infections is reported to be 90% or more.

C-reactive protein (CRP) forms a precipitate with the somatic C polysaccharide of the pneumococcus. First reported in 1930, and later found in a variety of other conditions, it is a sensitive but nonspecific indicator of inflammation of infectious or noninfectious origin. CRP is not demonstrable in normal serum, but it is present in rheumatic fever, myocardial infarction and postcommissurotomy syndrome. It is most useful in the diagnosis of rheumatic fever, the amount present being related to the degree of disease activity, and it can be used as a guideline to the efficacy of therapy. It is similar to the sedimentation rate in this respect.

A positive *rapid plasma reagin* (RPR) can be one of three things: (1) latent syphilis, treated or untreated; (2) a technical error; or (3) a false positive test. After the test is repeated to rule out technical errors, further studies such as the *Treponema pallidum* immobilization test or fluorescent treponemal antibody absorption test can determine if syphilis is present. False positive results can be obtained in a variety of conditions, including malaria, leprosy, connective tissue diseases and the common cold.

Also studied in the diagnosis of cardiovascular diseases are rubella titers, utilizing complement fixation and hemaglutination-inhibition tests; antinuclear antibodies and lupus erythematosus preparations. False positive results of LE tests occur in most patients receiving high doses of procainamide for a few weeks to a few months.[7] Complement fixation tests are positive in over 90% of patients with chronic Chagas' heart disease.

URINE

A freshly voided concentrated sample of urine should be used for examination.[8] Urine osmolality and specific gravity are increased in dehydration and in congestive heart failure with otherwise good renal function. Proteinuria and hematuria may be observed, especially with right-sided heart failure or constrictive pericarditis. Hematuria may be due to renal emboli originating from mural thrombi in transmural infarction or to bacterial endocarditis with renal involvement. Malignant hypertension with necrotizing arteriolitis, collagen vascular disease or excessive anticoagulation can result in hematuria. Myoglobinuria and myoglobinemia have been reported to be sensitive indicators of acute myocardial infarction.[9] Their significance and clinical application, however, are still to be verified. Urinary excretion of catecholamines and cortisol has also been shown to be increased during acute myocardial infarction.

The diagnosis of pheochromocytoma is dependent on the measurement of urinary levels of catecholamines or their metabolites or both.[10] The upper limit of normal for urinary excretion of free catecholamines is approximately 100 mg./24 hours, or less than 0.1 μg./mg. creatinine.[11] Most pheochromocytomas excrete more than 300 mg. catecholamines per 24 hours (0.3 μg./mg. creatinine). The major catecholamine metabolites, metanephrine and normetanephrine, and vanillylmandelic acid (VMA) are excreted in greater amounts and are more amenable to assay. Of the two, measurement of the metanephrines is preferable because a false positive test is less common. In practice, a normal level of total metanephrine excretion rules out pheocromocytoma, but an elevated level does not necessarily prove its presence.[10] In 80 to 90% of cases the biochemical diagnosis of pheocromocytoma can be made on the basis of an abnormal increase in VMA and total metanephrines in two urine specimens from a noncomatose patient. The specimens should be collected after discontinuation of all drugs for at least 2 days, and the patient should be on a diet containing known trypotophan and serotonin content.[7]

Urinary excess of hydroxyindoleacetic acid (HIAA), a metabolic product of serotonin, is usually diagnostic of the malignant carcinoid syndrome.

SERUM ENZYMES

Enzymes are the organic catalysts that mediate most of the chemical reactions in the body. They are found in essentially all body tissues and fluids and are assayed in terms of their activity in the medium under observation. Assays of enzymes found in the blood or serum are most commonly used. Some of these may gain access to the circulation from injured cells, and some may come from overproduction in "normal" cells. Literally dozens of enzymes have been identified and investigated. Clinically important enzymes are discussed later in this chapter.

Values used for the results of enzyme tests are either standard units or variations thereof. An enzyme unit is the amount of enzyme that catalyzes the conversion of 1 micromole of substrate or enzyme per minute under standard conditions of the test (temperature, pH and substrate concentrations).[12] Some enzymes used clinically exist as isoenzymes in the body; that is, there may be slight identifiable differences in the same enzyme produced by different body organs, allowing one to trace the source of that particular part of the enzyme activity. It should be noted that the level of any given parameter measured at a given time represents a balance between its production or release into the circulation and its clearance therefrom.

Lactic Dehydrogenase (LDH). LDH is the enzyme that catalyzes the oxidation of lactic acid to pyruvic acid. This is a reversible reaction involving both aerobic and anaerobic metabolism. LDH is found throughout the body, being especially rich in skeletal muscle, myocardium, kidney and liver. Normally, LDH activity is detectable in the serum, and the absolute value of the enzyme varies somewhat at different laboratories. Many conditions can cause increase of LDH; the highest value is observed in megaloblastic anemias and leukemia. Levels of LDH are commonly two to four times higher, or even slightly greater, in acute myocardial infarction, congestive heart failure and cardiogenic shock. Patients with myxedema also have increases in this enzyme. Increase in the enzyme level begins within hours after acute myocardial infarction, peaking during the first 24 to 48 hours, and may persist for up to two weeks.

Since various cardiac and noncardiac disorders can produce LDH elevations, identification of the five LDH isoenzymes can occasionally be of great value. Myocardium and RBCs are rich in isoenzymes 4 and 5, while liver and skeletal muscle are rich in isoenzymes 1 and 2. In LDH elevation in a patient without anemia, a high isoenzyme number (American numbering system) would be supportive evidence of its myocardial origin.

Glutamic Oxalacetic Transaminase (SGOT). SGOT is found in heart, liver, skeletal muscle, kidney, brain and other organs. Therefore elevations of SGOT levels may be found in diseases involving any organ rich in its content. In respect to cardiac disorders, elevation of the enzyme level may be observed in acute myocardial infarction, pericarditis, myocarditis, arrhythmias, congestive failure, trauma and postelectrical cardioversion (probably more related to skeletal muscle damage than cardiac). Elevation may also be seen in shock and pulmonary infarction. In addition, a wide range of hepatic and skeletal muscle disorders can cause an increase of this enzyme.

However, the determination of SGOT has been used traditionally to support the diagnosis of acute myocardial infarction. Enzyme activity in the serum begins to rise 6 to 12 hours after infarction, peaking around 24 hours and returning to baseline levels usually by the fourth day. An increase of more than ten times baseline has been reported to be correlated with a higher incidence of hemodynamic complications in myocardial infarction. When there is a question whether an increase in SGOT is cardiac or hepatic in origin, the serum glutamic pyruvate transaminase (SGPT) determination may be extremely valuable. The reason for this is that essentially SGPT is found only in liver and not in myocardium or skeletal muscle.

Creatine Phosphokinase (CPK). CPK catalyzes the reversible reaction of creatine phosphate with adenosine diphosphate (ADP) to produce creatine and adenosine triphosphate (ATP). The enzyme is found in high concentration in skeletal muscle, myocardium and brain. Little or no CPK is found in the liver. Recently CPK has had its greatest use in the diagnosis of acute myocardial infarction. In myocardial infarction, increases in CPK are detectable within coronary sinus blood in the most acute phases and in the peripheral venous blood within an hour of myocardial infarction. With uncomplicated myocardial infarction, the enzyme level usually peaks within 12 hours and returns to normal within 36 to 48 hours. As with SGOT, elevations greater than ten times normal are often found in patients with myocardial infarction associated with a significant hemodynamic derangement.

It should be remembered that the CPK level can also be greatly elevated in skeletal muscle disease, cerebral infarction, hypothyroidism and pulmonary infarction. Assay of the isoenzymes of CPK has greatly increased the value of CPK as an indicator of myocardial infarction. The M-B fraction of CPK originates essentially only from myocardium, and therefore its increase supports the diagnosis of myocardial damage. This is particularly important when coexistent skeletal muscle or brain damage contributes to total CPK increase.[13] CPK is the most specific serum enzyme clinically available at the present for the diagnosis of myocardial infarction.

FLUID AND ELECTROLYTES

The extracellular fluid, particularly the vascular compartment, and total body water and the electrolytes are extremely important in the management of cardiac patients. Because of the frequent use of potent diuretics, iatrogenic hypovolemia is often unavoidable. Total body water is approximately 60% of body weight. Body water is two-thirds intracellular and one-third extracellular. When volume depletion occurs, both water and sodium are lost in varying proportions. Frequently during diuretic therapy, more sodium than water may be lost. Sweating, hyperventilation and diarrhea may cause water loss to exceed sodium loss. The symptoms associated with volume depletion are thirst, weakness, orthostatic dizziness or syncope, nausea, vomiting and apathy. The patient may have recordable weight loss (2.2 pounds/liter of fluid loss), tachycardia, poor tissue turgor and orthostatic hypotension.

Body water cannot be readily measured outside the research laboratory, so that clinically one must estimate volume loss on the basis of weight loss, hemoconcentration, BUN increase in excess of creatinine and a low volume of urine of high specific gravity. Serum sodium is a reflection of the total body water and total body sodium and therefore cannot be used as a guide to fluid depletion.

Volume overload likewise cannot be measured by routine laboratory tests. There is usually an excess of both salt and water, especially when volume overload is due to congestive heart failure. Weight gain, low BUN concentration and hemodilution are some of the signs of simple volume excess.

Sodium. The normal plasma sodium concentration is 136 to 142 mEq./liter. This is usually measured by flame photometry. The sodium measurement can be falsely lowered as a result of elevation of the blood sugar level and by serum lipemia. There are rarely any symptoms due to hyponatremia itself unless the level of sodium becomes less than 115 mEq./liter. Hypernatremia rarely occurs as a result of sodium excess per se; it is usually due to water loss in excess of sodium. The volume of water necessary to restore the serum sodium concentration to normal may be calculated by the following formulas:

Normal volume body water (TBW)
$$(L.) = 0.6 \times \text{normal body weight (kg.)}$$

$$\frac{\text{Normal serum (Na}^+) \times \text{TBW}}{\text{measured serum (Na}^+)} =$$
$$\text{current TBW}$$

$$\text{Body-water deficit} = \text{normal TBW} -$$
$$\text{current TBW}$$

Potassium. Like sodium, potassium is measured with a flame photometer. Because K^+ is released from platelets and WBCs during clotting and retraction, the serum potassium level may be falsely elevated. Therefore, plasma potassium will reflect the true circulating concentration of the potassium ion. The daily K^+ requirement is approximately 1 mEq./kg. body weight, and a normal diet in the United States generally contains 80 to 200 mEq. potassium. The normal plasma potassium is 4 to 5 mEq./liter. It is intimately related to the plasma pH; K^+ increases about 0.6 mEq./liter for each 0.1 unit decrease in pH. For example, in a patient in whom pH is 7.40 and K^+ is 4.0 mEq./liter one could expect K^+ to increase 1.8 to 5.8 mEq./liter when the pH falls to 7.1. Under this circumstance, a normal K^+ finding in the presence of severe acidosis would represent true hypokalemia. Since the red blood cells contain about 90 mEq./liter K^+, K^+ will be increased in a hemolyzed specimen of blood. Thus it should be clear that measured hyperkalemia does not necessarily have hemolysis as its basis.

Clinically, most patients with hypokalemia usually are not symptomatic until serum potassium concentration falls to 3.0 mEq./liter or less. Common symptoms in hypokalemia include weakness, hyporeflexia, tetany, paralysis and cardiac arrhythmias. It is well known that hypokalemia frequently predisposes to digitalis-induced arrhythmias. The most common electrocardiographic findings in hypokalemia are prominent U waves; less common are peaking P waves (pseudo P pulmonale), inverted T waves and S-T segment depression. It should be remembered that normal excretion of K^+ may be 80 mEq./liter/day and that plasma potassium decreases slowly during progressive K^+ loss. Thus a plasma K^+ value of 2.0 mEq./liter (pH 7.4) could represent a potassium deficit of 200 to 400 mEq. under this circumstance. During potassium depletion, potassium replacement should be carried out slowly—no faster than 40 mEq./hour—because redistribution of potassium takes place slowly. Acute hyperkalemia may be produced if this is not done.

Hyperkalemia may be induced iatrogenically, or it may be due to renal failure, hemolysis or muscular crush injuries. The most common cause of hyperkalemia is overuse of potassium salts as sodium replacement in salt-restricted patients, in which case the most serious symptoms are the cardiac manifestations, which may result in ventricular fibrillation, cardiac arrest and even sudden death. These manifestations usually occur when the serum potassium level is more than 7.0 mEq./liter. The most common electrocardiographic findings in hyperkalemia are tall, peaked T waves with narrow bases during the early stage. Intraventricular conduction delay, A-V block, flat P waves, ventricular tachyarrhythmias and cardiac standstill may be observed in advanced hyperkalemia.

Calcium and Magnesium. It is uncommon for these two electrolytes to be involved in cardiac problems although their excess and deficiency states both cause electrocardiographic abnormalities. It has been reported that hypomagnesemia often coexists with hypokalemia and predisposes to digitalis intoxication. Hypomagnesemia is commonly found in patients with alcoholic cardiomyopathy, and the incidence of digitalis toxicity is often high. In addition, a synergistic action between digitalis and calcium is well known. Thus, digitalization should be carried out with special care when hypercalcemia is suspected. Hypercalemia produces shortening of the Q-T interval, whereas hypocalemia produces prolongation of it.

COAGULATION STUDIES

Many physicians are often involved in anticoagulation treatment of patients and in the evaluation of bleeding in postcardiotomy patients. Following is a short survey of the basic tests used in the coagulation schema.

Prothrombin Time. This test measures the time required for fibrin to form in plasma after calcium and tissue thromboplastin are added. The reaction involves successively factors VII, X, V, phospholipid, prothrombin and fibrinogen. This is the extrinsic system and is entailed in coagulation when tissue damage occurs, as in a laceration, with release of tissue thromboplastin. In patients receiving oral anticoagulant therapy, the vitamin–K dependent factors are reduced. In this case, prothrombin time is prolonged (normal: 12 seconds) because of decreases in factors VII, II (prothrombin) and X. The results may be expressed in comparison to a normal control (e.g., 2.3:1) or in comparison to dilutions of normal plasma. Because of the short half-time of factor VII (normal: 7 hours) the result may be significantly prolonged without appreciable decreases in the levels of factors II and X. Factor VII plays little part in coagulation in vivo, so that in the case of prolongation of the prothrombin time due to decrease in factor VII, clotting can still occur.

Partial Thromboplastin Time (PTT). The PTT is a means of evaluating the intrinsic clotting system. In the original method, phospholipids, or "partial" thromboplastin, are added instead of "complete" thromboplastin as in the prothrombin time. Contact with glass activates factor XII, and cascade occurs. In a modification of the original technique kaolin is used with the phospholipid as an activator; factors XII and XI are rapidly activated, and cascade continues. The activated PTT and PTT can test the activity of all factors except factors XIII, VII and III. The normal concentration of the individual factors must, in general, be reduced to less than 30% to cause prolongation of the test. Because the PTT and the activated PTT are reliable and reproducible methods, many laboratories utilize these tests to monitor heparin therapy, the object being to prolong coagulation time two to three times longer than normal.

Thrombin Time. This test measures the rate of fibrin formation in the presence of thrombin. The time is prolonged when the level of fibrinogen is less than 100 mg./100 ml.; it is prolonged by heparinization or the presence of fibrin split products. It is possible that a nonheparin inhibitor could be present to prolong the reaction.

Other coagulation tests exist, of course, but their applications in cardiac patients without specific hematologic disease are minimal.

SUMMARY

Various laboratory studies used in the diagnosis of cardiac diseases are described. No single laboratory study is absolutely diagnostic or confirmative of any particular cardiac disease because there is a significant incidence of false positive and false negative results as well as of laboratory errors. Furthermore, the results of a particular laboratory test may be normal in some circumstances and abnormal in different clinical circumstances and in cardiac and noncardiac disorders. Therefore, every laboratory test should be carefully interpreted in conjunction with clinical findings.

Parameters most commonly studied in the laboratory include complete blood counts, erythrocyte sedimentation rate, serology, urinary catecholamines, various electrolytes, serum enzymes (SGOT, LDH and CPK) and coagulation. Metabolic studies utilized in the diagnosis and assessment of degree of coronary heart disease are purposely omitted in this chapter because they are available only at medical teaching institutions with sophisticated laboratory facilities.

Other non-invasive diagnostic tests, including cardiographic methods, roentgenographic studies and serum determinations of digitalis and other antiarrhythmic drugs, are discussed elsewhere in this book.

REFERENCES

1. Reynolds, R. D., Coltman, C. H., and Beller, B. M.: Iron treatment in sideropenic intravascular hemolysis due to insufficiency of Starr-Edwards valve prosthesis. Ann. Intern. Med. 63:295, 1965.

2. Bush, J. A., and Dunger, L. E.: Congenital absence of the spleen with congenital heart disease: Report of a case with antemortem diagnosis on the basis of hematologic morphology. Pediatrics, 15:93, 1955.

3. Burch, G. E., and DePasquale, N. P.: The hematocrit in patients with myocardial infarction. J.A.M.A. 180:63, 1962.

4. Hershberg, P. I., Wells, R. E., and McGandy, B. B.: Hematocrit and prognosis in patients with acute myocardial infarction. J.A.M.A. 219:855, 1972.

5. Friedman, G., Klutsky, A. L., and Sigelaub, A.: The leukocyte counts as predictor of myocardial infarction. N. Engl. J. Med. 290:1275, 1974.

6. Hurst, J. W., Logue, R. B., Schlant, R. C., and Wenger, N. K.: The Heart, Arteries and Veins, ed. 3 New York, McGraw-Hill Book Co., 1974.

7. Swarbick, E. T., and Gray, I. R.: Systemic lupus erythematosus during treatment with Pronestyl. Br. Heart J. 34:284, 1972.

8. Sternheimer, R.: Urinalysis in cardiovascular disease. *In* Cardiology: An Encyclopedia of the Cardiovascular System, edited by A. A. Luisada. New York, McGraw-Hill Book Co., 1959, vol. 2 (Suppl.).

9. Kagen, L., et al.: Myoglobinemia following acute myocardial infarction. Am. J. Med. 58:177, 1975.

10. Gitlow, S. E.. Mendlowitz, M., and Bertain, L. M.: The biochemical techniques for detecting and establishment of the presence of a pheochromocytoma. Am. J. Cardiol. 26:370, 1970.

11. Hunter, R. B., Marshall, T. D., and Oram, E. J.: Catecholamine excretion in cases of pheochromocytoma. Q. J. Med. 32:225, 1963.

12. Davidsohn, I., and Henry, J. B.: Todd-Sanford Clinical Diagnosis by Laboratory Methods, ed. 15. Philadelphia, W. B. Saunders Co., 1974.

13. Konthinen, A., and Somer, H.: Determination of serum creatine kinase isoenzymes in myocardial infarction. Am. J. Cardiol. 29:817, 1972.

Index

Page numbers in *italics* refer to illustrations; page numbers followed by t refer to tables.

FEB